Health

Russell Whaley, M.P.H., Ph.D.

Slippery Rock State College
Slippery Rock, Pennsylvania

Health

Prentice-Hall, Inc.

Englewood Cliffs, New Jersey

To Holly, and to the kids—Jenifer, Margaret, Elizabeth, Clarissa, Candy, Joseph, and Adam

Library of Congress Cataloging in Publication Data
Whaley, Russell F.
  Health.

  Includes bibliographies and index.
  1. Health.   I. Title.
RA776.W468   613   81-21124
ISBN 0-13-384610-5   AACR2

Printed in the United States of America

10 9 8 7 6 5 4 3 2 1

PRENTICE-HALL INTERNATIONAL, INC. *London*
PRENTICE-HALL OF AUSTRALIA, PTY. LIMITED, *Sydney*
PRENTICE-HALL OF CANADA, LTD., *Toronto*
PRENTICE-HALL OF INDIA PRIVATE LIMITED. *New Delhi*
PRENTICE-HALL OF JAPAN, INC., *Tokyo*
PRENTICE-HALL OF SOUTHEAST ASIA PTE. LTD., *Singapore*
WHITEHALL BOOKS LIMITED, *Wellington, New Zealand*

Art Director: Florence Dara Silverman
Production Editor: Martha Goldstein
Book Designer: Bill Gray
Page Layout: Jack Meserole
Cover Designer: Florence Dara Silverman
Cover Art: Bill Longcore
Line Art: Danmark & Michaels, Inc.
Photo Researcher: Anita Duncan
Manufacturing Buyer: Ray Keating

ISBN 0-13-384610-5

Contents

Introduction   1

     Holistic Health   2   /   Change   2   /   Responsibility   2

Threats to Life and Wellness   3

     Causes of Death in Young Adults   3   /   Causes of Disease in Young Adults   3

Choosing for Health   4

     Tomorrow's Problems   4   /   A Step Beyond   5

UNIT ONE   Mental Health   8

1. Personality   10

Chapter Objectives   10

Profile of the Mentally Healthy   11

Threats to Mental Health   11

     Brain Damage   11   /   Stress   13

Mind and Body   14

    The Brain   14   /   The Nerves   14   /   How the Body and the Mind
    Affect Each Other   14   /   Levels of Awareness   16

Theories of Personality   17

    Freud   17   /   Erikson   19   /   Humanistic Psychology   22   /   Behavior   25

    Summary   26   /   Suggested Readings   27

2. Stress   28

  Chapter Objectives   28

  Stressors   29

    Stress and the Levels of Consciousness   32   /   The Nature of Stress   33   /
    Stress and Disease   36

    Summary   42   /   Suggested Readings   42

3. Coping   44

  Chapter Objectives   44

  Coping   45

    Unconscious and Conscious Coping   46   /   Problem Solving   46   /
    Defense Mechanisms   48   /   Time Structuring   48

  Not Coping: Dysfunction   50

    Five Levels of Dysfunction   50   /   Problems of the Mind   51

  Treatment of Dysfunction: Psychotherapy   54

    "Talk" Therapies   54   /   Nonverbal Therapies   57

    Summary   53   /   Suggested Readings   59

UNIT TWO Drugs   60

4. Illicit Drugs   62

  Chapter Objectives   62

  What Is a Drug?   63

Psychoactive Drugs   63

Young Adults and Drugs   65

The Effects of Drugs   66

    Stages of Drug Dependence   68

Categories of Drugs   68

    Marijuana and Hashish   69 / Stimulants   70 / Depressants   72 /
    Tranquilizers   72 / Psychedelics   73 / Narcotics   75

Preventing Drug Abuse   76

Rehabilitation   78

    Summary   79 / Suggested Readings   79

5. Alcohol   81

What We Drink   82

The Effects of Alcohol   83

The Costs of Alcohol   87

The Rise, Fall, and Rise of Drink   88

Kinds of Drinkers   89

Alcohol Abuse   89

Dynamics of Alcohol Dependence   90

Why People Misuse Alcohol   93

Diseases Connected with Alcoholism   93

The Impact of Alcoholism on Family Life   95

Treatments for Alcoholism   96

Student Drinkers   96

Responsible Drinking   99

Drinking Precautions   100

Recognize Irresponsible Drinking   101

    Summary   102 / Suggested Readings   102

6. Tobacco   103

    Chapter Objectives   103

    Anatomy of a Habit   105

      Why Do People Smoke?   105   /   Kinds of Smokers   105

    Effects of Smoking   107

      What Is the Smoke?   109   /   Diseases Associated with Smoking   109   /
      Pipes and Cigars   113   /   Quitting   113   /   Why Quit?   114   /
      How to Quit   115

    Smoking and Society   117

      The Government's Role   118

      Summary   120   /   Suggested Readings   120

UNIT THREE Physical Health   122

7. Exercise   124

    Chapter Objectives   124

    Advantages of Exercise   125

    The First Steps   127

      Measuring Your Fitness   127   /   Goals   131

    Kinds of Exercise   131

      Isometrics   132   /   Isotonics   133   /   Anaerobics   135   /   Aerobics   135

    A Way of Life   138

      Warm-Up   138   /   Cool-Down   143   /   Overload   143   /
      How Much?   144   /   Fatigue   144   /   Sustaining Interest   144   /
      When?   145   /   Exercise Logs   145

    Sleep: The Complement of Exercise   145

    How Much Do Students Sleep   146

      Summary   147   /   Suggested Readings   147

8. Nutrition   148

Chapter Objectives   149

Nutrients   149

Nutrients That Provide Energy   149   /   Nutrients That Do Not Provide
Energy   153   /   Essential Nutrients   159

Non-Nutrients   159

Additives   161

Flavor and Color   161   /   Food Processing   161   /   Nutrition   162

The Basic Four   162

Meats   163   /   Fruit and Vegetables   163   /   Grains   163   /   Milk   163

A Suitable Diet   165

Recommended Dietary Allowance (RDA)   165   /   Vegetarianism   165

Nutritional Fallacies   167

Misinformation   167   /   Food Quackery   167

Malnutrition   168

Undernutrition   169   /   Overconsumption   169

Shopping   170

Summary   171   /   Suggested Readings   172

9. Weight Control   173

Chapter Objectives   173

Dieting: A Way of Life   174

Causes of Overweight   176

Genetic Causes   176   /   Physiological Causes   177   /   Environmental
Causes   177   /   Psychological Causes   178

Diets and Dieting   178

Fad Diets: How to Go Nowhere Fast   180   /   A *Real* Diet   184   /
Other Ways to Lose Weight   187

Summary   190   /   Suggested Readings   190

10. Noncommunicable Disease 191

Chapter Objectives 191

Classifications of Disease 192

Incidence and Prevalence 192

Risk Factors 193

Inherited Diseases 194

Genetic Diseases 194 / Congenital Defects 195 / Late Appearing Genetic and Congenital Diseases 195

Disorders of Blood Flow: The Cardiovascular Diseases 196

Your Heart in Sickness and in Health 199 / Atherosclerosis and Essential Hypertension 201 / Stroke 202 / Heart Attack 203

The Dreaded Disease: Cancer 204

What is Cancer? 205 / How Cancers Grow 207 / Is Death Inevitable? 208 / The Warning Signs 209 / A Varied Assortment 209 / Is There a Cure in Sight? 214

Allergies 214

The C.O.L.D. That Kills 215

Arthritis: Crippler of the Young and Old 216

Diseases of the Digestive Tract 217

Diseases of the Nervous System 218

Summary 219 / Suggested Readings 220

11. Communicable Diseases 221

Chapter Objectives 221

It's Infectious, but Is It Communicable? 222

Americans: How Sick Are We? 222

The Process of Infection 223

The Invaders 224 / Human and Animal Reservoirs 226 / Direct and Indirect Transmission 227 / Etiology 227 /

Agent-Host-Environment Relationship   228   /   Factors in the Environment   228   /
The Protectors   229

Some Common Communicable Diseases   231

Viral Diseases   231   /   Rickettsial Diseases   235   /   Bacterial Disease/Sexually
Transmitted Disease   236   /   Fungal Disease   240   /   Protozoan Diseases   240
Arthropod Infestation   240   /   Worm Infestation   241

Controlling Communicable Disease   241

Summary   244   /   Suggested Readings   244

UNIT FOUR   Sexuality   246

12. Sexuality   248

Chapter Objectives   248

Sex Roles   249

Society Is Destiny   250   /   Role Conflict in Women   251   /   Sex-role
Pressures on Men   253   /   The Androgynous Personality   257

Physical Sexuality   259

Sexual Development   259   /   Intrapersonal Sexuality   261   /   Interpersonal
Sexuality   263   /   Homosexuality   264   /   Variation   264   /   Public Attitudes
and the Law   265

Summary   266   /   Suggested Readings   267

13. The Biology of Sex   268

Chapter Objectives   268

The Biological Man   269

External Sex Organs   269   /   Internal Sex Organs   269

The Biological Woman   271

External Sex Organs   271   /   Internal Sex Organs   272   /   Secondary Sex
Characteristics   274

Sexual Intercourse   274

Positions 275 / Lovemaking 276 / Stages of Sexual Response 276
Sexual Dysfunction 277 / Older People 279

Pregnancy: A New Life Begins   280

Heredity 280 / Fertilization 280 / The Three Trimesters
of Pregnancy 282

Birth   286

The Three Stages of Labor 286 / Fetal Positions 287 / Anesthesia during
Labor: Pros and Cons 288 / Education for Childbirth 288 / Where Should
the Baby Be Born 288 / New Methods of Delivery 289

The First Few Months of Life   291

Breast Feeding 291 / Post Partum Depression 291

Summary   292 / Suggested Readings   293

14. Birth Control, Sterilization, and Abortion   294

Chapter Objectives   294

Birth Control   295

Responsibility 296 / The Biological Basis of Contraception 296

Birth Control Methods   297

Natural Methods 298 / Mechanical Methods 301 / Hormonal
Methods 303 / IUDs 305 / Birth Control in the Future 305

Surgical Sterilization   306

Men 306 / Women 307

Abortion   308

Methods 308 / Debate over Abortion 310

Summary   312 / Suggested Readings   313

UNIT FIVE Life Cycles   314

15. The Family   316

The College Years   317

Marriage   319

    Advantages of Marriage   319   /   Why People Marry   320   /   Preparation for
    Marriage   320   /   Successful Marriages   323   /   Equal Marriage   323

Parenthood   324

    Should You Be a Parent?   324   /   Protecting a Relationship   326   /
    Adoption   326

Divorce   327

    "Splitsville"   329   /   Social Trends Encouraging Divorce   330

The Family Regroups   331

    One-parent Families   331   /   Remarriage   331   /   "Without Benefit of
    Clergy"   332   /   Staying Single   332

    Summary   333   /   Suggested Readings   333

16. Aging, Dying, and Death   335

Chapter Objectives   335

Trends   336

    Population and Society   337   /   Life Expectancies   338

Aging   340

    Diseases of Old Age   340   /   Personality and Aging   341   /   Poverty and
    Old Age   342   /   How to Live Forever   342

Death   343

    What Is Death?   344   /   Dying: Myths and Realities   345   /   Impact of
    Death on the Dying   346   /   Stages of Death   347   /   Grief   347

    Summary   352   /   Suggested Readings   353

UNIT SIX   Social Health   354

17. The Health-care Delivery System   356

Chapter Objectives   356

Medical Care: A 20th-Century Revolution   357

Medical Care Today: A Problem of Availability 357

The High Cost of Health 360

Third-party Payers 360 / Medical Technology 362 / Specialization among Physicians 362 / An "Imperfect" Market 363

The Consumption of Health Care 363

Stages of Care 363 / Place of Care 364 / New Ideas in Health Care 364

Health Insurance 366

Types of Health Insurance 366 / How to Shop for Insurance 366 / Private Insurance Companies 367 / The Government's Role: Medicare and Medicaid 367

Reducing Health-care Costs 368

Investor-owned Hospitals: Benefits as Business 368 / Physician Extenders 369

The Government's Responsibility 370

Socialized Medicine 370 / National Health Insurance 371 / Costs 371

Choosing a Physician 372

Communicating with a Physician 373 / Choosing a Dentist 375

Summary 376 / Suggested Readings 377

18. Health-care Products 378

Chapter Objectives 378

The Drug Industry 379

The Cost of Health-care Products 380 / Brand Names and Generics 380 Prescription and Over-the-Counter (OTC) Drugs 380

Using Drugs 381

Side Effects 381 / Drug Interaction 382 / How to Take Medicine 382

Drug Advertisements 383

Appraising Advertisements 383 / The Art of Half-truth 384 / The Truth, but Not the Whole Truth 384

Guidelines for Buying OTC Drugs 384

Specific OTC Products   386

For the Common Cold 386 / Cough Medicines 386 / Pain 387 /
Stomach Problems 387 / Itching 388 / "Feminine Hygiene" 389
Acne 389 / Allergy 390

Cosmetics   390

Mouthwashes 391 / Deodorants and Antiperspirants 391 / Eye
Makeup 391 / Hair-care Products 391

Quacks and Quackery   392

The Birth of Quackery 392 / How to Spot a Quack 392 / Nostrums 393
Controlling Quackery 398 / How to File a Consumer Complaint 398

Summary   399 / Suggested Readings   399

19: The Environment   401

Chapter Objectives   401

Environmental Pollution   402

Air Pollution 402 / Water Pollution 404 / Toxic Wastes 406 /
Solid Wastes 407 / Pesticides 408 / Heavy Metals 409 /
Radiation 410

The Urban Environment   412

The Social Environment 412 / Pests 412 / Noise Pollution 413

Social Action for the Environment   414

Conservationsim and Environmentalism 414

Future of the Spaceship Earth: Population and Other Problems   415

Too Many People 415 / Too Few Resources 416 / Too Few Solutions 416

Summary   418 / Suggested Readings   418

20. Violence   420

Chapter Objectives   420

The Roots of Violence   421

The Impaired Self-image 421 / Violence as a Learned Response 423

Kinds of Violence 423

Domestic Violence 423 / Street Crime 426 / Rape 428 / Violence in the Schools 429

The Cost of Violence 430

Collective Violence 432

Summary 434 / Suggested Readings 434

APPENDIX: First Aid and Safety 436

A Glossary of Specific First Aid Problems and Treatments 439

Bleeding 439 / Breathing Problems 440 / Broken Bones 442 / Burns 442 / Choking on Food or Other Objects (The Abdominal Thrust) 443 / Heart Attacks 445 / Overdose on Drugs 449

Safety at Home 451

GLOSSARY 458

INDEX 480

Preface

The writing of this book forced me to think about all the ways that college health courses have changed, while in many respects they have remained the same, since I was an undergraduate 30 years ago. They have changed because our society has changed, by getting rid of many old problems and by dealing—sometimes successfully, sometimes not—with many new ones. But these courses have *not* changed in the sense that many old problems still bedevil us. Even 30 years ago, most people died from cardiovascular diseases, cancer, and accidents. Then as now, drunken driving killed thousands each year. Sexually transmitted diseases, at that time called venereal diseases, were becoming more and more common. Hucksters, quacks, and phony drugs were sold in every town and city, and honest medical care was getting more costly.

Yet some things were different 30 years ago. Tuberculosis was still among the 10 leading causes of death. Polio struck thousands of people each summer. Cases of smallpox were reported in the United States. Marijuana was mainly for jazz musicians. Few people complained about cigarette smoking, and few understood its dangers. A visit to a physician's office cost $5 and a home visit—then still common—cost $10. The "Pill" was only a gleam in a researcher's eye, and what a small minority of people called "free love" was plain immorality to the rest. (A lot of people indulged in it nonetheless.) You could even assume that men and women who lived together were married.

The changes of the past 30 years showed me that writing a health textbook is no route to immortality, for any statement that may be true as I write it might not be true the day after; change makes liars of us all, despite our best intentions. So this book is intended for today; it is as up-to-date as possible.

About This Book

Health does not presume to instruct the instructors about what they should teach, or how. It is intended, on the contrary, to be used by teachers of many different outlooks and many different approaches to teaching. To make that possible I have included all those topics, principles, and concepts that are central to beginning courses in today's health education. I have stressed two main themes. The first is the connection between the social, mental, and physical aspects of health—an idea sometimes called "holistic" health. The second is our personal responsibility to preserve our own health by living healthy lives.

How The Book Is Organized

The material in this book has been divided into six basic units.

Unit One, Mental Health, introduces the reader to the workings of the mind and the brain, to the growth of the personality, to the concept of stress, and to our responses (successful and unsuccessful) to it. These topics come first because "high-level wellness" (see the Introduction) depends in great part on a positive self-image—the ability to feel good about yourself.

Unit Two, Drugs, examines one of the least successful ways of coping with stress: the use and misuse of psychoactive substances. Alcohol gets the longest chapter in this unit, since it is (and always has been) the most commonly used and misused psychoactive drug; tobacco and illicit drugs each get chapters of their own.

Unit Three, Physical Health, consists of chapters that focus on exercise, nutrition, weight control, noncommunicable disease, and communicable disease. The text shows how fitness and diet are related to overall health; and it explains the interaction between the physical and mental elements of health.

Unit Four, Sexuality, explores not only contraception and the biology of sex but also the emotional and social aspects of sexuality, especially sex roles. The text discusses as well the particular concerns of students about their own sexuality.

Unit Five, Life Cycles, reviews two matters of great recent interest: social relationships, and aging, dying, and death.

Unit Six, Social Health, examines the health-care system of the United States, health-care products and consumerism, the present and future of our environment, and violence. I believe that the chapter on violence is the first of its kind in personal health textbooks, and it is all too timely.

Key Features

1. *Objectives* alert the student, at the beginning of each chapter, to the most important topics they will be reading about.

2. *Boxes* supplement the basic text by presenting case studies and other items of high interest. Together with the marginal notes, the illustrations, and the photographs, they make the text a "friendly" one to the student.

3. *Self-assessment devices* are included in the body of the text so that readers can assess their own wellness and the risks to it. These devices raise the student's awareness of the need to change unhealthy behavior.

4. *Summaries* at the end of each chapter outline the major points in it.

5. An *appendix* on first aid and safety provides basic information on those subjects.

6. A *glossary* of technical terms appears at the end of the book.

7. An *index* makes it easy to find any topic discussed in the text.

Acknowledgments

Writing a textbook is rather like playing the piano in a Beethoven concerto—it requires strength as well as skill, and it can succeed only with the help of the orchestra and its conductor. The conductor in this case was Roger Samuel Draper, development editor. I am also grateful to Ray O'Connell, of Prentice-Hall's College Editorial Department, who recruited me for this project; to Alice Dworkin, his assistant; to Ray Keating, manufacturing buyer for Prentice-Hall; and to Cecil Yarbrough, the director of Prentice-Hall's Book Project Division.

Early drafts of this book were helped along by the writing, editorial, and research skills of Jane Barrett, David Conti, David Crook, Terry Dugan, Toni Goldfarb, Susan Joseph, Allen Kimbrell, Kenneth Kimmel, Walter Kroczak, Rita Maidat, Virginia Muhlenberg, and Margaret Scal. Martha Goldstein, the managing editor of Prentice-Hall's Book Project Division, copy edited the manuscript with skill and enthusiasm and saw the project through its production stages with the aid of Walter Saxon. Florence Dara Silverman, the division's art director, and Bill Gray, book designer, worked to embody the manuscript in a handsome physical product, as did Anita Duncan, who researched the photographs. Marc Anderson used much ingenuity in tracking down permissions; Robert Mony coordinated the fine glossary; and Paula Bradley put a good deal of effort into her excellent index. My own team of researchers deserves heartfelt thanks, too: Janet Redmond gave me much able assistance in the early going; and Laurie Debelak, Linda Losiewicz, Sheila Peters, Joan Tarquino, and Melba Tomeo all made important contributions later on.

I am also indebted to my colleagues at "the Rock," among them Emil Bend, Charlie Bish, Bernie Freydberg, Stan Kendzorski, and George Mihalik. I owe a special word of thanks to Lois Thompson, who reviewed two chapters. Ken Lowry, Larry Lowing, and Joyce Murray gave me moral support and valuable information.

Early drafts of this manuscript were reviewed by a number of colleagues at other institutions. I offer sincere thanks to these dedicated (and at times, I'm sure, frustrated) seekers of truth:

John P. Allegrante, Teachers College, Columbia University
Ruth Ann Althaus, George Williams College
Winslow J. Bashe Jr., M.D., School of Medicine, Wright State University
Richard A. Berger, Biokinetics Research Laboratory, Temple University
Gerald Braza, University of Utah
Andrew J. J. Brennan, Center for Health Help, Metropolitan Life Insurance Company
Janet Curtis, Long Beach City College
George S. Everly Jr., Loyola College; University of Maryland
Robert Kertzer, University of New Hampshire
Patricia A. Kreutler, Simmons College
Richard A. Fee, Psychophysiology Research Lab, University of Louisville
Larry Olsen, Arizona State University
Bernard Pollack, Brooklyn College, City University of New York
Dorothy Slack, University of Vermont
Andrew Sorensen, Department of Preventive, Family, and Rehabilitation Medicine, University of Rochester.

Of course, any errors that managed to elude them are strictly my own.

For my wife Holly, who did most of the chores on the farm while I scribbled away the hours, I cannot express enough admiration and thanks. To the kids—Jenifer, Margaret, Elizabeth, Clarissa, Candy, Joseph, and Adam—whose time with me was sacrificed to the writing of this book, I can only say that I'll do better next year. I dedicate this book to them and to my wife.

Russell Whaley, M.P.H., Ph.D.
Slippery Rock, Pennsylvania

Introduction

To understand human health, you must understand human beings. Human bodies, like those of all living things, are magnificent works of physiology: Our cells, tissues, organs, and systems are marvels of chemistry and engineering. But merely as biological machines we do not cut a great figure among the creatures of the earth. Many animals are bigger, stronger, and faster than we are, and certain plants live longer than we do. Yet we rule over the oldest of plants and the strongest of animals because we are more intelligent than they are. Our intelligence is our ability to see problems and solve them, on the one hand, and to have strong and complex emotions, on the other.

These qualities make us human, for better or worse. And sometimes it is for the worse, since we often try to solve the *wrong* problems, and our emotions are often futile and destructive. Not even the most stupid of animals make war on each other; murder and race hatred are known only among human beings. These evils should make us feel ashamed. They should also make us think.

Despite the problems that our intelligence creates for us, human beings might have died out long ago, like the mastodon and the woolly mammoth, had intelligence not been useful to us, on balance. Since you yourself are human, there is no need to explain its benefit to individuals. But the greatest benefit of intelligence is that it helps to free us from our individual limitations. The other members of the animal kingdom must face life pretty much alone: Each fly, each lion, each sparrow

1

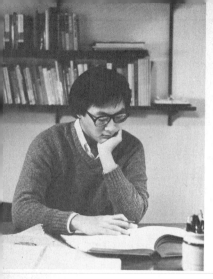

Deborah Chu/Photo Researchers

can make use only of its own abilities, and the cooperation that may occur within these species is instinctive and therefore limited. The cooperation of human beings is more planned, more flexible, more extensive, more wonderful.

Cooperation has made people far more different from each other than the members of any other species are. We rely on one another for food, for clothing, for shelter, and for a good many other things, and it is this mutual reliance that makes us individuals; without it, we would all have to do more or less the same things to survive, as flies, lions, and sparrows do. And cooperation has made the many *groups* of human beings, living in widely separated places, far more different than the geographically separate groups of other species: A dog in India lives in pretty much the same way as a dog in America does, but the people of the United States live by customs and ideals very different from those of India. These differences divide human beings into separate societies.

Holistic Health

Because human life has physical, mental, and social aspects, human health has physical, mental, and social dimensions. Health is like a circle; each dimension runs into the others, and a change in any one part changes the whole. Physical illness affects our mental and social outlook, social stresses upset the mind and the body, and mental illness has physical and social symptoms. So health, or wellness, should be seen as *holistic*, since it deals with the whole person—mind, society, and all. As the U.N. World Health Organization said in 1947, health is "a state of complete mental, physical, and social wellbeing, not merely the absence of disease or infirmity." It is a positive quality, the development of each human being's potential, not just a negative quality, the absence of sickness. These positive qualities are called "high-level wellness."

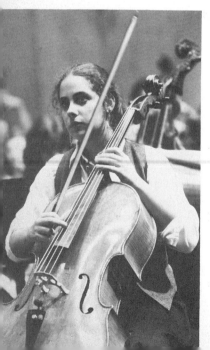

Jan Halaska/Photo Researchers

Change

No one has ever achieved health in the holistic sense, or in any other, and then stayed healthy forever. On the contrary, our minds and bodies constantly move between health and sickness. Our environment—physical and social, internal and external—changes moment by moment. To achieve wellness you, too, must be able to change, since there is only one unchangeable condition for human beings: death. But changes can be made only within narrow limits, limits that permit the mind and body to maintain homeostasis, or balance (see Chapter 3). Beyond these limits lie discomfort, disease, and death.

Responsibility

Some threats to health are largely beyond our control—genetic diseases (see Chapter 10), for instance. Some are partly controllable, like the place where you live. Some are completely controllable—those that

2

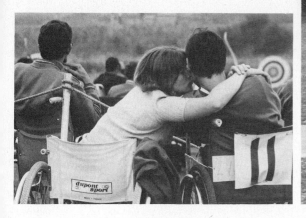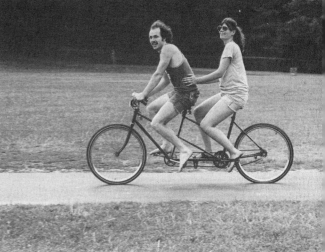

result entirely from personal behavior, like smoking. People with a genetic disease (see Chapter 10) do not have a responsibility to discover a cure for it, *but we are all responsible for knowing what kinds of behavior are healthy or unhealthy—and for acting on that knowledge.* The chief aim of this book is to help you learn how to know and do the things that will help you to preserve your wellness.

Health does not mean the same thing for all. Disabled people who manage to have work and active social lives are healthy—because health is the ability to respond to challenges.
Left: Stan Goldblatt/Photo Researchers
Right: Lily Solmssen/Photo Researchers

Threats to Life and Wellness

As a whole, the American people have never been more healthy, yet the death rate for American teenagers and young adults (people aged 15–24) is higher today than it was 20 years ago. This paradox is not a statistical illusion; it is real. Why?

Causes of Death in Young Adults

About 75 percent of all deaths of young adults result from accidents (see Appendix), murder (see Chapter 20), and suicide (see Chapter 3). If you think about accidents, murders, and suicide you will see that, unlike genetic diseases, they are avoidable. They are part of a way of life—a violent and destructive way of life, one that could be changed. Most of the time, this way of life is a not-very-successful way of coping (see Chapter 3) with the changes that come with adolescence and young adulthood: physical growth and maturity, and the move from dependence to independence. These changes create stress (see Chapter 2), and some people respond to stress in unhealthy ways: mental illness (Chapter 3), drug taking (Chapter 4), violence (Chapter 20), and suicide Chapter 3). Mentally healthy people respond to stress by coping with the problems that caused it.

Causes of Disease in Young Adults

Since the deaths of young people most often result from their way of life, it seems to follow that their diseases and infirmities should also reflect that way of life, right? Right!

One important aspect of this life style is sex. Sex is one of life's greatest pleasures, but it is also the means of transmitting a whole category of diseases—the sexually transmitted diseases (STDs, see Chapter 11)—and young people contract about 9 million cases of them each year, 75 percent of the total. Also as a result of sexual activity, about 1 million teenage women become pregnant each year—1 of 4 aged 19.

The start of active sexuality (see Chapter 12) is one of the many sources of stress in the lives of young people. Stress can provoke many kinds of responses—from mental illness (see Chapter 3) to stress-related disease (see Chapter 2), such as high blood pressure, gastrointestinal (GI) problems (see Chapter 10), nervousness, and headaches.

Yet another kind of response to stress—and another important aspect of the life style of young people—is drug taking. Levels of drug use and drug dependency vary from year to year, but they are very high, and most drug abusers are young. Alcohol abuse is less concentrated among young people, but about 3.5 million of them have drinking problems.

Of course, the life styles of young people do not cause all their health problems. Mononucleosis, infectious hepatitis, respiratory and GI infections, and other infectious ailments (see Chapter 11) all stalk the ranks of the young, and so do such noninfectious diseases (see Chapter 10) as allergies, heart diseases, and cancer.

Choosing for Health

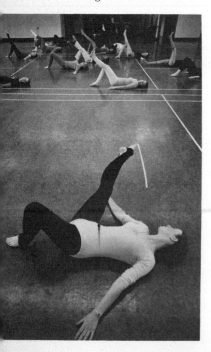

Ellis Herwig/Stock, Boston

Since so many threats to health stem from your way of life, you can to some extent choose to be healthy. That means, first of all, caring about yourself. In all the many years of human life, no one has ever been just like you; you can make your own unique contribution to mankind, and no one else can make it for you. If you do not choose to make it, it will be lost forever.

Choosing to be healthy means caring about other human beings as well as about yourself, for they too have unique contributions to make—to your own life and to humanity as a whole.

Choosing for health means learning to live with your body—using, developing, and enjoying its physical abilities (by eating sensibly, exercising, and resting) and its capacity for shared sexual pleasure.

Choosing means using good sense: "If you can't be good, be careful," as the proverb sadly but wisely has it (see Chapter 14). Prevent disease when you can (see below), and seek professional care (see chapter 17) when you fall sick. Do what your physician tells you to do.

Tomorrow's Problems

After the age of 25, your health problems usually change, first slowly, then dramatically. The age of 40 is something of a milestone. Heart disease (see Chapter 10) then becomes the leading cause of death (about 953,100 deaths in the United States in 1979), followed by cancer

(403,780 deaths in 1979). Strokes, too, emerges as a prominent cause of death (169,350 deaths in 1979). You may be able to avoid these diseases in the future by the way you live now. Let us take a closer look.

Some diseases, like measles, tetanus, whooping cough, and polio, are entirely preventable because you can be vaccinated (see Chapter 11) against them. Other diseases, like arthritis (Chapter 10) and brain tumors (see Chapter 10), cannot now be prevented at all. Many diseases fall between these two extremes: They are caused, in part, by behavior, but in part by genetic predisposition (see Chapter 10).

An Ounce of Prevention. Diseases are preventable on various levels. Primary prevention means avoiding disease in the first place, by eating carefully (see Chapter 8), getting enough exercise and rest (see Chapter 7), creating favorable conditions at home and at work, and other general measures. It also includes specific protective measures, like vaccination and the use of protective devices (seat belts, for example). Secondary prevention means discovering diseases early, through physical examinations (see Chapter 17); treating diseases in the early stages, when they are easiest to cure; and taking measures to prevent their transmission to others (see Chapter 11). Tertiary prevention means limiting the consequences of disease and the rehabilitation of its victims.

Applied Prevention. Diseases like stroke and cancer—those that usually strike people after they reach the age of 25—generally are long in developing. What can you do right now to stay more healthy later on? One thing is to understand and act on the idea of "risk factors." These are physical conditions and forms of behavior that are statistically related to disease (see Chapter 10 for a longer explanation); smoking, for example, is statistically related to lung cancer (see Chapter 6).

You can lower the risk of getting a disease by eliminating controllable risk factors from your life—using primary prevention.

A Step Beyond

Some forms of behavior—like smoking—are controlled by individuals. Some are not. For instance, in the 1950s houses were built at Love Canal, in Niagara Falls, New York, on land once used as a chemical dump (see Chapter 19). Those who lived in these houses suffered from high rates of many diseases. They might have ended their problems by moving; but moving is not easy. The whole problem might have been avoided if the chemical company had disposed of its wastes safely, but private individuals could not have forced it to do so.

The point is that some kinds of health can be ensured only by collective action—politics. A health book should not lecture on politics, but organized interest groups, many with very selfish viewpoints, do much to injure the health of others. But no such group is as strong as the voting power of our people.

David Powers/Stock, Boston

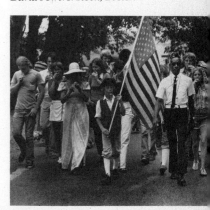

SELF-ASSESSMENT DEVICE: A TEST FOR BETTER HEALTH

Smoking

	Almost Always	Sometimes	Almost Never

If you never smoke, enter a score of 10 for this section and go to the next section on *Alcohol* and *Drugs*.

	Almost Always	Sometimes	Almost Never
1. I avoid smoking cigarettes.	2	1	0
2. I smoke only low tar and nicotine cigarettes *or* I smoke a pipe or cigars.	2	1	0

Smoking Score: _____

Drinking

	Almost Always	Sometimes	Almost Never
1. I avoid drinking alcoholic beverages *or* I drink no more than 1 or 2 drinks a day.	4	1	0
2. I avoid using alcohol or other drugs (especially illegal drugs) as a way of handling stressful situations or the problems in my life.	2	1	0
3. I am careful not to drink alcohol when taking certain medicines (for example, medicine for sleeping, pain, colds, and allergies).	2	1	0
4. I read and follow the label directions when using prescribed and over-the-counter drugs.	2	1	0

Alcohol and Drugs Score: _____

Eating Habits

	Almost Always	Sometimes	Almost Never
1. I eat a variety of foods each day, such as fruits and vegetables, whole grain breads and cereals, lean meats, dairy products, dry peas and beans, and nuts and seeds.	4	1	0
2. I limit the amount of fat, saturated fat, and cholesterol I eat (including fat on meats, eggs, butter, cream, shortenings, and organ meats such as liver).	2	1	0
3. I limit the amount of salt I eat by cooking with only small amounts, not adding salt at the table, and avoiding salty snacks.	2	1	0
4. I avoid eating too much sugar (especially frequent snacks of sticky candy or soft drinks).	2	1	0

Eating Habits Score: _____

Exercise/Fitness

	Almost Always	Sometimes	Almost Never
1. I maintain a desired weight, avoiding overweight and underweight.	3	1	0
2. I do vigorous exercises for 15–30 minutes at least 3 times a week (examples include running, swimming, brisk walking).	3	1	0
3. I do exercises that enhance my muscle tone for 15–30 minutes at least 3 times a week (examples include yoga and calisthenics).	2	1	0
4. I use part of my leisure time participating in individual, family, or team activities that increase my level of fitness (such as gardening, bowling, golf, and baseball).	2	1	0

Exercise/Fitness Score: _____

Stress Control

	Almost Always	Sometimes	Almost Never
1. I have a job or do other work that I enjoy.	2	1	0
2. I find it easy to relax and express my feelings freely.	2	1	0
3. I recognize early, and prepare for events or situations likely to be stressful for me.	2	1	0
4. I have close friends, relatives, or others whom I can talk to about personal matters and call on for help when needed.	2	1	0
5. I participate in group activities (such as church and community organizations) or hobbies that I enjoy.	2	1	0

Stress Control Score: _____

Safety

	Almost Always	Sometimes	Almost Never
1. I wear a seat belt while riding in a car.	2	1	0
2. I avoid driving while under the influence of alcohol and other drugs.	2	1	0
3. I obey traffic rules and the speed limit when driving.	2	1	0
4. I am careful when using potentially harmful products or substances (such as household cleaners, poisons, and electrical devices).	2	1	0
5. I avoid smoking in bed.	2	1	0

Safety Score: _____

After you have figured your scores for each of the six sections, circle the number in each column that matches your score for that section of the test.

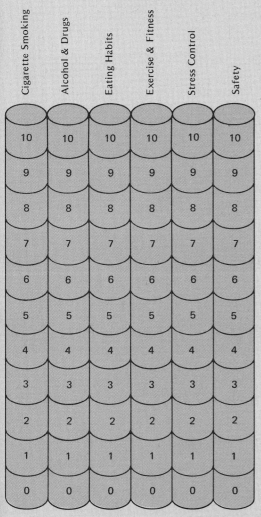

Remember, there is no total score for this test. Consider each section separately. You are trying to identify aspects of your lifestyle that you can improve in order to be healthier and to reduce the risk of illness. So lets see what your scores reveal.

What Your Scores Mean to You

Scores of 9 and 10

Excellent! Your answers show that you are aware of the importance of this area to your health. More importantly, you are putting your knowledge to work for you by practicing good health habits. As long as you continue to do so, this area should not pose a serious health risk. It's likely that you are setting an example for your family and friends to follow. Since you got a very high score on this part of the test, you may want to consider other areas where your scores indicate room for improvement.

Scores of 6 to 8

Your health practices in this area are good, but there is room for improvement. Look again at the items you answered with a "Sometimes" or "Almost Never". What changes can you make to improve your score? Even a small change can often help you achieve better health.

Scores of 3 to 5

Your health risks are showing! Would you like more information about the risks you are facing and about why it is important for you to change these behaviors. Perhaps you need help in deciding how to successfully make the changes you desire. In either case, help is available.

Scores of 0 to 2

Obviously, you were concerned enough about your health to take the test, but your answers show that you may be taking serious and unnecessary risks with your health. Perhaps you are not aware of the risks and what to do about them. You can easily get the information and help you need to improve, if you wish.

Source: U.S. Department of Health and Human Services. Public Health Service, Office of Disease Prevention and Health Promotion.

Mental Health

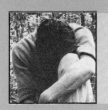

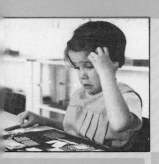

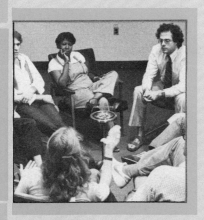

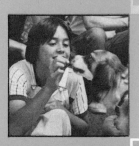

UNIT ONE

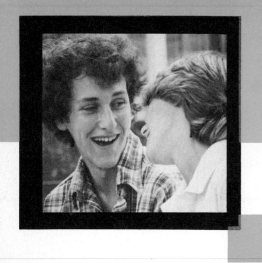

Personality

chapter objectives

When you have finished reading this chapter you should be able to:

1. Define self-esteem and relate it to mental health
2. Explain Freud's concepts of id, ego, and superego; conscious, preconscious, and unconscious
3. Understand Erikson's eight stages of personality development
4. Understand the levels of Maslow's Hierarchy of Needs and recall their order of development
5. Understand the concepts of Glasser's Reality Therapy
6. Explain how behaviorism may change harmful behavior patterns through negative and positive reinforcement

Health is described in the Introduction as a state of complete well-being—physical, mental, and social. Physical health can be defined and measured by such standards as energy, endurance, and freedom from disease. Mental health is hard to define and hard to measure. But it is basic to general good health.

Mental health can be defined as being able to adjust to one's society. Being mentally healthy starts with having self-esteem—feeling good about your *self*. This means making the best use of your talents and skills for both yourself and society.

Profile of the Mentally Healthy

People who feel good about their lives can laugh at their faults but keep their sense of self-respect. They may enjoy success and recover from setbacks. They do not set goals that are too easy or too hard. When problems arise they can face them.

Those who have mental health have good feelings about others as well as themselves. They can form friendships that last. They can trust and be trusted to do what they are supposed to do. They do not bully others and they do not let others bully them. They tolerate, respect, and even cherish the fact that people differ in many ways.

The mentally healthy deal well with life's demands. Mental health, after all, is not the absence of problems, but the ability to resolve (or "cope" with) them. Mentally healthy people are not obsessed by problems; they cope with them as they arise, not before or after. They try to solve any problems without the use of threats or force.

Mentally healthy people try to make pleasant conditions where possible, but accept those that cannot be changed. They seem to achieve more in life than others do—because they see that the key to achievement is planning ahead, setting goals that are ambitious but which they can attain. They are realists and optimists, and they look forward to each day and to new life events.

Threats to Mental Health

Mental health is not constant; it changes as our needs change. Mental health, like physical health, can be undermined in quite a few ways. Like physical health, mental health needs nurturing, protection, and, sometimes, treatment. There are always threats to our mental health, from inside as well as from outside the body. Two of the worst threats are brain damage and stress.

Brain Damage

Some mental disorders have an "organic," or physical, base. Infections, brain tumors, head injuries, and gene patterns can damage the

Work and Love—these are the basics. Without them there is neurosis.
—*Theodore Reik*

Being mentally healthy starts with self-esteem—feeling good about yourself.
Mimi Forsyth/Monkmeyer

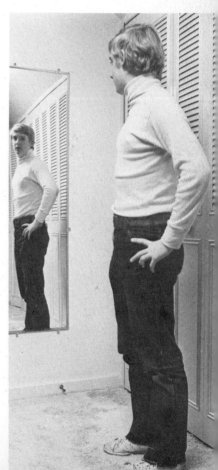

SELF-ASSESSMENT DEVICE 1-1: PUZZLES HAVE PIECES

As people grow and mature, they develop feelings and attitudes toward themselves. This is referred to as "self-image." This exercise has been developed to aid you in the identification of your "self-image."

Listed below are groups of words that are descriptive of personal characteristics that you may exhibit or that are related to you. Please circle all the words that you feel are most descriptive of yourself and your behavior.

loud	clumsy	prudish	gentle
artistic	petite	mouthy	hard-working
dishonest	peaceful	envious	sloppy
smart	mean	concerned	funny
quiet	slim	creative	loving
talented	hostile	muscular	complaining
competitive	charming	naive	firm
poised	happy	conceited	good-humored
cautious	well-dressed	generous	lazy
clever	crabby	sad	unique
responsible	polite	attractive	warm
skinny	heavy	aggressive	energetic
mature	outspoken	friendly	absent-minded
reckless	two-faced	nervous	respectful
committed	moody	talkative	kind
thoughtful	husky	impatient	articulate
proud	rebellious	loyal	sympathetic
tall	forthright	organized	accepting
sophisticated	spiritual	athletic	honest
shy	selfish	narrow-minded	unselfish
reflective	stubborn	sensitive	spiteful
well-built	dependent	short	intellectual
bossy	prejudiced		

Look over the words you have chosen. Do you notice any pattern about your feelings about yourself?

Are you satisfied with your self-image? Please explain your answer. Is there anything you can do to reinforce or change it? List your ideas.

Do you think you have a positive self-image or a negative self-image? What has influenced the development of your image?

Source: The Center for Learning, Inc. 1972. Adapted for classroom use.

brain and so affect the mental state. If a pregnant woman drinks large amounts of alcohol, her unborn child's brain may not develop properly. Genetic and pregnancy counseling, immunizations, and periodic health screenings may help to prevent and detect such problems.

Older people sometimes have physical disorders that can lead to mental disorders. For instance, not enough of the right food or hardened blood vessels (causing less of a blood flow to the brain) often lead to senility or other mental problems. Some problems with blood vessels and blood flow can be controlled with drugs. Some problems caused by poor nutrition can be found and corrected by counseling. Often, funds may be sought from public welfare agencies to ensure a good diet.

Stress

We can all tolerate some stress (see Chapters 2 and 3). The ability to do so varies from person to person and from time to time. But prolonged stress can lead to what has been called a "nervous breakdown." The stress may be physical or social in nature, or both at once. Some people may become depressed while struggling with a major disease or general ill health; some people have mental distress after the death of a spouse or parent, failing at school or work, losing at love, or retiring. Denying these problems, or panicking, may increase the pain and the pressure. Each further crisis may then become harder to handle.

Poverty—with its bad housing, poor schools, racism, and other social ills—can cause stress that damages our mental health.

Poverty can cause stress that damages our mental health.
Nick Sapieha/Stock, Boston

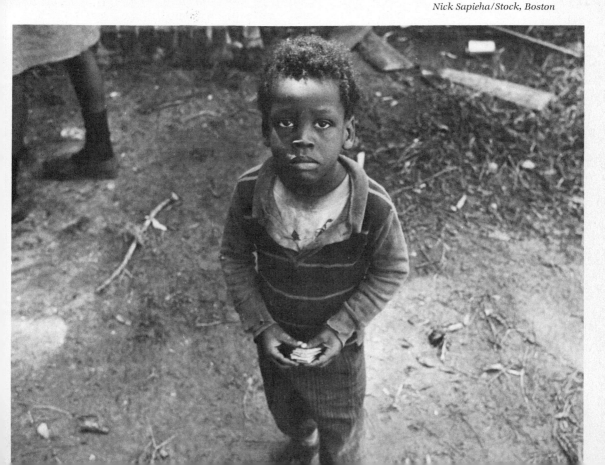

Mind and Body

The way that the mind relates to the body fascinates philosophers, physicians, poets—in fact, all of us—and it has through all the ages. The division between the functions of the mind—thought and feeling—and the functions of the body—like breathing and digesting—may be complex and often blurred. The functions of the mind and body overlap and affect each other at all times. So the concept of "total" health must embrace both mental health and physical health.

Since the same organ, the brain, controls both physical and mental functions through the nervous system, the brain is the starting point for our study of health.

The Brain

The brain consists of four parts: the *cerebrum,* which directs thought and judgment; the *medulla* and *cerebellum,* which direct the body's physiological functions; and the *limbic system,* which is the source of emotion. The brain is part of a larger network, the *nervous system,* whose function is to protect the body and allow it to adjust to the environment. The nervous system collects and sends out messages through a system of nerves, which go to all parts of the body.

Nerves called sensory receptors are found in the eyes, the ears, the nose, and the skin of the body. They transmit vital messages to the brain about conditions in the environment. The brain reacts to these data by sending out directions on how the organs should cope with the changing conditions. If, for instance, a light shines in your eyes, you will blink automatically to protect them. But your response to someone's words requires thought—first to interpret and then to respond.

The Nerves

Although the body only has one set of nerves, it has been found to work in two distinct ways. The *autonomic* nervous system controls the "automatic" bodily actions, like the heartbeat, breathing, and digestion. The *voluntary* nervous system controls conscious mental action, like thought, motion, and language. The two "systems" work together to help us adjust to the environment.

How the Body and the Mind Affect Each Other

Mind and Matter.   The body affects the mind in many ways. A high fever may cause us to become weak and to hallucinate. Cancer, heart disease, and other disorders can all alter mental outlook and personality. So, too, can the use of alcohol or drugs. Even a common headache, cold, or stomach upset can make us feel annoyed or depressed.

The mind can also affect the body in many ways. Mental attitude can affect digestion; eating while tense is a common cause of gas or heart-

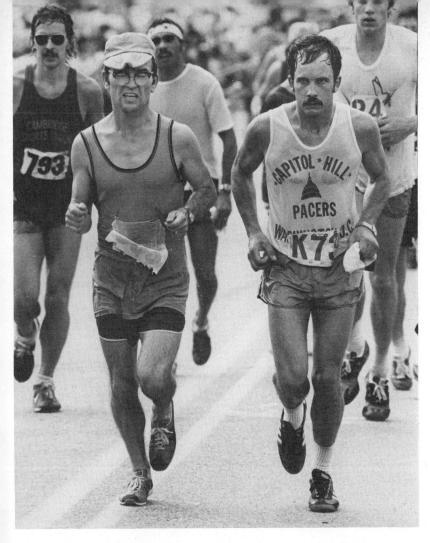

Mens sana in corpore sano: A sound mind in a sound body (from the Latin).

Peter Southwick/Stock, Boston

burn. Peace of mind and contentment show up in both posture and sleep habits, as well as in regular voiding of body wastes. Fear, worry, and frustration often cause physical problems, among them ulcers, migraine headaches, bowel disorders, sleepless nights, and high blood pressure.

The way the mind and the body affect each other may be quite dramatic. People who believe in voodoo—a form of witchcraft—may become sick and even die when they learn that certain rituals were practiced against them. Losing the desire to live may also result in physical changes that can bring on death. During the Korean war (1950–1953) some U.S. prisoners of war, with no apparent physical disorders, despaired of life to the point that they gave up and died.

The mind may also affect the body in helpful ways. When we hear music or see a beautiful painting, the mind responds with contentment, and thus affects the body's well-being. Looking at scenery, hearing rain fall, reading a good book—all these may soothe and comfort the mind. When we are pleased and we relax we may promote that elusive quality of life, peace of mind. This, in turn, can help the body feel well and function well.

The Adaption Mechanism.   Another example of the complex way that the body and the mind affect each other is the *adaption mechanism.* This consists of a fixed sequence of reactions that begin when the nervous system receives data about the body's environment. Stimuli (or signals) like pain, bright light, or cold weather are dealt with quickly, without the help of the mind. This reaction is called a reflex. But other signals are more complex; they call forth a second stage, one of feeling/ emotion. Then the mind helps us react to the signal. At the third stage, of thought, we reflect on the collected data and then plan our course of action. Think about an adaption mechanism in action: A driver *sees* a car out of control, *feels* fear, *thinks* of a way to avoid an accident, and *acts* to avoid it. All this happens within fractions of a second.

Ideally, the adaption mechanism works in a continuous stream; but it can be blocked at any of its stages. The driver might not see the other car. Or the driver might (at the stage of emotion) panic and become confused. In either of these cases the driver will fail to take the right action (in this case swerving or braking), so an accident might occur.

Levels of Awareness

Some researchers think that thinking and feeling take place on a few levels of awareness. Sigmund Freud (1856–1939), a Viennese physician, was the first to develop this idea. He argued that there were three such levels: the *conscious,* the *preconscious,* and the *unconscious.* He felt that these three levels cannot always work together in harmony and that this could harm one's mental health (see Chapter 2).

The Conscious. A conscious thought is one of which we are aware at any given moment; at *this* moment *you* are aware of the definition of a conscious thought. Perception, judgment, memory, and attention all belong to the domain of the conscious. The conscious mind helps us adjust to the demands of the world more directly than the other two levels of awareness. When conscious, we are awake to life. We deal with others and use the knowledge built up over thousands of years of human thought to solve problems and make judgments.

The Preconscious. Thoughts and feelings that can become conscious but are not conscious at a certain time were called the preconscious by Freud (and the *subconscious* by some other researchers). Humans can focus attention on just one idea or thought at a time. When our attention shifts to other matters, what was preconscious then becomes conscious. For instance, a student's conscious attention in an English class might be focused on *Hamlet*. But in the next class, say in art, the student thinks about Greek statues.

The Unconscious. You already knew about the conscious and preconscious levels of awareness before those labels were attached to them. But now let us consider Freud's third level, the unconscious. For Freud, this was a level commonly unknown to us, a vast region of the mind that affects us profoundly although it is normally "blocked from consciousness"—that is, repressed. The unconscious holds childhood wishes, impulses, and emotional events. These are repressed, Freud claimed, because most of us "unconsciously" fear their full release. The contents of the unconscious are governed by their own set of laws, laws that are not subject to the logic of the world in which we live. The instincts, wishes, and impulses of the unconscious—like those of a child—demand instant fulfillment. As children, he said, humans have drives—aggression, exhibitionism, bisexuality, even a desire for sex with the parent of the other sex—that, socially, we would not accept. As the conscious comes to reject such drives, they become sources of anxiety. But it would be dangerous to fulfill them, so most adults seek to do so only in fantasy, dreams, images, and in hallucinations.

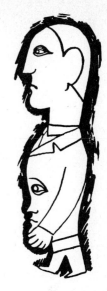

The Unconscious. Freud believed that potent inner forces determine human behavior.

Woodcut by Jean Cocteau/The Bettmann Archive

Theories of Personality

Freud

Freud's concept of the unconscious was the base for his theory of personality, one that stresses the importance of the repressed drives of sex and aggression. In fact, Freud claimed that these drives shape the personality from earliest infancy.

Just as Freud divided awareness into three levels, so too did he divide personality into three "systems," the *id,* the *ego,* and the *superego.* He thought of these not as three structures, but as mental tendencies, or forces. Although Freud's theory of personality cannot be proved, it may still offer some insights into human behavior.

The Id. For Freud, the id was the source of our most basic drives, the life forces we need for survival: sex and aggression. Both drives demand instant fulfillment whatever the consequence, a demand that Freud called the *pleasure principle.* The id is the engine, the source of energy for the personality as a whole. From it develop the ego and the superego. Unlike the ego and the superego, the id is present from birth. It works on the unconscious level of awareness.

The brain is viewed as an appendage of the genital glands.
        —*Carl Jung on Freud*

The Ego. Freud held that this second system of personality, the ego, emerged from the id through experience. The quest of the ego is not pleasure, but to survive, to be secure, and to master. The ego screens information from the outside world to protect us from the drives of the id, which may be destructive. At the same time the ego must attempt to *satisfy* the id, in a socially acceptable way.

For instance, while in class you may be attracted to someone. If you try to make physical contact quickly—as the id would have you do—you will be censured, perhaps even arrested. You can, however, express this feeling of attraction in a socially acceptable way, by asking the other person for a date. The ego is always doing things of this sort, always testing reality, on the one hand, but always serving the demands of the id, on the other. Unlike the id, which is impulsive, the ego acts by imposing reason and order. Each of our lives is unique, and so are the lessons drawn by each of us from life's events. Each ego is thus unique as well.

The Superego. Freud thought that the ego must also take into account the demands of his third system of the personality: the superego. And that is no easy task. The superego is the opposite of the pleasure-loving id; it strives to be moral and perfect. The superego holds for us the values of our parents and their culture; it seeks to preserve the social order so that humans can live together. The superego forbids and warns us. It often acts as a critic. Yet the superego also rewards the ego for a job well done.

Personality Dynamics. Freud's theory of how the personality develops and grows stresses how the id, ego, and superego affect one another. Each of us must somehow strike a balance between the fulfillment of the sex and the aggression drives (or instinct), on the one hand, and our social restraints, on the other. For Freud, these two forces, instinct and society, are always in conflict—and personality is the sum or the end product of the compromises that must be made between them.

Freud's theories are still in hot contest. No matter what is said about them, it is quite clear that the mind is subject to pressures from both inside and outside—work, love, disease, to name but three. Somehow, our minds must try to respond to them in a way that is not only real but also fulfilling to us. We do not have to apply the name "ego" to the aspect of the mind that tries to make that response. We do not even have to accept Freud's theories in whole or in part. But we do need to have a name for this reality-testing aspect of the mind, and the name that has been accepted is the ego. In this sense, a healthy ego is needed for mental well-being. If egos are weak people cannot balance the conflict of the instincts with the demands of society. Weak egos have difficulty coping with stress because the demands made upon them are too great (see

Chapters 2 and 3). People with weak egos also have feelings of low self-esteem and low self-worth, which may undermine the making of safe and smart decisions.

Erikson

Erik Erikson (1902–   ), a *neo-Freudian* (one who attempts to do research and to build theory on Freud's ideas), studied the ego's development. For Erikson, the ego moves through a sequence of eight stages that overlap. In each stage the ego needs to overcome a conflict between growth and stagnation; it also needs to master a certain social role. Each stage has a new level of ego development that needs a new set of coping skills. Failure to complete the early stages with success causes trouble in the later ones. For, as Erikson saw it, feelings of failure in the early stages may lodge in the unconscious. At a later stage, such feelings can surface in the conscious mind; there they can keep the ego from coping well with problems like those that caused the first failure. Erikson saw that the longer the trail of failures, the more power each new one would have.

Erikson's scheme of development is identified below by the conflict that characterizes it.

Stage One: Trust versus Mistrust. Babies show trust through physical acts: deep sleep, good appetite, and regular bowel movements. Babies learn to trust the steady process of the body's urges and the love and comfort given by those who care for them. The creation of trust is the first task of the ego, its first step in the making of ego-identity. The successful completion of this stage hinges on care. Those who were not cared for well cannot create this sense of trust. They may grow up to become adults who are not trustworthy and who do not expect this from others. For Erikson, trust is the basis for all mental health.

Stage Two: Autonomy versus Shame and Doubt. In this stage the child masters toilet training and body control. The child's ego must now develop "a sense of self-control without loss of self-esteem," leading to a "lasting sense of good will and pride." Strict toilet training deprives the child of a natural sense of self and self-regulation; it leads, as well, to deep-rooted feelings of guilt and shame. Those who pass through this stage with success learn how to work with others without a loss of their sense of self. They learn how to tell individuality from willfulness.

Stage Three: Initiative versus Guilt. Knowing how to tell individuality from willfulness now deepens. The ego should cease acts that merely defy and protest to join with others in new projects and forms of play. The joyful child builds on growing powers of movement and thought,

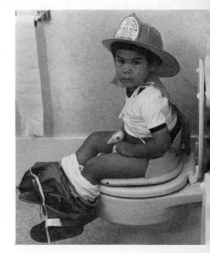

In the stage of "autonomy versus shame and doubt" the child masters toilet training and body control.

Peter Menzel/Stock, Boston

Erikson's model of development may treat the unfolding of *men's* lives as the norm and largely ignore the life events and problems faced by women. In *Passages*, Gail Sheehy looks at the stages in the lives of women. Here are some of her comments on those stages:

> *Pulling Up Roots.* The tasks of this passage are to locate ourselves within a peer group role, a sex role, an anticipated occupation, an ideology, a world view. As a result, we gather the impetus to leave home physically and the identity to *begin* leaving home emotionally.
>
> Even as one part of us seeks to be an individual, another part longs to restore the safety and comfort of merging with another. Thus one of the most popular myths of this passage is: we can piggyback our development by attaching to a Stronger One. But people who marry during this time often prolong financial and emotional ties to the family and relatives that impede them from becoming self-sufficient (p. 27).
>
> *The Trying Twenties.* Doing what we "should" is the most pervasive theme of the twenties. The "shoulds" are largely defined by family models, the press of the culture, or the prejudices of our peers. If the prevailing cultural instructions are that one should get married and settle down behind one's own door, a nuclear family is born (p. 27).
>
> *Catch-30.* Impatient with devoting ourselves to the "should," a new vitality springs from within as we approach 30. Men and women alike speak of feeling too narrow and restricted . . . The woman who was previously content at home with children chafes to venture into the world . . . If the discontent doesn't lead to a divorce, it will, or should, call for a serious review of the marriage and of each partner's aspirations in their Catch-30 condition (pp. 28–29).
>
> *The Deadline Decade.* The loss of youth, the faltering of physical powers we have always taken for granted, the fading purpose of stereotyped roles by which we have thus far identified ourselves, the spiritual dilemma of having no absolute answers—any or all of these shocks can give this passage the character of crisis . . . Women sense this inner crossroad earlier than men do. The time pinch often prompts a woman to stop and take an all-points survey at age 35. Whatever options she has already played out, she feels a "my last chance" urgency to review those options she has set aside and those that aging and biology will close off in the *now foreseeable* future. For all her qualms and confusion about where to start looking for a new future, she usually enjoys an exhilaration of release. Assertiveness begins rising. There are so many firsts ahead (pp. 30–31).
>
> *Renewal or Resignation.* If one has refused to budge through the midlife transition, the sense of staleness will calcify into resignation . . . If we have confronted ourselves in the middle passage and found a renewal of purpose around which we are eager to build a more authentic life structure, these may well be the best years (pp. 31–32).

Gail Sheehy, *Passages: Predictable Crises of Adult Life.* (New York: Dutton, 1974), pp. 25–32.

powers that are focused on new challenges. Success in this stage helps the child develop a sense of duty, to care for younger children, to play games and use tools.

Stage Four: Industry versus Inferiority. The child is now ready for school. This is the time when the ego learns to act in the outside world, to use its tools, to play by its rules. Seeing that the family does not provide a permanent home, children turn outside it for new direction. Being able to "perform" in school gives children a sense of worth. They learn to carry out projects with instructions from their teachers. They become aware of social lines drawn between rich and poor or white and black and learn that there is a division of labor. They weave this knowledge into a growing self-identity. But those who are held back from trying to master new skills now may withdraw to the dream-like world of family rivalries.

Stage Five: Identity versus Role Confusion. This stage is commonly called adolescence. As childhood ends, sexual urges and rapid body growth make youths feel confused and full of self-doubt. They are obsessed with how others, mainly their classmates, view them; they wonder how they will fit into the adult world; they struggle to create a new self from fragments of their earlier years. Their struggle is intense, sometimes desperate. In the effort to forge an identity, young people idolize heroes, join cliques, and fall madly in love. They try one thing, then another, then sometimes the opposite. Social rules seem to be "out of synch" with their inner feelings and needs. Great pressures are put on them to choose careers, deal with parents, with friends, and with their blossoming love lives. Great decisions are called for, yet the knowledge of how to make those decisions is limited. One of life's most difficult tasks is to build on early achievements while going on to create adult selves.

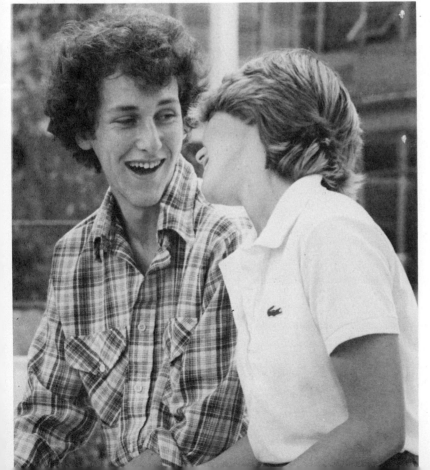

Adolescents must learn how to live in the adult world, for example, by forming romantic relationships.
Paul Conklin/Monkmeyer

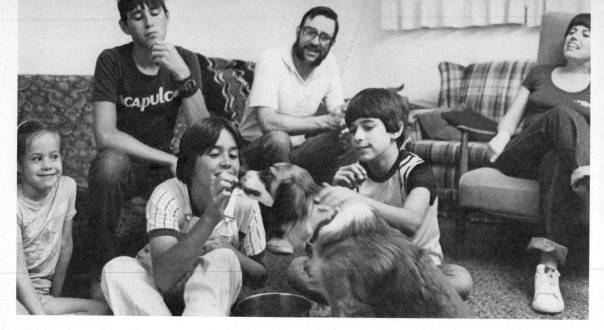

Adults need links with young people, and young people need adults to guide and teach them.

Mimi Forsyth/Monkmeyer

Stage Six: Intimacy versus Isolation. Young adults in this stage form sexual and romantic bonds, complete with ethical commitments, physical and emotional pleasure and pain, and self-sacrifice. Loving another person in this way compels them to expose their egos and newfound senses of self, since it is hard to love and still stay a separate person with separate feelings, problems, and triumphs. People with weak egos, whose selves are not well forged, fear romantic closeness and often isolate themselves.

Stage Seven: Generativity versus Stagnation. Adults need links with young people as much as infants need care from adults. In this stage the growth of the ego comes from closeness and sharing with a lover. Adults who complete this stage with success can be trusted to guide and teach the young.

Stage Eight: Ego Integrity versus Despair. In this last stage, the aging adult reviews the victories and defeats of life. Older adults should feel a sense of fulfillment and dignity, without regrets for missed chances, regrets about the lives they have led. Older people who fail to achieve this inner peace are thrown into despair, sorrow, and the fear of death or the desire for it.

Humanistic Psychology

Maslow.   Abraham Maslow (1908–1970) was an American psychologist who objected to Freud's focus on those aspects of personality that are not healthy or normal. Freud, he argued, had developed his theories in the course of treating the sick, so the result was limited and negative.

Maslow saw that happy children can cope with guilt, tension, and other problems. Freud's theory failed to explain this. So, Maslow, in fact, helped change the focus of research from the abnormal to the normal.

Hierarchy of Needs. Maslow found that humans progress in life through a "hierarchy of needs," needs that unfold in a fixed sequence over a long span of time. The "lower" (or early) needs must be fulfilled before the more complex needs. For instance, the need for food is felt and must be dealt with before the need for esteem. Children who live in violent neighborhoods, where their very safety is not certain, cannot devote themselves to mental growth. A person who must scrounge for food cannot be concerned about status.

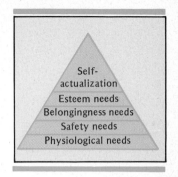

Figure 1–1. Maslow's Hierarchy of Needs.

Data (for diagram) based on Hierarchy of Needs in "A Theory of Human Motivation" in Motivation and Personality, *2nd Edition by Abraham H. Maslow Copyright © 1970 by Abraham H. Maslow Reprinted by permission of Harper & Row, Publishers, Inc.*

The lower needs must be resolved, to some extent, each day. This may not be so of the higher needs, however. As people grow from one stage to the next, they can satisfy the lower needs as they acquire the more complex skills needed for the higher ones. The highest level of human growth, for Maslow, was *self-actualization,* or the reaching of full human potential. Most people do not reach this stage—some because they are kept from it, others because of the choices they have made. But every person may reach self-actualization, and many people have glimpses of this state during what Maslow called *peak experiences.*

Growth and Development. The most basic human needs, the first needs that any child has, are for food, water, and shelter. These let us function. For some time all children must have these needs satisfied by adults.

For adults, of course, the lower needs are still basic to life and growth, but most adults can have them satisfied by their own efforts. Once these needs are satisfied, the next level of need is for safety, safety from known and imagined threats, both social and physical. As we achieve a certain level of safety, we begin to search for love and, what is similar, a sense of belonging to a group. To satisfy such needs, we must feel *worthy* of love.

A sense of belonging leads us to feelings of self-esteem—the belief that we enjoy the respect of others and that we are worthy of that respect. This feeling increases self-confidence, which leads us to want to know and to understand. When we feel a sense of mastery over the world, only then may we seek to fulfill our artistic and creative needs.

Self-actualization. The highest state of development is self-actualization. People at this stage can make use of all their potential, their skills, and their talents. Self-actualized people differ from other people. They are highly individual and always growing. All the aspects of their personalities are in harmony.

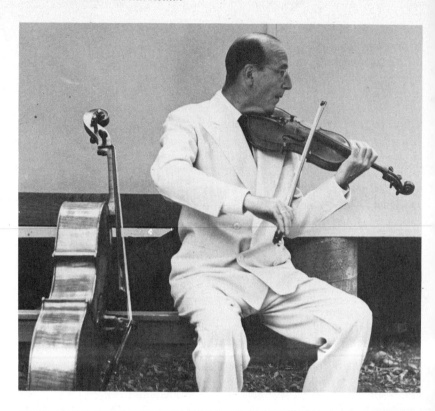

Music is one of the ways in which people use their talents—or achieve self-actualization.

Fred Grunzweig/Photo Researchers

Maslow named Abraham Lincoln, Thomas Jefferson, and Eleanor Roosevelt as self-actualized people. Albert Schweitzer (1875–1965) is another. As a young man, Schweitzer earned the degree of Doctor in Theology, and he wrote some classic studies in religion. At the same time he became a renowned organist devoted to J. S. Bach. At age 30, Schweitzer began to study medicine, then went to Africa to spend the rest of his life as a mission doctor, while devoting his evenings to writing huge works on the philosophy of culture. While few of us can aspire to this level of diverse achievement, we can all seek to use those gifts that we do have to the utmost.

Glasser.   Like Maslow, William Glasser was not satisfied with Freud's focus on what had been "done" to people with psychological problems. He felt that they should be encouraged to confront their own decisions and mistakes. His humanistic approach to personality development is the basis of a method of psychotherapy known as *reality therapy* (RT).

Reality therapists see two basic human needs: to love and be loved, and to feel worthwhile. Instead of searching out the complex history of a patient, as Freudians do, reality therapists help patients explore their present lives.

Reality and Responsibility. The central premise of reality therapy is that people with emotional handicaps deny the real world. They cannot fulfill the basic needs of giving and receiving love, of feeling that they are worthwhile to themselves and to others. We all have these needs, but we vary in being able to fulfill them in a responsible way—one that lets others fulfill *their* needs as well.

Responsible behavior is the base of RT. Glasser urges that labels like neurotic, psychotic, and schizophrenic (see Chapter 3) be dropped, and that the term "irresponsible" replace them. RT promotes responsible behavior by teaching patients to stop denying the real world and to see that they must fulfill their needs within its framework. Patients are led away from the habit of blaming present sadness on the past—on a loveless or deprived childhood. They are encouraged to give themselves credit when they do right and to correct themselves when they do wrong.

Glasser feels that parents should teach responsibility to their young children, since the younger we are when given love and discipline, the easier for us to learn responsibility. Yet he feels that responsibility can be learned at any time. Glasser urges therapists and counselors to set an example that is open, truthful, and has integrity—to get involved with patients in responsible ways, not remain remote as some traditional analysts do.

Behaviorism

Not all who have studied the human mind feel (as Freud, Erikson, Maslow, and Glasser do) that it should be thought of as something apart from (though part of) the body. Some have argued that thought is simply one of the functions of the body, like breathing. This point of view is now called *behaviorism*.

Behaviorists say that labels like "consciousness," "id," and "mental life" are false. Thinking, they say, amounts to "speaking to oneself" within, and they see emotions as the product of hormones (chemical substances produced in the body). Behaviorists deny that conscious or unconscious thoughts are the moving force for behavior; to them behavior is in fact the product of *conditioning*. Conditioning is a process of learning in which a human or an animal is taught to react to a stimulus by making a certain response. There are two kinds of conditioning: *classical* and *operant*.

In classical conditioning, the subject learns to associate a stimulus—which before conditioning would *not* have caused a response—with one that automatically gets a response. In operant conditioning, the subject is more active than in classical conditioning and behavior is changed through *reinforcement*—by rewards for what the researcher wants to encourage but punishment for anything else.

Operant conditioning is used widely to modify human behavior, to

---

Traits of the Self-actualized

Self-actualized people are characterized by:

A clear perception of reality

High acceptance of self, others, and nature

Great spontaneity

Marked detachment and desire for privacy

Significant autonomy and resistance to inculturation

Renewable sources of appreciation

Richness of emotional reactions

Many peak experiences of ecstacy

Strong identification with the human species

Positive interpersonal relationships

Democratic character structure

Enhanced creativity

Data from "Self-Actualizing People" in Motivation and Personality, *2nd Edition by Abraham H. Maslow* Copyright © 1970 by Abraham H. Maslow. Reprinted by permission of Harper & Row, Publishers, Inc.

break habits like smoking or eating or drinking too much. The method works by *negative reinforcement,* by punishing behavior that the subject wants to stop. For instance, the drug antabuse (disulfiram) causes a nasty reaction each time a person who takes it drinks some alcohol, so few will risk a drink after taking the drug. Drinkers then learn to associate alcohol with the nausea that the drug causes.

Behaviorism is socially meaningful. In contrast to the Freudians (and those who think that inborn drives are most important), the behaviorists think that *social conditioning* is most important. If we could change our environment, by changing the sort of conditioning that people get, the behaviorists think that we could change human social behavior.

SUMMARY

Health is as much a mental state as a physical one, but the concept of "mental health" is hard to define. In trying to do so, Freud said that the mind functions on three levels of awareness: the conscious, the preconscious, and the unconscious. On each level, life events are stored with the feelings that go with them. Not all researchers agree with this concept of the conscious, since events and memories come into play and affect our actions. The function of mental action is to help humans make good adjustments in their lives. Freud called the mental system that controls and orders adjustments the ego. The ego strives to balance the inner drives that come from the id with the moral demands of the superego. The ego must also cope with social realities. For the mind to function well, the ego must be strong. If the ego is weak, the id's and the superego's demands will cause it great stress. Some researchers, like Maslow, suggest that human behavior is a response to needs. But for Erik Erikson, a neo-Freudian, the ego grows through a series of life stages, from infancy to old age. When a stage is not achieved with success, the result can be lifelong psychological damage. Non-Freudians, like Maslow and Glasser, have done important work on the theory of personality.

But remember, you do not have to learn any one theory of personality to understand and change your own behavior for the better. One thing that you can change if you want to improve your mental attitude is the amount and impact of the stress in your life. Although you may not be aware of stress, it greatly modifies how you adapt to the world. When you become aware of the causes and sources of stress, you can help to reduce its impact, and this will enhance your mental and even your physical well-being.

Suggested Readings

Cassimatis, Emmanuel. "Mental Health Viewed as an Ideal." *Psychiatry* 42 (1979): 241–253. Discusses health and mental health in terms of the medical model, the psychoanalytic model, and the existential model. From this is derived a definition of mental health.

Egbert, Emily. "Concept of Wellness." *Journal of Psychiatric Nursing and Mental Health Services* 18 (1980): 9–12. A review of the literature in an attempt to define the concept of wellness. Offers a list of traits of wellness as described by the various authors.

Forgus, Ronald, and Shulman, Bernard H. *Personality: A Cognitive View.* Englewood Cliffs, N. J.: Prentice-Hall, 1979, pp. 22–52. Discusses the personality theories of Freud, Erikson, and the behaviorists. Contains a good diagram of Freud's concept of personality structure.

Monte, Christopher F. *Beneath the Mask: An Introduction to Theories of Personality.* New York: Praeger, 1977, pp. 480–516. A concise overview of the work of Abraham Maslow, Carl Rogers, and other humanistic psychologists.

Schaffer, Kay F. *Sex-role Issues in Mental Health.* Reading, Mass.: Addison-Wesley, 1980, pp. 1–48. A discussion of sex-role stereotypes in our society and the effects of these on the behavior and attitudes of American women and men.

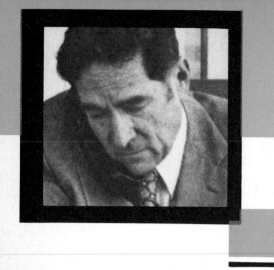

Stress

chapter objectives

When you have finished reading this chapter you should be able to:

1. Understand what stress is, where stress comes from, and how it affects you
2. Compare Freud, Maslow, and Erikson on inner and outer sources of stress
3. Explain the difference between specific and nonspecific responses to stress
4. Discuss how stress is related to disease
5. Identify stress-prone personalities

Your personality—your mental self-image—lives in your memories. Your self-image affects the way you respond to each event in life; and each event in life affects your self-image. To some of these events you react with stress—a feeling that we usually describe as one of anxiety. As we shall see, however, that is not its scientific meaning.

Stressors

Sources of stress, called *stressors,* can come from inside or outside. Stress from within might be caused by personality conflict; stress from without might be caused by a contagious disease or by rush hour traffic. Stressors are not just psychological. They may be chemical, environmental, biophysical, and psychosocial. There are many types of stressors and they affect us all at all times.

For most people, social pressures are the most common stressors—and the least pleasant. School, jobs, social status, race, ethnic group, and family are all sources of social pressure. Not only do they affect your social role and the respect you get from others, they are critical when you define your own sense of self-esteem—a basic building block of mental health.

Stress and College Students. Among the most stressful life stages are the teen years and young adulthood, the time from puberty to full maturity. Most college students are passing through these stages. They must "get it all together" by uniting the personality traits that emerged before their teens, like trust in others, self-confidence, and good work habits. If they succeed, they will be able to pull together their attitudes about their parents and other adults; their sexual selves; their mental and emotional capacities; and their varied social roles (as citizens or as members of a certain ethnic group).

The effort to pull together identities that differ and sometimes conflict makes the teen years and young adulthood a time of quite heavy stress.

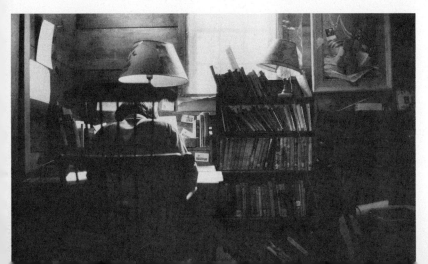

Donald Wright Patterson, Jr./ Stock, Boston

SELF-ASSESSMENT DEVICE 2-1: HOLMES-RAHE STRESS TEST

Which of the following events have you experienced within the last two years?

Event	Points	Event	Points
1. Death of spouse	100	24. Trouble with in-laws	29
2. Divorce	73	25. Outstanding personal achievement	28
3. Marital separation	65	26. Spouse begins or stops work	26
4. Jail term	63	27. Begin or end school	26
5. Death of close family member	63	28. Change in living conditions	25
6. Personal injury or illness	53	29. Revision of personal habits	24
7. Marriage	50	30. Trouble with boss	23
8. Fired at work	47	31. Change in work hours or conditions	20
9. Marital reconciliation	45	32. Change in residence	20
10. Retirement	45	33. Change in schools	20
11. Change in health of family member	44	34. Change in recreation	19
12. Pregnancy	40	35. Change in church activities	19
13. Sex difficulties	39	36. Change in social activities	18
14. Gain of new family member	39	37. Mortgage or loan less than $10,000	17
15. Business readjustment	39	38. Change in sleeping habits	16
16. Change in financial state	38	39. Change in number of family get-togethers	15
17. Death of close friend	37	40. Change in eating habits	15
18. Change to different line of work	36	41. Vacation	13
19. Change in number of arguments with spouse	35	42. Christmas	12
20. Mortgage over $10,000	31	43. Minor violations of the law	11
21. Foreclosure of mortgage or loan	30		
22. Change in responsibilities at work	29		
23. Son or daughter leaving home	29		

What is your total score? A total below 150 indicates low stress, between 150 and 199 mild stress, between 200 and 299 moderate stress, and above 300 major stress.

Source: Adapted from T. H. Holmes and R. H. Rahe, "The Social Readjustment Rating Scale," *Journal of Psychosomatic Research* 11 (1967): 213-218. Copyright © 1967. Reprinted with permission from Pergamon Press, Ltd.

The 5 Most Stressful College Situations

1. *Stress of Separation from Family.* Most people look forward to leaving home, but many aren't really prepared for what it means. For a lot of students off to college, it's their first extended period of time away from home. No Mom and Dad around to talk to you, get you organized, tell you what to do and when to do it. No loving family to support and reward you. In order to survive, the student is required to reorient herself, to take charge of her own life and to develop new relationships to replace the everyday support network of family and old friends, a process that may take months or even years.

2. *Stress of Freedom.* In the old days, before the sexual revolution and coed dorms, rules on most campuses were very clear—you couldn't have members of the opposite sex in your room, you had to be in at a certain time, you couldn't drink liquor on campus. Today, on many campuses across the country, the idea of *in loco parentis* is dead. You don't have anyone telling you how to behave nor do you have anyone to lean on. Some universities don't even require class attendance; in seminars of 300 to 400 students, grades depend solely on how well you do on the final exam. So you have to figure things out for yourself—and making the inevitable mistakes leads naturally to feelings of failure and a lowering of self-esteem.

3. *Stress of Competition.* With the increasing competition for places in grad schools and jobs after graduation, today's college is a kind of academic pressure cooker. A student may feel compelled to decide between an academic or a social life: "Either I spend all my time studying and get good grades or I spend time making friends and risk not getting into med school." Or she may find her friends becoming deadly enemies as they all compete for the same grad school slot. Either way the result is a tremendous sense of isolation.

4. *Stress of Peer Pressure.* The desire to be accepted by one's peers leads to extreme pressure to conform. Along sexual lines, everyone feels the compulsion to perform. The young woman entering college may feel everyone will have more experience; if she's a virgin she may be embarrassed and hope no one will find out before she can "remedy" the situation. Men also may worry about their inexperience and being compared to everyone else, fears that can result in impotence. A person also may feel compelled to adopt the attitudes of her friends toward drugs and alcohol, regardless of how she really feels. A different kind of peer pressure arises when a student finds herself in a group that expresses disdain toward going to the counseling service that could help her.

5. *Stress of Choosing a Career.* While the late teens and early twenties should be a time of discovery and experimentation, the student who is unsure of what her major and career will be may feel guilty about her inability to make a quick decision; since her parents are spending all this money, she reasons, she should know what she's doing (at the same time her parents—consciously or unconsciously—may be sending out a similar message). If she chooses a major against her parents' wishes, she'll feel she's letting her parents down; if she chooses a certain major because her parents expect it, she'll feel like she's letting herself down. People may also find themselves studying not what they enjoy but what they believe will get them a job after graduation—their lives are geared entirely to the future, which creates more stress.

Those who succeed in pulling their identities together feel good about who they are. They know where they are going and have a set of values that guide them. But college students cannot always develop a whole and complete identity with ease. As a result, many suffer from the effects of stress in damaging amounts. While none of us can meet all the challenges of life with complete success, some have more success than others have.

Stress and the Levels of Consciousness

As you read in Chapter 1, Freud thought that the personality has three "systems": the id, or the forces of instinct; the ego, or the conscious mind; and the superego, or the rule enforcer. As Freud viewed it, these systems often come into conflict. Their conflict is an important source of inner stress.

The demands of the id are powerful and also dangerous, since the id is not concerned with the real world. The id wants pleasure and wants it now. The superego, too, is not concerned with the real world, but with morals and principles. It rejects compromise and demands duty to ideals, no matter how futile or destructive. The id and the superego, then, are two powerful sources of inner stress.

The ego must somehow reconcile the demands of the id and the superego while it responds to the many sources of stress from the outside. Let us see how the ego does this. Consider the case of a student doing badly in an important course. The course is so important that failing it could threaten the student's career. This threat involves the student's present and future and the demands of the outside, the real world. These are not, however, the only demands that the ego must deal with. The student (like most of us) is also being tempted by the demands of social and sexual life. This seeking after pleasure, said Freud, comes from the id. The ego must decide—to study or to date. Moral demands fight pleasure demands. Following one course of action must be at the expense of the other.

How may such a conflict be resolved? A neo-Freudian, like Erik Erikson (see Chapter 1), might argue that earlier life events, earlier goals, will decide it. Erikson described middle childhood as a time marked by inner conflict between useful action (industry), on the one hand, and feelings of inferiority, on the other. Children who passed through this conflict with success acquired a sense of duty and good work habits. But those who had rarely been praised for their work did not expect much of themselves. They grow up poorly prepared to face this kind of conflict, and if it arises, stress must be the outcome.

The student's conflict can be examined from other points of view. Abraham Maslow, a humanist psychologist whose ideas are described in Chapter 1, believed that we must all fulfill certain basic needs. Only when the lower, the physical needs are satisfied can we go on to fulfill

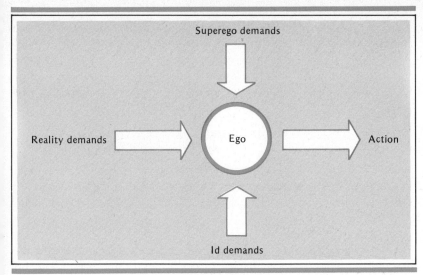

Figure 2-1. The Relation of Id, Ego, and Superego in the Psychoanalytic Model. This diagram shows the concept of the ego as the central core of the personality, which mediates between inner demands and outer demands. *Source:* From *Abnormal Psychology and Modern Life*, 4th edition by James C. Coleman. © 1972 Scott, Foresman and Company. Reprinted by permission.

the higher needs, those that are purely human, like the need for love and the need to understand the world around us. A humanist psychologist might then suggest that the student's conflict will be ended by that student's success (or failure) in fulfilling this order of needs: the need for food, for safety, for love and belonging, and for self-esteem. Past success in fulfilling those needs will allow the student to deal with the problems of the present.

The Nature of Stress

Stress is a word and an idea that is common to us. Yet, it is often misused. If we say we are "under stress" we imply that at other times we are free of stress. In fact, we are always under some stress. The mind and the body are always adapting to both inner and outer changes, even during sleep. Only the dead are free from stress.

Stress is thought to be unpleasant. But, research shows that pleasant events cause stress, too. What exactly is this thing called stress that is caused both by happy and sad events?

The Nonspecific Response.   Defined simply, stress demands the body to adapt to something—to mobilize its defenses. Dr. Hans Selye, a leading researcher in the field of stress, has shown in a series of tests that *all* causes of stress, no matter what they are, produce the same biochemical changes in the body. Selye's own definition of stress was "the nonspecific response of the body to any demand made upon it." The response is not specific because it is the same for any kind of stress.

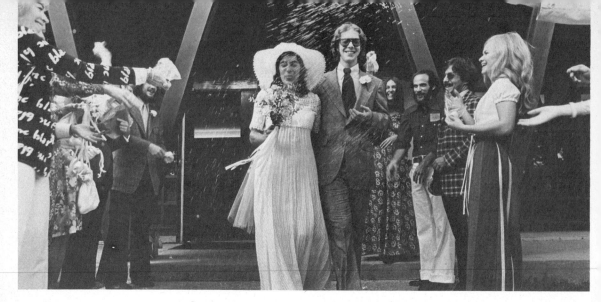

Pleasant events—like marriage—cause stress, just as unpleasant ones do.

Frank Siteman, 1980/Stock, Boston

Remember that sources of stress (stressors) can produce many kinds of physical and mental responses. Some of them—*not* the stress response—are specific (the immune system that responds to a polio virus, for example). But all stressors produce a nonspecific response as well, one that is the same for all stressors. Like the specific responses, this nonspecific one—stress—is not just a state of mind; it is a real response of the body's biology to real pressures placed on it. We cannot avoid stress, says Selye, but we can understand it, learn how to live with it, and even make it productive.

The Alarm Reaction for Fight-or-Flight

- Stored sugar and fats pour into the bloodstream to provide fuel for quick energy
- The breath rate shoots up, providing more oxygen
- Red blood cells flood the bloodstream, carrying more oxygen to the muscles of the limbs and the brain
- The heart speeds up and blood pressure soars, insuring sufficient blood supply to needed areas
- Blood-clotting mechanisms are activated to protect against injury
- Muscles tense in preparation for strenuous action

- Digestion ceases, so blood may be diverted to muscles and brain
- Perspiration and saliva increase
- Triggered by the pituitary gland, the endocrine system steps up hormone production
- Bowel and bladder muscles loosen
- Adrenalin pours into the system, as do the hormones epinephrin and norepinephrin
- The pupils dilate, allowing more light to enter
- All senses are heightened

Source: Philip Goldberg, *Executive Health* (New York: McGraw-Hill, 1978), pp. 26–27.

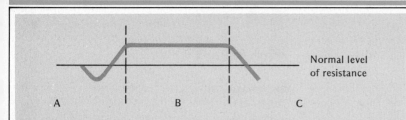

Figure 2–2.   The Three Phases of the General Adaptation Syndrome (G.A.S.)
Source: Reprinted by permission of the publisher and author Hans Selye: *Stress in Health and Disease,* Wobwin: Butterworth Publishers, Inc., 1976.

Normal level of resistance

A   B   C

A. Alarm reaction. The body shows the changes characteristic of the first exposure to a stressor. At the same time, its resistance is diminished and, if the stressor is sufficiently strong (severe burns, extremes of temperature), death may result.

B. Stage of resistance. Resistance ensues if continued exposure to the stressor is compatible with adaptation. The bodily signs characteristic of the alarm reaction have virtually disappeared, and resistance rises above normal.

C. Stage of exhaustion. Following long-continued exposure to the same stressor, to which the body had become adjusted, eventually adaptation energy is exhausted. The signs of the alarm reaction reappear, but now they are irreversible, and the individual dies.

The General Adaptation Syndrome.   The knowledge that both pleasant and not-so-pleasant events produce the same response came from Selye's 1936 tests. Selye observed animals' responses to injections of poisons and nonpoisons, as well as their responses to cold, heat, infection, and other stimuli. It turned out that some (though by no means all) of their responses were the same. He named these responses the *General Adaptation Syndrome* (G.A.S.).

The G.A.S. has three stages:

1.   First comes the alarm reaction. The subject responds to a stressor with surprise and alarm—an intense call-up of the body's resistance.
2.   Second, there is resistance. The subject learns to cope with the stressor.
3.   Third, there is exhaustion. The subject's energy is gone—is exhausted.

Eustress and Distress.   Selye called the positive stressors *eustress* and the negative ones *distress.* Most of us use the word "stress" when we refer to distress; but as we now know, positive events cause that same response—the G.A.S.

In distress, the overload of negative stressors causes us to be weak and makes us prey to other stressors. In eustress, the positive stressors (achievements) result in growth, strength, and resistance to distress. The G.A.S., however, is the same for both distress and eustress. Natural

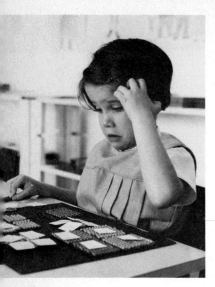

Frustration causes exessive stress on the mind or body, and this creates distress.

Suzanne Szasz/Photo Researchers

human drives, said Selye, require some sort of fulfillment. When they are blocked, it causes frustration. Frustration, in turn, causes stress in parts of the body or mind, and this creates distress. But success over the blockage creates eustress.

The causes of frustration may be quite simple—as when we lack the money to buy something we want. But Selye pointed out that frustration can result from a lack of self-esteem, too, from lack of regard for our own accomplishments. People who lack self-esteem are frustrated, even tortured, by a sense that they have failed. This makes day-by-day events hard to bear, so they become sources of distress.

There is some common ground between Selye's theory of eustress and distress, Maslow's hierarchy of needs, and Erikson's theory of ego development. All three hold that some basic needs must be fulfilled for us to function at our best. All suggest that the need for self-fulfillment and the growth of the emotions is not an empty concept; rather, it is the base for sound mental and emotional growth. Their agreement shows how important this is for coping with stress.

Conditioning.   Although stress, in the sense of the G.A.S., is the same in all cases, each of us differs in how we react to each kind of stressor. Some of us respond strongly to all stressors, while some of us respond strongly to only certain stressors, like the death of a parent.

Selye said that one lesson we can learn from the G.A.S. is that our bodies can deal with only a certain amount of stressors and stress. At some point fatigue sets in; then the body breaks down in some way.

Conditioning helps to explain why some of us react to a stressor more or less strongly than others do, for conditioning can help or hinder the impact of stressors. Conditioning factors can come from within the body or from the outside. Outside factors may be treatment with drugs, hormones, or diet. Some hormones and drugs can reduce the effect of stressors, others can increase it. As for inner conditioning, some of us are born with a way to cope with stressors—sometimes for the best, sometimes for the worst. Our age, too, may be an important inner factor.

Stress and Disease

At some point stressors may lead to a breakdown of the body, and thus to disease. Moreover, disease and debility are stressors, and stress (from sources other than illness) helps to determine the course of each disease. Sometimes, stress may help us recover, but at other times it may make the disease more harmful.

Although no two of us react in the same way to a stressor, certain things occur when resistance is weakened by stressors. In the case of stress-related diseases, you may be nervous, but fatigued and sleepless,

SELF-ASSESSMENT DEVICE 2-2: THE SIGNS AND SYMPTOMS OF STRESS DISORDERS

Have you noticed any of these problems during the past two (2) months? Use the following symbols in responding on the checklist:

- X — haven't had this problem at all
- C — constant or nearly constant occurrence
- F — frequently
- O — occasionally

1. Tension headaches _____
2. Sleep-onset insomnia _____
3. Fatigue _____
4. Overeating _____
5. Constipation _____
6. Lower back pain _____
7. Allergy problems _____
8. Feelings of nervousness _____
9. Nightmares _____
10. High blood pressure _____
11. Hives _____
12. Alcohol/nonprescription drug consumption _____
13. Low-grade infections _____
14. Stomach indigestion _____
15. Hyperventilation _____
16. Worrisome thoughts _____
17. Dermatitis _____
18. Menstrual distress _____
19. Nausea or vomiting _____
20. Irritability _____
21. Migraine headaches _____
22. Early morning awakening _____
23. Loss of appetite _____
24. Diarrhea _____
25. Aching neck and shoulder muscles _____
26. Asthma attack _____
27. Colitis attack _____
28. Periods of depression _____
29. Arthritis _____
30. Common flu or cold _____
31. Minor accidents _____
32. Prescription drug use _____
33. Peptic ulcer _____
34. Cold hands or feet _____
35. Heart palpitations _____
36. Sexual problems _____
37. Angry feelings _____
38. Other _____

© 1978 Sally J. Nelson/Don Isbell/Mitchell Clionsky in Philip Goldberg, *Executive Health* (New York: McGraw-Hill, 1978), p. 37.

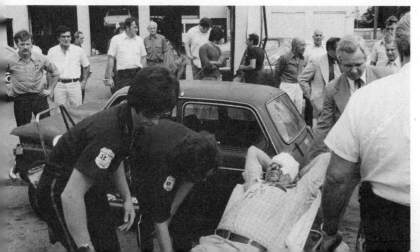

Accidents are stressors that can help create various stress-related conditions.

Donald Dietz/Stock, Boston

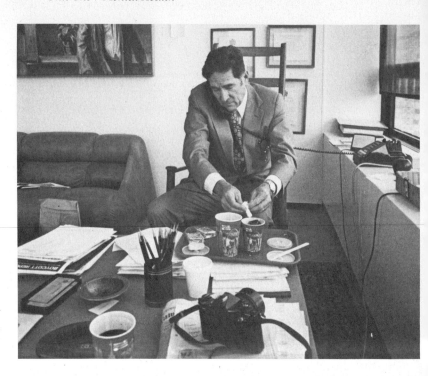

Type A people often try to do more than one thing at a time.

George W. Gardner, 1979/Stock, Boston

have bowel trouble and indigestion, and be depressed and irritable. Physicians cannot measure the extent of such symptoms, but they can measure its signs, which are objective measurements that something is wrong with the body's functioning. Such signs of stress-related diseases can be nonspecific or specific. Nonspecific signs are those that are common to *most* stress conditions, like a fast pulse rate and shortness of breath. Specific signs—high blood pressure, ulcers, cold hands and feet, low-grade infections—go with specific stress-related disorders.

Stress-prone Personality.   Some kinds of personality traits cause some of us to suffer from stress-related diseases more than others do. If we study the traits of stress-prone personalities, we can learn to find them in ourselves—and, perhaps, learn how to control them.

Type A Behavior Pattern.   Two researchers, Meyer Friedman and Ray H. Rosenman (1974), showed that some kinds of behavior tend to promote stress-induced medical problems, like heart disease. They called these kinds of behavior the *Type A* behavior pattern.

Type A people are obsessed by a sense of urgency. They try to do more and more work in less and less time. They seem to struggle with deadlines that are not real and seem to think that work done at a fast

SELF-ASSESSMENT DEVICE 2-3: SELF-EVALUATION—THE GLAZER-STRESSCONTROL LIFE-STYLE QUESTIONNAIRE

As you can see, each scale below is composed of a pair of adjectives or phrases separated by a series of horizontal lines. Each pair has been chosen to represent two kinds of contrasting behavior. Each of us belongs somewhere along the line between the two extremes. Since most of us are neither the most competitive nor the least competitive person we know, put a check mark where you think you belong between the two extremes.

		1 2 3 4 5 6 7	
1.	Doesn't mind leaving things temporarily unfinished	— — — — — —	Must get things finished once started
2.	Calm and unhurried about appointments	— — — — — —	Never late for appointments
3.	Not competitive	— — — — — —	Highly competitive
4.	Listens well, lets others finish speaking	— — — — — —	Anticipates others in conversation (nods, interrupts, finishes sentences for other)
5.	Never in a hurry, even when pressured	— — — — — —	Always in a hurry
6.	Able to wait calmly	— — — — — —	Uneasy when waiting
7.	Easygoing	— — — — — —	Always going full speed ahead
8.	Takes one thing at a time	— — — — — —	Tries to do more than one thing at a time, thinks about what to do next
9.	Slow and deliberate in speech	— — — — — —	Vigorous and forceful in speech (uses a lot of gestures)
10.	Concerned with satisfying himself, not others	— — — — — —	Wants recognition by others for a job well done
11.	Slow doing things	— — — — — —	Fast doing things (eating, walking, etc.)
12.	Easygoing	— — — — — —	Hard driving
13.	Expresses feelings openly	— — — — — —	Holds feelings in
14.	Has a large number of interests	— — — — — —	Few interests outside work
15.	Satisfied with job	— — — — — —	Ambitious, wants quick advancement on job
16.	Never sets own deadlines	— — — — — —	Often sets own deadlines
17.	Feels limited responsibility	— — — — — —	Always feels responsible
18.	Never judges things in terms of numbers	— — — — — —	Often judges performance in terms of numbers (how many, how much)
19.	Casual about work	— — — — — —	Takes work very seriously (works weekends, brings work home)
20.	Not very precise	— — — — — —	Very precise (careful about detail)

SCORING: Assign a value from 1 to 7 for each score. Total them up. The categories are as follows:

Total score = 110–140: Type A_1.

If you are in this category, and especially if you are over 40 and smoke, you are likely to have a high risk of developing cardiac illness.

Total score = 80–109: Type A_2.

You are in the direction of being cardiac prone, but your risk is not as high as the A_1. You should, nevertheless, pay careful attention to the advice given to all Type A's.

Total score = 60–79: Type AB.

You are an admixture of A and B patterns. This is a healthier pattern than either A_1 or A_2, but you have the potential for slipping into A behavior and you should recognize this.

Total score = 30–59: Type B_2.

Your behavior is on the less-cardiac-prone end of the spectrum. You are generally relaxed and cope adequately with stress.

Total score = 0–29: Type B_1.

You tend to the extreme of non-cardiac traits. Your behavior expresses few of the reactions associated with cardiac disease.

This test will give you some idea of where you stand in the discussion of Type A behavior. The higher your score, the more cardiac prone you tend to be. Remember, though, even B persons occasionally slip into A behavior, and any of these patterns can change over time.

Source: This questionnaire was designed by Dr. Howard I. Glazer, director of behavior management systems at EHE Stresscontrol Systems, Inc., in Philip Goldberg, *Executive Health* (New York: McGraw-Hill, 1978), pp. 98–100.

pace is better than work done with care. They need to score what they do in numbers and then try to exceed that score the next time. Although they may seem confident and self-assured, often, they are not secure at all, but desperate to be noticed. Since they compete all the time, they are always in conflict with those around them. They are easily hurt and often angry—without a real base for either feeling.

Type A Behavior and Heart Disease. Friedman and Rosenman's research suggests that those with Type A personalities tend to suffer from heart disease (see Chapter 10) about twice as often as others do. And they develop heart disease early—in their thirties and forties—not in their sixties. Type A behavior may not cause heart disease, but statistics do correlate heart disease and Type A behavior.

Type B Behavior Pattern. Friedman and Rosenman also found a personality type that is the opposite of Type A. Although *Type B* people do not lack ambition and drive, they are less likely than Type A people to suffer the ill effects of stress, since they are simply not obsessed by the desire to achieve endlessly.

Most people have at least some of the traits of Type A and some of Type B. Friedman and Rosenman think that most urban Americans fall into one or the other of these groups; only a small number of people seem to have an equal number of the traits of both groups.

Our culture values those who compete, achieve, and "keep up with the Joneses." This makes for much stress-related disease.

A 1978 study found that teaching in college is one of the lowest-pressure jobs in the United States.

Sepp Seitz/Woodfin Camp & Associates

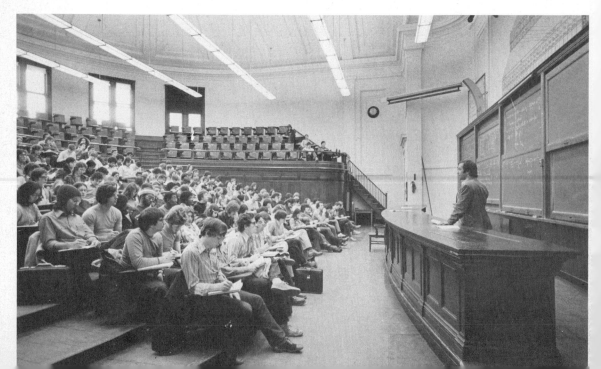

Highest-pressure and Lowest-pressure Jobs in the United States

In a 2-year study conducted by the National Institute for Occupational Safety and Health in cooperation with the Tennessee Department of Mental Health and Mental Retardation, over 22,000 health records of workers in 130 jobs were studied for stress-related diseases. The frequency of these diseases in the various jobs resulted in the following lists of highest- and lowest-stress jobs.

Highest	*Lowest*
1. Manual laborer	1. Clothing sewer
2. Secretary	2. Checker, examiner of products
3. Inspector	3. Stockroom worker
4. Waitress/waiter	4. Craftsman
5. Clinical lab technician	5. Maid
6. Farm owner	6. Heavy equipment operator
7. Miner	7. Farm laborer
8. Office manager	8. Freight handler
9. House painter	9. Child care worker
10. Manager/administrator	10. Packer, wrapper in shipping
11. Foreman	11. College or university professor
12. Machine operator	12. Personnel, labor relations
	13. Auctioneer/huckster

Source: U.S. Department of Health, Education and Welfare, National Institute for Occupational Safety and Health, *Occupational Stress* (Washington, D.C.: Government Printing Office, 1978).

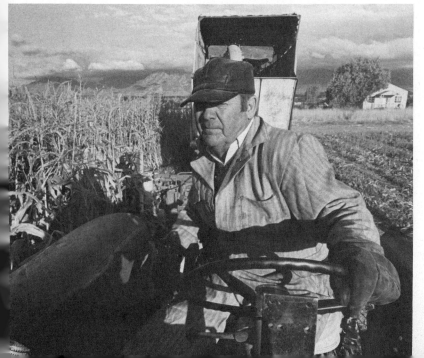

The same 1978 study found that owning a farm is one of the highest-pressure jobs in the United States.
John Running/Stock, Boston

SUMMARY

Stress is a word we hear often, one that may mean to us something like anxiety. But research done by Dr. Hans Selye in 1936 showed that both pleasant and not so pleasant events may produce the same symptoms of stress: the general adaptation syndrome (G.A.S.) of alarm, resistance, and exhaustion. Selye found that there are positive sources of stress (eustress) and negative ones (distress). Eustress lets us develop and grow and resist negative stressors. Distress leaves us weak, so that we cannot deal with too many stressors.

The works of the major personality theorists—among them Freud, Maslow, and Erikson—suggest that life's stresses shape the growth of personality, or self-image, and that personality in turn largely shapes our response to stress. They show, as well, that to strive for self-fulfillment is not just an ideal or a dream, but a basic need for health.

Physical health, like mental health, can be lost because of severe or prolonged stress. Among the symptoms of stress-related diseases are fatigue, sleepless nights, depression, and migraine headaches. People who have the so-called Type A behavior pattern suffer more than others do from stress-related diseases, mainly heart disease.

Only death frees us from stress. Instead of seeking freedom from stress, we should seek to master it, to understand the way it works and affects us. Only then can we learn the ways to cope with it that lessen its impact. That will be the substance of Chapter 3.

Suggested Readings

Cox, Tom. *Stress.* Baltimore: University Park Press, 1978, pp. 91–111. The cost of stress is expressed in terms of its effect on physical and psychological well-being.

Friedman, Meyer, and Rosenman, Ray H. *Type A Behavior and Your Heart.* New York: Knopf, 1974. This is the study that described the Type A and Type B behavior patterns and their link with stress and disease.

Kjervik, Diane K., and Martinson, Ida M., eds. *Women in Stress: A Nursing Perspective.* New York: Appleton-Century-Crofts, 1979. Chapter 5 (pp. 89–95) "Male and Female Response to Stress." This chapter deals with the sex differences in response to stress. Chapter 9 (pp. 144–156) "The Stress of Sexism on the Mental Health of Women." The mental health of women has been harmed by the sexism in our society. Stages through which women pass in confronting the stress of sexism are discussed, along with methods that therapists can use to help them.

Kobasa, Suzanne C. "Stressful Life Events, Personality, and Health: An Inquiry into Hardiness." *Journal of Personality and Social Psychology* 37 (1979): 1–11. This article considers the importance of personality in the illness-provoking effects of stress.

Selye, Hans. *Stress in Health and Disease.* Boston: Butterworths, 1976. At present, the most definitive work on stress.

Warheit, George J. "Life Events, Coping, Stress, and Depressive Symptomatology." *American Journal of Psychiatry* 136 (1979): 502–507. This study illustrates the complex nature of life events, coping resources, and depressive symptomatology. The findings suggest that while life-event losses and the lack of personal and social resources are related to high-depression-scale scores, other factors are more important sources to explain depression.

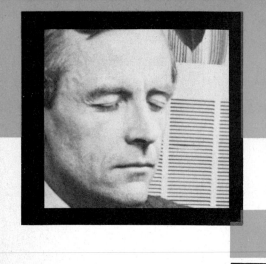

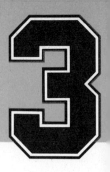

Coping

chapter objectives

When you have finished reading this chapter you should be able to:

1. Describe some of the successful means of coping
2. Understand the way that conscious coping differs from unconscious coping
3. Describe the way that problem solving differs from the use of defense mechanisms
4. Recognize Menninger's levels of dysfunction
5. Discuss the problems of the mind and whether or not they can be treated
6. Distinguish between the treatments for the mind and which disorders can be treated by each

Humans learn to adapt to the changing demands of the world around them. This outer world consists of both natural factors—like heat and humidity—and social factors, like work and school. Because it changes all the time, and rapidly, the inner world of body functions must change to adjust to its demands.

Homeostasis is the term used for the adjustments your body makes to keep itself working in a balanced way. While the range of adjustments that let your body maintain its homeostasis is very narrow, the changes that cause such adjustments are often very great. When the body must adjust beyond the narrow range of homeostasis, it is under stress.

Coping

Attempting to make all the adjustments that maintain homeostasis is called *coping*. When you cope you are dealing with an event and its effects. There are two ways of coping. When they believe themselves to be at the mercy of events, crises, obstacles, and trying demands, people cope in a *reactive* way. Fight or flight are the basic devices of reactive coping. But they often lead to frustration, self-blame, annoyance,

What You Can Do to Prevent Stress	How to Know When to Get Help
There are certain steps a student can take to alleviate the problems and stresses of this age group. —Freshmen should find at least one support system on campus: get involved in a group of friends or a dorm committee, or join an academic or social club. —Become involved in one activity outside of your academic pursuits: this way you won't be basing all your self-esteem on your grades. (But don't overdo it and spread yourself *too* thin.) —Take advantage of the various counseling services available on most campuses—sex counseling clinics, test anxiety programs, women's groups, career workshops, etc.	Anyone experiencing any of the following stress warning signs should get professional help: —if you find yourself panicked at the first mid-term period. —if you constantly berate yourself for letting yourself and your parents down. —if "I can't do it!" is your first reaction to everything. —if you can't sleep, eat, or start eating too much. —if you're so paralyzed with fear and anxiety that you've stopped working. —if you feel isolated, without anyone to turn to, or if your feelings of isolation become so overwhelming that you find yourself crying or depressed a lot. —if your feelings of self-worth are based entirely on how well you do academically or on other external sources.

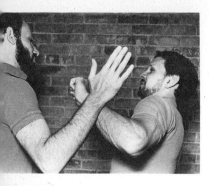

When the mind receives a stimulus it reacts by trying to protect the body.

Ken Karp

chronic fatigue, tension, depression, and stress-induced illness. They may also lead to acts of self-indulgence—like overeating, drug abuse, alcohol, smoking, or violence.

Active ways of coping assume that you can control your own behavior and your patterns of interaction—that you can decide what needs to be changed and how you will do it. Active ways of coping are problem solving, relaxation techniques, exercise, good nutrition, therapy, and work.

Unconscious and Conscious Coping

Much coping is unconscious. When the weather becomes hot and humid, we do not cause sweating in response. The autonomic nervous system, which works without the help of the conscious mind, directs the sweat glands to give up more moisture. Also, our basic response to stress, the General Adaptation Syndrome—alarm, resistance, and exhaustion—is automatic, and it is largely independent of our conscious thoughts. Part of the mind's coping (as opposed to that done by the autonomic nervous system) takes place unconsciously as well.

Conscious Coping. Most of the mind's coping is partly conscious, but partly not. When a stimulus reaches the conscious mind, the mind must decide what to do about the stimulus. The mind draws on its "memory bank" for something that might be relevant to this one. Then it reviews the emotions that went with it. Some conscious coping just involves a simple response for a simple stimulus. Hunger for food is, normally, a simple stimulus. Often the best response to it is equally simple. But sometimes the mind must confront difficult problems with no simple, single, obvious solution. How does the mind cope then?

Problem Solving

The best way to cope with a complex problem is to solve it. Since there are so many ways to solve problems, we can only present a few.

1. *Define the problem.* People with problems often think that they know what they are. But often they do not. A student who is having trouble with a course might see the course itself, or the teacher, as the problem. The student might well be right. But sometimes something outside the course—the student's family or love life—is really to blame. The symptoms of a problem—the ways it comes to our notice—are not the problem itself.
2. *Assess your skills for coping with the problem.* Let us again look at a student having trouble with a course. Suppose that this student does not have the background to do well in it. This, and not the professor, is the real problem. In this case the student will have to change goals. Do not forget that people often overestimate their

Stress Management

1. *Talk/Share.* It has been stated by Dr. William Menninger that every person needs someone with whom he can talk at a trusting sharing level. This provides multiple benefits. It is healthy fight response to stress. It also provides opportunities to test reality, to get feedback from someone whose opinion we trust without becoming defensive or secretive.

2. *Anticipation.* One of the mature adaptive mechanisms referred to in George Vaillant's interesting, informative book, *Adaptation To Life,* is anticipation. I interpret this to mean that you have got to know the territory. Or, in Boy Scout terms, "Be prepared." If public speaking causes you stress, it is extremely helpful to know the audience, the subject, the equipment you will use and the physical environment as well as to rehearse the speech and try to anticipate the questions that will be asked by the audience.

3. *Find Enjoyment.* Whatever specific technique you decide to use on a regular basis should be calculated to bring enjoyment now or in the reasonable future. It makes no sense to take up jogging if you find that activity boring. Find another aerobic exercise that will have the same cardio-vascular benefit and that you enjoy. The same is true of relaxation exercises. If you find meditation difficult, try yoga or affective guided imagery.

4. *Sublimate.* We all possess aggressive, hostile and competitive energies. These need to be uncapped at regular intervals, in positive rather than negative ways. It is much better to hit a racquetball than a boss or child. It's better to bang around in a wood working shop or on your car engine than on a family pet.

5. *Exercise/Sports.* I find this category particularly helpful to me, but I would caution those who have not actively engaged in sports continuously throughout their lives to have a physical examination and a talk with their physician before undertaking an exercise program. It can have multiple benefits in terms of stress reduction. It also relieves hostile, competitive energies in a positive way. It improves physical conditioning. It burns calories. And it provides a diversion from work life. It may also provide fresh air, sunshine and friendships.

6. *A Philosophy of Life.* This method might be satisfied by religion. It might be satisfied by a deep personal sense of understanding that there are not always rational answers to the complex problems of life. Whatever, it is important to have an overriding positive sense about life and our part in it.

Source: Jerry W. Johnson in *Journal of School Health,* January 1981, pp. 41–42. Copyright 1981, American School Health Association, Kent, Ohio 44240.

skills. Doing so undermines solving problems just as much as ignoring them or underestimating them.

3. *Decide on a real course of action.* Alas, it would not be possible to list in this book every problem and its solutions. One thing is clear, though: Plans must be *devised;* most complex problems do not right themselves without help.

4. *Know what you want.* To take an advanced course, you should know the facts taught in the basic course. If you do not, you may not care enough about the advanced course to take the basic one. Do not embark on a project if you do not want success enough to make the effort.

To solve a problem you have to know what you want and be able to make choices.

Christa Armstrong/Photo Researchers

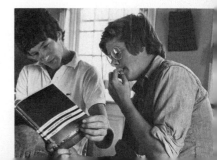

Defense Mechanisms

Problem solving is the best way to cope with stress, but few people can cope with each problem this way. *Defense mechanisms* are short-term means of coping (or coping strategies) for stressors that attack a weak point in the make-up of the personality. To some extent, the use of defense mechanisms is quite normal. But sometimes they lead to harmful actions, for yourself and others. The stronger your sense of self-esteem, *the less likely* you are to use the defense mechanisms described here.

There are many defense mechanisms. They include *regression* (to revert to childish behavior), *rationalization* (to wrongly blame circumstance for personal failure), *segregation* (to divide thought into groupings that have no base in logic), and *projection* (to attribute one's own faults to someone else). Great harm may come to those who employ *repression* (a forceful form of forgetting, one that may lead to mental conflicts that cannot be resolved) and *conversion* (when the stress of life's problems is turned into physical signs and symptoms). When used too often and for too long, defense mechanisms can become a form of *not* coping.

Time Structuring

If defense mechanisms work, they work for the short term—on certain problems only. Long-term coping is a way of life, though, a pattern that forms for how we try to cope with most problems. One kind of long-term coping, first found by Dr. Eric Berne, is called *time structuring*. Time structuring takes six forms: *withdrawal, ritual, pastime, activity, games,* and *intimacy*. Withdrawal means the smallest amount of involvement with other people; the other forms mean more and more involvement, going from ritual to intimacy.

Games

One kind of time-structuring is called a "game." These are not games we play for fun but forms of social push and pull. There are many games. Eric Berne calls one of them "See What You Made Me Do." It can be played between roommates, spouses, parents and children, and those who work together. In one of its versions, a "player" who does not desire social contact starts an isolated task. When someone—a spouse or co-worker, say—walks in, the player's task is disrupted. The player then turns and says, "See what you made me do!" The intruder is, in fact, blameless; the player simply uses the scene to repel the intruder and confirm the isolation.

   Withdrawal means to remove oneself from contact with others, either physically or mentally. Rituals and pastimes are no more than shallow forms of exchanges between people. Games (see box) are forms of interaction whose real meanings are concealed; and activities are what people do to meet real life demands. Intimacy is the level reached when people care; it means shared insights, or "soul touching." It occurs in friendships, marriage, work, or between people in times of great stress. It is an adult relationship in which people are honest and open. It means far more than just sexual intimacy. It is the most self-involving form of time structuring, has the most risk, and may have the greatest rewards.

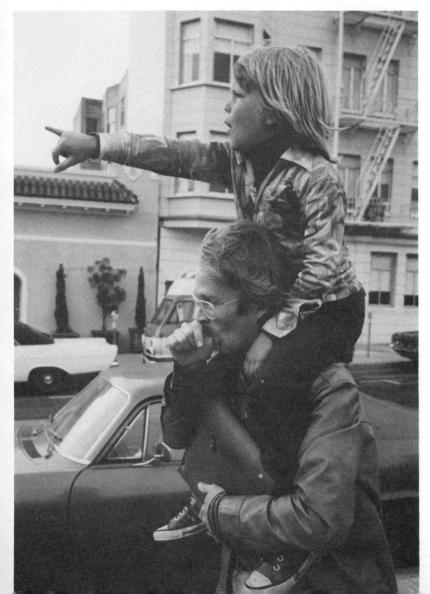

When we regress we revert to childish behavior.

R.S. Uzell, III 1980/Woodfin Camp & Associates

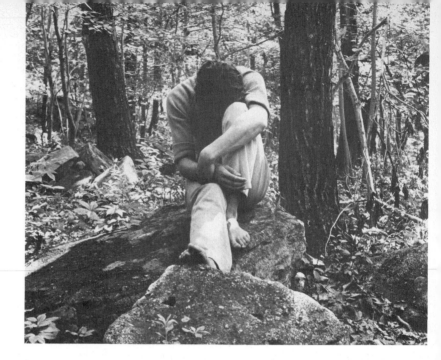

Not Coping: Dysfunction

When you feel more stress than you can cope with, your mental balance may be thrown off. Karl Meninger, a famous psychiatrist, called this *dysfunction.* He suggested that there are five levels of dysfunction.

Five Levels of Dysfunction

At the first level, the ability to cope with stress is slightly, but clearly, reduced. One may have the "jitters," talk and laugh too much, often lose one's temper, feel restless, and worry. Sometimes ailments like sleeplessness or loss of appetite occur. People may seek relief in smoking, drinking, sleeping pills, and visits to physicians. But, for the most part, normal life goes on.

The second level is something like what has been called *neurosis.* (The American Psychiatric Association has recommended that this term be dropped.) Living a normal life is somewhat affected by *phobias* (intense fears of certain things), by a strong sense of anxiety, or by *obsessive–compulsive behavior* (checking your door over and over to make sure it is locked, for example). On the whole, though, basic perceptions of the real world remain intact.

On the second level, people are directing their aggressions mostly at themselves; in third-level dysfunction they direct them mostly at others. They still try to control themselves, but they often act aggressions out openly. If people on the third level are no longer fully in touch with reality, at the fourth level the effort to try to seem normal is given up. This fourth level is sometimes called *psychosis.* (In the past, its names were "lunacy" and "insanity.") The mind can no longer control aggressive and regressive impulses; behavior is not predictable—neither is action based on real-world needs. The person withdraws from work, friends, and family into a fantasy world. The fifth and last level is marked by the end of the will to live and by a resolve to end life, to commit suicide.

Problems of the Mind

Depression. Many students—and many who are not students—complain that they are exhausted or bored much of the time. They work too hard and achieve too little; or they ignore their work but worry about it. Their feelings toward school, their teachers, their lives in general are negative and hostile. These are classic signs of depression.

Loss: Forerunner of Depression. Any kind of loss can start depression: the death of a parent or a close friend; the end of a friendship or of a stage of life (such as childhood); or the loss of self-esteem. Sometimes an event causes a feeling of depression way out of proportion to the event itself—which may even be an imaginary one. But that is not important: Lack of self-confidence can turn any event, real or imaginary, into a cause for depression.

At times, depression may develop into a medical condition called *clinical depression.* This has such symptoms as stupor and lack of movement.

What to Do When a Friend Is Blue

When people are depressed they can be self-centered and trying. Those who care about them should remember that this behavior is due to: (1) their wanting to put others off because they fear rejection, (2) their bad feelings about themselves, and (3) their groping for ways to cope with anguish. Try to understand the behavior, and then consider some things to try to do to help a friend:

- Do not suggest that a depressed person should be happy, or even try to act happily; let the person express feelings of depression.
- Listen with sympathy and fellow-feeling, so that depressed friends know that you care about what they are going through.
- Do what you can to boost your friend's self-esteem; do not criticize or argue now—save it for a time when your friend can handle it.
- Use tact and subtly convey the idea that you can foresee a time when your friend's depression, and its cause, will have passed.
- Help your friend to achieve some kind of success, however small—perhaps by making use of a talent or a skill. A success in a small area of life can create a better feeling about all aspects of life.
- If necessary, help your friend to find help.

Warning Signs

Suicide is a real threat when you:

- talk about death or suicide often;
- say things that imply thoughts of suicide, such as "I can't take it anymore" or "No one understands how alone I feel";
- give away valued possessions;
- express a desire to "get even" with parents;
- purchase means for suicide (guns, pills);
- talk about the same personal or domestic troubles over and over again;
- show such symptoms of deep depression as constant fatigue, lack of interest in life, loss of appetite.

If you know someone who seems to be suicidal, ask that person whether he or she feels an urge to die; take the answer seriously; be sympathetic; try to implant the idea that "where there is life, there is hope"; urge the person to seek help from the local mental health or suicide prevention center.

Suicide.   The modern study of suicide began with the work of Emile Durkheim (1858–1917), a famous French sociologist. Durkheim found four kinds of suicide. People who do not achieve their worldly ambitions sometimes commit *egoistical suicide,* out of disappointment. *Altruistic suicide* is a trait of large groups, like armies, and of primitive cultures; here the victim lacks the individuality to resist the impulse to suicide. *Anomic suicide* is a trait of modern cultures, which (as Durkheim saw it) are *anomic,* or lacking in rules. When the rules of traditional cultures—which prescribe how to behave in every part of life— are lost to "modern" ways, feelings of confusion grow. With the loss of rules went one of the strongest of all rules—the one against suicide. Finally, there is *fatalistic suicide,* caused by being trapped. Here people kill themselves to escape restraints, like prison and slavery.

Durkheim explained suicide as the product of social forces. He resisted psychological explanations. Karl Meninger, a well-known psychiatrist, explained suicide as the product of personal intentions: the wish to kill, the wish to be killed, and the wish to die. The wish to kill, he said, is a form of suicide—but a form that goes outward. Suicidal people, who often blame others for their own failures or their suicidal feelings, try to kill them by killing themselves—a kind of revenge motive. A jilted lover might be moved to such a deed. The wish to be killed afflicts those who want to be punished for crimes or other things that have escaped the notice of others. The wish to end life's problems and pressures—as if life were an incurable disease—is the wish to die.

Young Suicides.   In America today, more and more people are losing the will to live: In the 1970s, about 25,000 suicides were reported each year. But many deaths involving drugs or cars are "disguised" suicides, so the number may be as high as 75,000 a year. Even more shocking is that large numbers of them are committed by young people. Of the 25,000 official victims, about 4,000 were between the ages of 15 and 24. Now think about this amazing fact: *Suicide is the third leading cause of death among people between 15 and 24.*

Young suicides result both from sudden crises—the death of a parent—and from long-term problems like loneliness and family tensions. The death itself often creates new tensions in the family, so that the parents of youths who commit suicide often deny that their children killed themselves on purpose. These parents are quite hostile toward those who confront them with the truth. They are often overcome by guilt and suffer from severe depression.

Psychoses.   Most of the problems of the mind discussed so far are *functional disorders;* they are created by the victim's past and present life events. But the causes of psychosis can be functional or *organic,* that is, physical. Among the physical causes are injury to the brain before or

SELF-ASSESSMENT DEVICE 3-1: THE HOPELESSNESS SCALE

Apply the following statements to yourself and mark each one true or false (T or F).

_____ 1. I look forward to the future with hope and enthusiasm.
_____ 2. I might as well give up because I can't make things better for myself.
_____ 3. When things are going badly, I am helped by knowing they can't stay that way forever.
_____ 4. I can't imagine what my life would be like in 10 years.
_____ 5. I have enough time to accomplish the things I most want to do.
_____ 6. In the future, I expect to succeed in what concerns me most.
_____ 7. My future seems dark to me.
_____ 8. I expect to get more of the good things in life than the average person.
_____ 9. I just don't get the breaks, and there's no reason to believe I will in the future.
_____10. My past experiences have prepared me well for my future.
_____11. All I can see ahead of me is unpleasantness rather than pleasantness.
_____12. I don't expect to get what I really want.
_____13. When I look ahead to the future, I expect I will be happier then than I am now.
_____14. Things just won't work out the way I want them to.
_____15. I have great faith in the future.
_____16. I never get what I want so it's foolish to want anything.
_____17. It is very unlikely that I will get any real satisfaction in the future.
_____18. The future seems vague and uncertain to me.
_____19. I can look forward to more good times than bad times.
_____20. There's no use in really trying to get something I want because I probably won't get it.

Key: You are expressing feelings of hopelessness if you have marked T for items 2, 4, 7, 9, 11, 12, 14, 16, 17, 18, 20; or F for items 1, 3, 5, 6, 8, 10, 13, 15, 19. The more items you have answered that match the key, the more hopeless you feel.

Source: Adapted from Table 1 of "Hopelessness: An Indicator of Suicidal Risk." by M. Kovacs, A. T. Beck, and M. A. Weissman, *Suicide and Life Threatening Behavior*, Vol. 5, #2, 1975, pg. 100, Human Sciences Press.

A Case History to Alleviate Self-doubt

If you ever doubt that perseverence can overcome obstacles, or that greatness is often preceded by adversity, consider this biographical sketch of a politician:

1832-lost job
1832-defeated for legislature
1833-failed in private business
1834-elected to legislature
1835-sweetheart dies
1836-nervous breakdown
1836-defeated for house speaker
1843-defeated for nomination to Congress
1846-elected to Congress
1848-lost renomination
1849-ran for land officer and lost
1854-defeated for Senate
1856-defeated for nomination for Vice-President
1858-defeated for Senate again
1860-elected President of the United States.

The politician was, of course, Abraham Lincoln.

Source: Philip Goldberg, *Executive Health* (McGraw-Hill, 1979), p. 112.

---

during birth, drug and alcohol abuse, and atherosclerosis, or "hardening of the arteries." Some cases of psychosis may be *genetic* in origin.

Unlike neurosis, psychosis distorts the victims' *sense* of the real world, and not only their coping with it. The two kinds of psychosis are *manic-depressive illness* and *schizophrenia*.

Manic-depressive Illness. Manic-depressive illness is marked by mood swings that go from joy to sadness or from sadness to joy. They are not always related to outside causes. During the depressive (or sad) phase, victims may lose self-esteem and withdraw in despair from the real world. During the manic phase, they are very active in their movements, talk too much, and are too assertive.

The length of the illness cycles can vary—lasting from 9 to 15 months. Although cures can just occur, the illness tends to return to the sufferer.

Schizophrenia. Some disorders of the mind, included under the term *schizophrenia,* are marked by at least some of the following symptoms: retreat from the world into a self-enclosed dream place; the belief that one's thoughts are "tapped" or are controlled by others; reduced ability to think (not coherent, vague, etc.); delusions (such as persecution); mood disturbances that include anxiety, confusion, and depression; odd movements or postures; violence and threats of violence.

Most researchers now think that schizophrenia is caused in part by one's genes and in part by one's life events. It is hard to cure, but many of its symptoms can be controlled.

Chemotherapy is the main treatment. The drugs used do not cure the illness but do control the symptoms. Psychotherapy, skilled counseling, social support, and restraint are used along with drugs. Shock (electroconvulsive) therapy is used in very withdrawn, depressed, or excited patients, but never alone.

Treatment of Dysfunction: Psychotherapy

Sometimes people cannot cope with stress by themselves—and this should not be any cause for shame. If help is needed, you can turn to a few forms of *psychotherapy.* They are divided into two categories: "talk" therapies and nonverbal therapies. In the "talk" therapies people try to find their sources of stress by talking to a therapist. Such therapies include *psychoanalysis,* based on the work of Sigmund Freud, *existential therapy, gestalt therapy, transactional analysis, encounter-group therapy, assertiveness training,* and *family therapy.* Nonverbal therapies may also have some amount of talk, but they rely on it less. These include the following: *Reichean therapy, primal therapy, behavior therapy,* and *nutrition therapy.*

"Talk" Therapies

Psychoanalysis. The best-known traditional psychotherapy is *psychoanalysis,* based on Freud's theory that symptoms of mental disturbance come from repressed sexual or aggressive urges. Psychoanalysis tries to help patients deal with their problems by finding the unconscious motives that cause them. Two common methods used in psychoanalysis are *free association* (the patient is encouraged to say whatever comes to mind, no matter how irrelevant it may seem) and *dream*

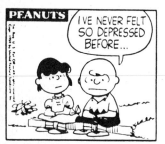

PEANUTS

I'VE NEVER FELT SO DEPRESSED BEFORE...

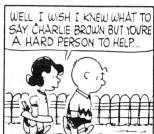

WELL, I WISH I KNEW WHAT TO SAY, CHARLIE BROWN, BUT YOU'RE A HARD PERSON TO HELP...

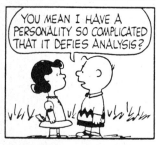

YOU MEAN I HAVE A PERSONALITY SO COMPLICATED THAT IT DEFIES ANALYSIS?

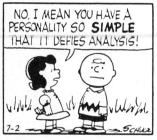

NO, I MEAN YOU HAVE A PERSONALITY SO **SIMPLE** THAT IT DEFIES ANALYSIS!

7-2   SCHULZ

(© 1959 United Feature Syndicate, Inc.)

analysis (in which the patient's dreams are discussed in terms of symbols for disguised urges or wish fulfillments).

In a classic psychoanalysis, patients see their analysts four times a week and lie on couches facing away from them. Analysts strive to be neutral (hence distant) to make possible what Freudians call *transference*, a pattern of behavior in which patients behave toward their analysts as they do toward authority figures—like their parents. Many forms of treatment inspired by the work of Freud are far less formal than this. In these the patient meets the analyst just once or twice a week and sits (rather than lies) facing the analyst, who behaves with less distance than a classical analyst does.

Existential Therapy. Existentialists view life as an arbitrary existence in a godless universe. Since humans feel anxiety about the ever-present threat of death, and since they also need to feel "authentic," to create meaning within a meaningless existence—these became the ground for *existential therapy*. The therapist, who serves as a model of "authenticity" and caring, attempts to help patients find meaning and values, and so lessen the anxieties in life.

In a classic psychoanalysis the patients see their analysts four times a week and lie on couches facing away from them.

Van Bucher/Photo Researchers

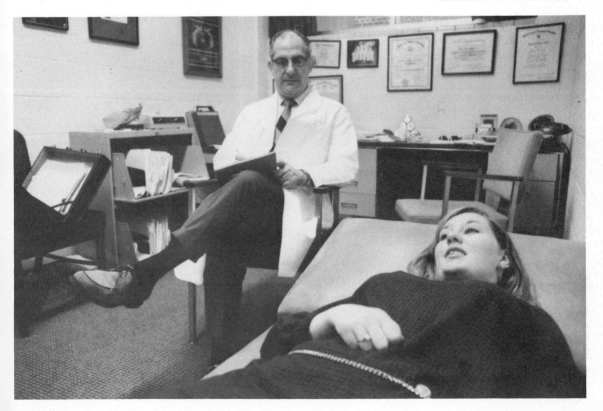

Have you ever felt that you needed help with a certain life problem, or with life in general? Most people have. If and when you feel you need help, that is reason enough to seek it.

Some people do not think that they need help even when they do. Among the problems that might indicate such a need are:

- Thoughts or feelings that life is meaningless, not worth living
- Trouble in getting along with parents, or brothers and sisters
- Trouble in getting along with your teachers, and problems in school
- Difficulty in holding a job
- Strained relationships with friends
- Problems with members of the opposite sex
- Trouble in making decisions

When you decide that you need help, what's next?

For college students the answer is probably a trip to the college health clinic, most of which have mental health specialists. Another source of advice is your family physician, who may be able to refer you to such a specialist. Finally, many organizations, such as city or county mental health associations and local mental health clinics refer people who seek help to private therapists.

How do you choose among the great variety of therapies?

That question cannot be answered in a book like this one, which cannot advertise one therapy over another. But you *can* study the section of this chapter called Treatment of Dysfunction: Psychotherapy. If you decide that you agree with one of these therapies, or feel comfortable with it, that in itself might be a reason to seek help. Again, your college health service or family physician may be able to refer you, or you may have to get in touch with an organization devoted to the kind of therapy you want.

Gestalt Therapy. The German word *"gestalt"* means a pattern or a whole. *Gestalt therapy* seeks to have patients create a sense of wholeness in their lives by integrating their thoughts, feelings, and actions within day-to-day living. The emphasis placed on the wholeness of patients' present life events makes gestalt therapy differ from psychoanalysis, in which the past is uncovered and dissected.

Transactional Analysis. Transactional analysis (TA) is based on Berne's study of human interaction and time structuring. TA helps patients understand and master the ways in which they deal with others and structure time. From this they can get "positive strokes" (reinforcement for their egos) from life and create a "winning life script"—a life style that is self-assertive and free from being controlled by others.

Encounter-group Therapy. An encounter group commonly includes between 6 and 20 people. They focus on their relations with each other, under the direction of a group leader. They pour out their feelings, disclose themselves frankly, without defenses, and often "confront" one another—in the hope of changing both attitudes and behavior inside and outside the group.

Assertiveness Training.   Some people lack confidence, so they cannot express their desires and feelings. Assertiveness training seeks to help them (1) see how assertion differs from aggression, politeness from nonassertion; (2) identify rights; (3) dispel ideas and feelings that prevent assertiveness; and (4) practice the skills of assertiveness.

Family Therapy.   Some problems are best understood and treated within the context of the family. Family therapy tries to treat all the members of the primary family group, at times together, at times one by one. It often makes use of some other kind of therapy, like TA.

Nonverbal Therapies

Reichean Therapy.   According to the philosopher-psychologist Wilhelm Reich, life systems and the universe both receive a biophysical fluid that Reich termed the Orgone. When the flow of Orgone is held back, in some way, illness and neurosis result. *Reichean therapy* tries to dissolve the block in the flow of Orgone.

Primal Therapy.   In *primal therapy* theory, neurosis is thought to be caused by a buildup of "primal" pain—that is, pain left over from childhood. Primal therapy seeks to let patients get in touch with this pain and then leave it behind, by helping them to act out the childhood experience that caused it.

Nutrition Therapy.   Some researchers believe that many mental problems really result from metabolic problems, and that these can be treated with a change in diet. No one suggests that this should replace all other treatment. Rather, they report some success in treating schizophrenia, alcoholism, drug dependency, and depression. In treating people who are jittery, overanxious, overweight, underweight, or overtired they also report some dramatic success. These ideas are still in the testing stage.

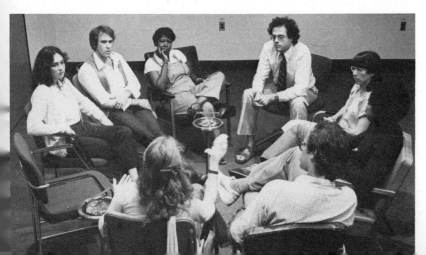

The members of an encounter group try to use their relations with each other to understand their behavior and change it.

Bohdan Hrynewyck/Stock, Boston

Meditation

Meditation began in India as a mystico-religious technique, but a Harvard heart researcher named Herbert Benson discovered that it is based on a real physical process, which he called the relaxation response. The form of meditation recommended by him, which is described below, has no religious significance, and it reduces tension very nicely.

1. Find a quiet room. If you cannot find one that is completely free of sound, play a recording of soft instrumental music or of soothing natural sounds.
2. Sit comfortably and in a straight-backed chair, with your head and back erect, your feet on the floor. Your hands should rest on your thighs, with fingers slightly open. Or sit on the floor as in the photo below.
3. Stretch and relax your neck muscles: lower your chin to your chest and raise it back up three times; bend your neck toward your back and return it to the upright position three times; rotate your head clockwise three times; rotate it counterclockwise three times. Then let your head hang slightly forward. Sit quietly. Close your eyes. Relax your muscles, especially the hands, face, and tongue.
4. Quiet your mind. Do not think about yourself, or even about how well you are meditating. Concentrate on your breathing: as you inhale through your nose, think "in"; as you exhale through your mouth, think "out."
5. Breathe softly, but now without thinking about your breathing. Repeat a "mantra"—a mind-calming word, such as *om* (in English, *one*) to yourself. Try to make your mind quiet. If distracting thoughts intrude upon your meditation, concentrate on the mantra.
6. The meditation session should last from 10 to 20 minutes.

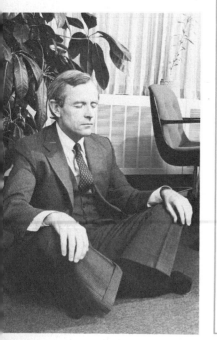

Ken Karp

SUMMARY

Our bodies and minds can only adjust to some of the demands and changes that occur. The narrow range of balance needed for good health is called homeostasis. Some adjustments are fairly simple—sweating when you get hot. Changes that threaten the homeostasis of the mind are harder for us to cope with. When we fail to cope with them the result is dysfunction—ranging from mere nervousness all the way to the loss of the will to live. The best way to cope with the sources of stress is by changing them or removing them by rational action—problem solving. Defense mechanisms are less healthy, but they are used commonly for short-run coping. The forms of time structuring are used widely for long-run coping.

Most people who have trouble coping still manage to keep a hold on the real world and live more or less normal and useful lives. But those who suffer from depression or from psychosis may at times end as suicides.

Some people who have trouble coping with stress can manage on their own. But some cannot. In that case the right coping strategy might be to seek out help.

Suggested Readings

Genevay, Bonnie, and Simon-Gruen, Dawn. "A Group Approach to Working with Stress." *Social Casework: The Journal of Contemporary Social Work* 60 (1979): 368–371. A review of the work of the staff at Family and Child Service of Metropolitan Seattle. They wanted to reach a broad base of people who did not feel the need for counseling, but who could use some basic human relations skills in facing stress and change in daily life. As a result, groups to teach people how to cope with stress were designed, formed, and called "Learning to Live with Stress."

Monat, Alan, and Lazarus, Richard S., eds. *Stress and Coping; An Anthology.* New York: Columbia University Press, 1977, pp. 141–149. This section deals with the ways that people handle stress, their coping style. The readings deal with coping processes and styles—regulation of one's emotions, the degree of threat, disposition and how they affect daily life and health.

Pittner, Mark S., and Houston, B. Kent. "Response to Stress, Cognitive Coping Strategies, and the Type A Behavior Pattern." *Journal of Personality and Social Psychology* 39 (1980): 147–157. A study of whether Type As respond with more arousal to threat to self-esteem than to threat of shock; of differences between Type A and Type B under high and low stress; and of how Type A and Type B differ in coping with stress.

"Stress." [symposium] *American Journal of Nursing* 79 (1979): 1953–1964. This symposium discussed the bad effects of stress, the Type A person, relaxation therapy in a clinic, a relaxation technique, and using relaxation.

Zacks, Hanna. "Self-actualization: A Midlife Problem." *Social Casework: The Journal of Contemporary Social Work* 61 (1980): 223–233. Based on new findings about midlife, an educational program is suggested to develop problem-solving techniques useful in dealing with issues of this stage and its focus on self-actualization.

Drugs

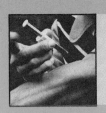

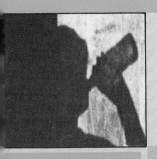

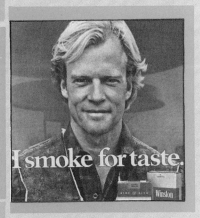

I smoke for taste.

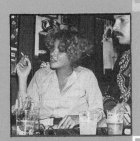

UNIT TWO

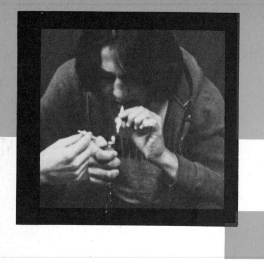

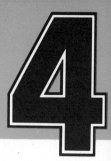

Illicit Drugs

chapter objectives

When you have finished reading this chapter you should be able to:

1. Discuss the extent of drug use in the United States
2. Discuss the reasons for drug use among college students
3. Distinguish between drug use and abuse
4. Discuss the impact of drugs (marijuana, stimulants, depressants) upon the body
5. Recognize the dangers of drugs and drug abuse on the body and the mind

In Unit One, we saw that people sometimes respond to stress by deal-ing with its causes and, sometimes, by becoming victims of physical or mental problems. In Unit Two, we will read about yet another response to stress: the taking of drugs.

What Is a Drug?

A drug is a substance, other than food (see Chapter 8), that can affect the workings of the body or the mind. Even in the most primitive cul-tures, people use herbs and other natural products to relieve pain, cure symptoms of illness, and feel the change in mood called *intoxication*—a "high" in today's slang. In ancient times, medicinals were a business, for merchants and traders traveled far and wide to find them. The search for spices, herbs, and medicines spurred on explorers and helped create huge empires; when Columbus discovered America he was look-ing for the Spice Islands. Today, drugs have created even bigger busi-ness—indeed, two big businesses—one legal and the other illegal.

Many drugs are now *controlled*; in other words, their use has been made legal in some instances but not in others. The extent of this con-trol varies a good deal from drug to drug and from country to country. Some drugs, like Heroin, are illegal; others, like aspirin, are legal. Mor-phine is legal only when prescribed by a physician. But alcohol can be bought from licensed dealers by anyone over a certain age (which var-ies from state to state). An *illicit drug* is one that is not used in a legal way, even if it is not an illegal drug. Finally, over-the-counter drugs (see Chapter 18) are legal and can be bought and used by anyone.

Illicit drugs are for the most part *psychoactive*—they change the user's chemistry, to affect mood or perception. This effect is often de-sired and so they may become *drugs of abuse*. Such drugs, when used often to cope with stress, have harmful effects on the user. Any psycho-active drug—even one that has many legitimate uses—can become a drug of abuse when used too often. But drugs that do not change mood or perception do not commonly become drugs of abuse.

Psychoactive Drugs

The drug problem consists chiefly of the abuse of psychoactive drugs. Many people do not understand the true extent of this problem because they do not know what the word "drug" really means. Some substances, like penicillin, are called drugs because they are prescribed as cures. But two drugs, tobacco and alcohol, have been accepted for so long that most of us do not view them as drugs at all. This shows only that atti-tudes on such questions are influenced by our culture, for alcohol and tobacco are indeed drugs, and dangerous ones at that. In fact, our in-take of caffeine, nicotine, and alcohol far exceeds our intake of illicit drugs. A study funded by the National Institute of Health (NIH) showed that in the early 1970s about 85 percent of adult Americans drank coffee, that 37 percent of the men and 29 percent of the women smoked tobacco, and that 55 percent of the men and 32 percent of the women were moderate to heavy drinkers of alcohol. Far fewer Americans used prescription drugs, let alone illegal ones. By any standard, caffeine, nicotine, and alcohol are *the* most widely used drugs in our society.

These statistics put the problem of psychoactive drugs in a better perspective. Above all, they make it clear that the line between illicit drugs, on the one hand, and legal drugs like alcohol, on the other, is really drawn to serve certain purposes; the fact is that misuse of alcohol has created more social problems and suffering than misuse of any other single drug. Even so, we cannot overlook this line drawn between illicit and legal drugs, because the law insists on it, and it is therefore an important part of our culture.

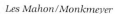
Les Mahon/Monkmeyer

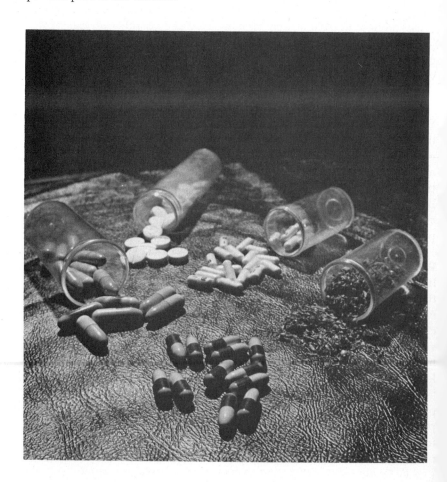

Table 4–1.   Percentages of People Aged 18–25 Who Have Used Drugs

Category	Drug	% for All Users Present and Past
controlled	alcohol	84
	cigarettes	68
	prescription stimulants	21
	prescription sedatives	18
	prescription tranquilizers	13
	cocaine	19
	opiates other than Heroin	14
illegal	marijuana, hashish	60
	hallucinogens	20
	Heroin	4

Source: 1977 U.S. Government Survey.

Young Adults and Drugs

In 1977 the U.S. government sponsored a study of drug use among people between the ages of 18 and 25. The study showed that alcohol was by far the most popular psychoactive drug used, followed by marijuana. (See Table 4–1.)

Drug Trends.   The smoking of marijuana still seems to be slightly on the increase among college students. The illicit drug in fashion at present is cocaine. Heroin seems to be making a comeback among young adults, after a decline in the early and mid-1970s. Hallucinogens, amphetamines, and barbiturates are being used less than they were in the late 1960s and early 1970s. Imaginative duos have also been created recently, such as the Ts and Blues (Talwin and pyribenzamine) currently popular "on the street."

Why Drugs?   You saw in Chapters 2 and 3 that stress is an element of life and that people must try to cope with it, on the conscious level or the unconscious level. Now, college is a very stressful time, and so too is early adulthood, for students must try to cope with course work and social pressures, while at the same time, they become adults. It is not a surprise that many college students, like many of their parents, turn for help to alcohol, cigarettes, and pills. It is not a surprise that other college students rebel against their "straight" parents by using drugs like "pot." The very fact that adults, whom students often blame for all their problems, by and large condemn marijuana seems to heighten its appeal. Those students who seek to solve their problems by withdrawing into a rich and meaningful inner world may look to drugs as a means of access to such a world.

In the United States, certain conditions tend to promote drug taking. One is the fact that our society subjects its members to very high levels of stress—more of it than many people know how to deal with intelligently. Another is the fact that people who attempt to cope by using drugs find them very easy to get hold of.

Many people, besides, are confused about our society's attitudes toward drugs and drug use. After all, we value progress in chemistry and the other sciences, and even our government approves and promotes the sale and use of drugs—as long as they have been accepted by scientists as "cures." Many people therefore fail to see the distinction between a licit and an illicit drug. They believe that some pill or liquid or ointment can be found to cure any physical problem at all; they believe anything that they are told about any drug (see Chapter 18).

The Effects of Drugs

Drugs achieve part of their effect by playing on our attitudes toward them and on our expectation about their physical and emotional impact. But for the most part, they work by affecting the action of the nervous system, which (as we saw in Chapter 1) consists of the brain and also of a network of nerves spread throughout the entire body. The nervous system's function is to help us respond to changes in the internal and external environment. Drugs actually become a part of the internal (biochemical) environment, and they influence the user's *perceptions* of the external (natural and social) environment. In both ways they influence our behavior, sometimes most profoundly.

The effect of a drug can vary from person to person and from time to time—with the dosage of the drug, the physical condition of its user, the way it is taken, the drug's strength, the user's former or current drug usage, the drugs that are used together at any one time, and the spacing of the doses.

Dose Response.   For the most part, the effects of a drug continue to increase as you take more of it and as you take it more often. The *threshold dose* of a drug is the amount needed to produce any effect at all on the user. As the dosage of a drug increases, the effects increase too, until the drug becomes harmful and, further down the road, lethal.

In the case of some drugs, the difference between a threshold dose and a lethal dose is very great. For example, only a small amount of alcohol will make you "happy" or even drunk; but you would have to drink a great deal of it at any one sitting to kill yourself from an excess of alcohol alone (as opposed to foolish behavior while under its influence). For many other drugs, however, the difference between a threshold dose and a lethal dose is quite small; people often overdose and die on these drugs because they cannot calculate how much they can take.

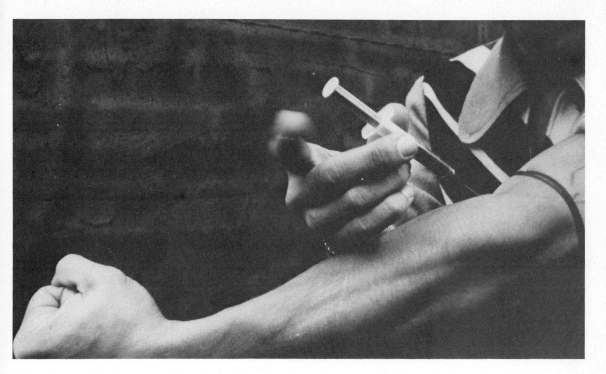

Mainlining.
Nicholas Sapieha/Stock, Boston

Biological Variability.   Each person's response to drugs varies from time to time. Suppose, for example, that in a test two people were given the same drug dose and then an increased dose. Each might differ in response to the drug, because of differing biological constitutions and their former use of the same drug. That is why it is very hard to say how anyone will respond to any one drug dosage. Also, two people who *for the most part* respond to a drug in the same way may really not respond to it the same way in one respect. For instance, they might reach the threshold dose response with the same dose, but their lethal dose might differ.

Method of Administration.   The way a drug is taken (or administered) can also influence its effect. In general, when a drug is injected into a vein ("mainlined") it takes effect rapidly. When drugs are taken by mouth (orally) or injected beneath the skin ("skin popped") the effects occur more slowly, though they sometimes last longer. When drugs are inhaled through the nostrils ("snorted") or when they are smoked, their effects are somewhat milder than with mainlining or skin popping, but their effects are felt earlier than when they are swallowed. Many psychoactive drugs can be (and are) taken in a number of ways.

Potency and Tolerance.   The *potency* of a drug is the amount that must be taken to produce the desired response; the smaller the amount needed, the more potent the drug. For many drugs, the response to a given potency (or dose) changes over time, for the effect of the dosage decreases each time the drug is taken. The drug taker is then said to have developed *tolerance* to the drug and, to restore the effect gotten at first, more and more of it must be taken. A Heroin addict, for example, might start out with a daily shot that costs, say, $20. Within a month, that same addict might need five a day, costing $100, just to get the same high. Tolerance to some drugs, like LSD, develops rapidly; tolerance to other drugs, like barbiturates, develops slowly.

Synergy.   Many drug users take more than one drug at a time. Sometimes the effect of two or more drugs taken at the same time simply equals the combined effect of each drug (effect of drug A + effect of drug B = effects of drugs A + B). But sometimes the effect of taking two or more drugs at the same time is *greater* than you would expect from each one—even when combined. This is called *synergy*.

Stages of Drug Dependence

Drug dependence is the need to take a drug regularly, in order to feel its effects or to avoid the discomfort of not taking it. Dependence on drugs may be mental, or both mental and physical. The first, the least compulsive, stage of drug dependence is a mental craving for a drug. The second stage is tolerance, which means that the effect of a drug lessens each time it is taken, so that the dosage must constantly be increased. *Addiction,* the most compulsive stage of drug dependence, means that the body requires the drug. When addicts try to quit they develop *withdrawal symptoms,* which differ for different drugs but are always so unpleasant that it is hard to quit.

Withdrawal.   Although the symptoms of withdrawal from each drug differ somewhat, they are almost the same for all drugs. When addicts cannot get the drugs they need, they first become anxious; then they become weak and may tremble; their muscles twitch and contract. Cramps in the abdomen, nausea, and vomiting often occur. An extreme drying out of the body may follow the vomiting, with rapid weight loss, and increased heart and respiration rates.

Categories of Drugs

Each drug shares certain features with other drugs, and these enable us to place it in a larger group, a category. The same drug may, in fact, fall into several groups. Heroin, for instance, is an opiate (derived from opium), but it is also an analgesic, in other words, a painkiller. Analgesics include many drugs that are not opiates, but all opiates are analgesics. The grouping that follows is therefore not the only possible one, but it is the most common one. It includes marijuana, stimulants, depressants, tranquilizers, psychedelics, and narcotics.

Marijuana and Hashish

Let us start with marijuana (street names: grass, pot), a drug that is really in a group by itself. Marijuana deserves this place, in part because it does not fall clearly into any of the others and because it is by far the most popular of the illicit drugs. Another popular illicit drug, hashish, is derived from the same plant and has the same active ingredient—tetrahydrocanabinol (THC)—and similar (though usually more powerful) effects. Marijuana is usually smoked in cigarettes (or "reefers" or "joints"), as is hashish, but both can also be eaten.

Marijuana—To Legalize or Not?

A great deal has been said about whether or not marijuana should be decriminalized. Here are some of the statements made by those who favor and those who oppose legalization.*

In Favor:

- decriminalization (the ending of criminal penalties for using marijuana) is not legalization
- decriminalization would reduce law-enforcement costs and contribute to taxes
- used moderately, marijuana is not very injurious
- the use of marijuana in states where it has been decriminalized is not significantly different from its use in states where it is still illegal
- current laws do not deter marijuana users
- people should be free to decide whether they want to use the drug
- marijuana is at worst a health problem, not a legal problem
- unlike alcohol, which is legal, marijuana does not usually prompt aggression
- marijuana is not physically addictive
- there is no evidence that marijuana use leads to the use of other drugs

Against:

- studies have shown that marijuana has harmful effects on the body
- it distorts sense perceptions and heavy, even regular, users suffer various mental impairments
- the availability of a drug promotes its use
- marijuana use is a "stepping stone" to the use of more dangerous drugs even if only for social, rather than physical, reasons
- the drug has increased in potency in recent years
- decriminalization would hurt the economy, because an increase of on-the-job smoking would decrease performance and output
- legalization might increase the number of auto accidents
- decriminalization would increase the use of marijuana

*Based on "An Overview of Marijuana Usage." *Congressional Digest* (Washington, D.C.: Government Printing Office), vol. 58, no. 2 (February 1979), pp. 34–62.

Marijuana has probably been used for thousands of years, but it only became common in the United States in the 1960s. Since then it has been widely used, widely debated, and widely tested. The debate over it has even changed its legal status. The U.S. government first passed a law to discourage its use in 1937. (Most states had done so before.) In 1951 it was placed under the jurisdiction of the federal narcotics laws. But marijuana, whatever its dangers, is not a narcotic in the medical sense, and in the early 1970s the Comprehensive Drug Abuse and Control Act broke the link between the two.

Research into the effects of marijuana has yet to produce conclusive or accepted findings. Some researchers think that the THC in marijuana and hashish can harm the brain and the reproductive system, and that it lowers resistance to infection, impairs short-term memory, and slows down motor functions (as when driving a car). It may create feelings of apathy, depression, and isolation from friends and family. Some think that the marijuana used today is more dangerous than that of the 1960s. Kids start smoking it at younger ages now, and there are reasons to think that the earlier it is used, the more harmful it is. In fact, the amount of THC in the marijuana reaching the United States seems to be rising, and this too may increase the risks. Finally, people who smoke it may now be smoking it more often. The burn products in the smoke, it seems, have even more harmful effects on the body than cigarette smoke has (see Chapter 6).

Marijuana is still illegal in most states. That does not deter people from smoking it, but if you are caught there may well be a price to pay. Price or not, most young people—including, in all probability, many of the readers of this book—have tried it. Although it does not lead straight to addiction or to madness, it still is not quite harmless.

Stimulants

As a group, the stimulants include some of the most common and respectable drugs, such as caffeine and nicotine, and one of the most fashionable, cocaine (street names: snow, coke). These three drugs are derived from natural substances. But the amphetamines (street name: benny, upper, speed) are synthetic (or manmade) prescription drugs. These are sometimes used to help lose weight, but they are a poor way to do so.

Stimulants excite the central nervous system. At first, users feel high (euphoric), talky, and very alive. They have little appetite for food, resist fatigue, and stay awake for days. The long-term effects of misuse include being restless and irritable, weight loss, paranoia (feelings of persecution), and an increased tendency to violence. Users often become abusers, often develop a dependence, then often develop tolerance, and therefore need larger and larger doses to get the high they crave.

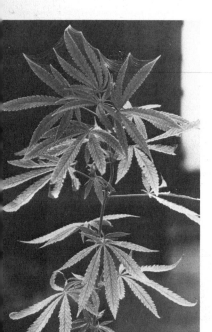

The marijuana plant (*Cannabis sativa*).

Anna Kaufman Moon/Stock, Boston

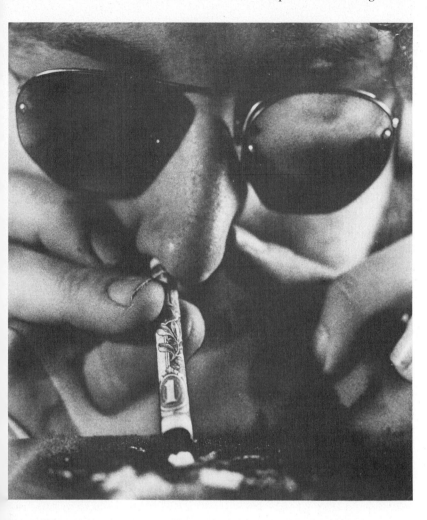

"Snorting" cocaine

Peter Simon/Stock, Boston

Cocaine.   Cocaine is a natural stimulant, one that has become more and more popular in recent years. It produces a powerful short-term high and also, at times, hallucinations (or visual distortions). Most users "snort" cocaine (inhale it), but it can also be injected. Since the body does not develop a noticeable tolerance to cocaine, the effects of a certain dose remain constant over time. But the user does become mentally dependent and driven to feel, yet again, the stimulation, the euphoria, and the illusion of great mental and physical power that the drug creates. When cocaine's effects fade, users sometimes get depressed, and this may drive them to take yet another snort. A coke habit can soon become an expensive one since the cost is high and the effects are quite short-term.

Caffeine.   One quite legal stimulant is caffeine, which is present in coffee, tea, and cola drinks. Caffeine is mildly addictive and too much can make us feel anxious and irritable, as it increases blood pressure, heart rate, and oxygen needs. Coffee, America's most common source of caffeine, also contains oils that may irritate the stomach and aggravate, even cause, ulcers. Caffeine is found in some amounts in many products. The standard dose of Vivarin has more than a cup of coffee; but the following have less (in descending order): tea, No-Doz, Dr Pepper, Excedrin, Coca-Cola, Vanquish, Anacin, and cocoa.

Depressants

The *barbiturates* (street names: downers, pills) along with alcohol are the most used kinds of drugs in the group called *depressants,* drugs that depress the nervous system. They are in some ways quite similar. Both barbiturates, which are drugs prescribed for anxiety and sleeplessness, and alcohol produce symptoms commonly called "drunkenness." Both can be addictive. When deprived, those addicted to alcohol or to the barbiturates suffer the same withdrawal pains—and abrupt withdrawal from either can kill. Indeed, the effects of the barbiturates and of alcohol are so similar that researchers who study both call barbiturates "solid alcohol," and alcohol a "liquid barbiturate." The relationship between the two drugs is not limited to similar effects. People who take large amounts of one of them develop a "cross tolerance" to the other. Barbiturates, though, are more dangerous than is alcohol, because they usually come in pill form, and it is easier to die from swallowing too many pills than from drinking too much alcohol.

Because users of barbiturates develop a tolerance for them, they are usually taken in doses that become greater and greater with time. The abuse of barbiturates is the most dangerous kind of drug abuse, since withdrawal from them is even more severe than withdrawal from narcotics. Also, the effects of barbiturates on the mind, the emotions, and the body are less predictable than the effects of narcotics like morphine.

Tranquilizers

Tranquilizers are legal when used by prescription, and they are among the most prescribed of all drugs. Like barbiturates, they are used to treat anxiety and tension. Valium, the most widely used, is typical of the *minor tranquilizers,* the ones most often sought and prescribed. *Major tranquilizers,* such as Thorazine and Compazine, are used in the treatment (see Chapter 3) of severe psychotic disorders, often in hospitals.

In recent years, the frequency with which some physicians prescribe minor tranquilizers has been criticized and put under study. After all, as we saw in Chapter 2, anxiety and tension are part of life, and to some extent useful. But if people take tranquilizers for long periods of time, they can become both mentally and physically dependent on them. Also, depression—and other signs of withdrawal—have been known to occur when their use has been discontinued for any reason.

Psychedelics

Psychedelics (also called hallucinogens) produce distortions of the real world and, sometimes, hallucinations. The best known psychedelics are lysergic acid diethylamide, or LSD (street name: acid), peyote, mescaline, and Phencyclidine hydrochloride (street names: PCP and "Angel Dust"). Psychedelics alter the working of the mind in a way that sometimes resembles a psychosis (see Chapter 3). The physical effects of a typical psychedelic, like LSD, include tremors, rapid heartbeat, dilation of the pupils of the eyes, and sleeplessness; the mental effects include changes in perception and mood—swings from elation to depression or the reverse.

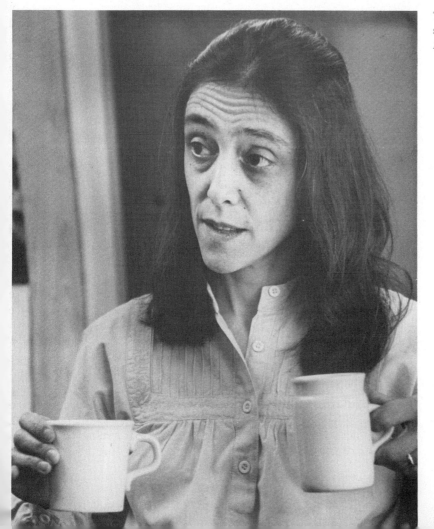

The other addiction: "One sugar or two?"
David S. Strickler/Monkmeyer

Table 4–2. Major Effects of Hallucinogens and Marijuana

	Hallucinogens	Marijuana
Physical	Dizziness	Dizziness
	Dilation of pupils	Reddening of eyes
	Weakness	Nausea and vomiting
	Tremor	Drowsiness
	Dry mouth	Increased appetite
	Nausea and vomiting	
	Decreased appetite	
Cognitive	Decreased concentration	Decreased concentration
	Inability to express thoughts	Inability to express thoughts
	Rapid thoughts	Rapid thoughts
	Poor judgment	Poor judgment
	Poor memory	Poor memory
	Sense of time passing slowly	Sense of time passing slowly
Emotional	Altered mood	Altered mood
	Tension relieved by laughing	Euphoria
	or crying	Uncontrolled laughing
	Euphoria	
	Depression	
	Anxiety	
Perceptual	Blurred vision	Blurred vision
	Altered, often exaggerated	Altered, often exaggerated
	shapes and colors	shapes and colors
	Increased acuity of hearing	Increased acuity of hearing
	Distortion of space	Distortion of space
	Organized visual illusions	Poor self-perception
	and hallucinations	Hallucinations
	Colors may be "heard"	Colors may be "heard"
	and sounds "seen"	and sounds "seen"

Source: Robert E. Silverman, *Psychology,* 4th ed. (Englewood Cliffs, N.J.: Prentice-Hall, 1982), p. 257. By permission.

In a typical LSD trip the user may feel a seemingly increased level of awareness and mental clearness, a distorted sense of perception, and a weakening of self-control. Common statements or notions take on profound meanings that seem spiritual or philosophical. The effect, or "trip," brought on by LSD will seem horrid to some and very worthwhile to others. The effect from a single dose of LSD sometimes recurs in "flashbacks" days, weeks, or even months later. Little is known about the cause of flashbacks or about the long-term problems of LSD use.

The psychedelics do not seem to be addictive. No deaths have been attributed to overdoses of LSD, for instance. But people under its influence have committed suicide or died in accidents.

PCP, a psychedelic that has just become quite popular, was developed as an anesthetic. It is no longer used for that purpose because of its bizarre side effects, including hallucinations, even death. It is now often sprinkled on parsley or on marijuana and smoked, to enhance the effect.

Narcotics

Narcotics both excite and depress the nervous system. At first they create in the user a euphoric rush, an elation, and then a numbness, a suppression of hunger, sexual desire, and anger. Though not all users become addicted to narcotics, they are among the most mentally addictive of all drugs. They are mostly mainlined or popped by users, although they may be smoked or snorted.

Besides being drugs of abuse, such narcotics as opium, morphine, and codeine also have a medical use, as analgesics (or painkillers). Narcotics reduce pain by changing our perceptions of it, not by blocking its transmission through the nervous system.

The most important subgroup of narcotics consists of the *opiates,* the drugs derived from *opium,* a natural substance. These include *morphine, codeine,* and *Heroin* (street names: H, horse, smack, shit). Heroin, the most powerful opiate and the one most often abused, was trademarked at the turn of the century and used as a treatment for morphine addiction. A synthetic narcotic, *Methadone,* is now used to treat addiction to Heroin. Among the other synthetic narcotics are *Darvon* and *Demerol.* Darvon is commonly prescribed by physicians as a pain reliever for such problems as menstrual cramps and severe muscle sprains. But in recent years its effect as a painkiller has been questioned, while its effect as a euphorant has made it a drug of abuse. Re-

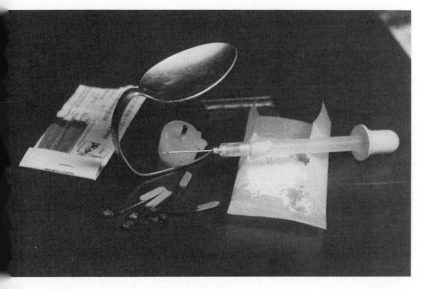

Heroin paraphernalia.
Charles Gatewood/Stock, Boston

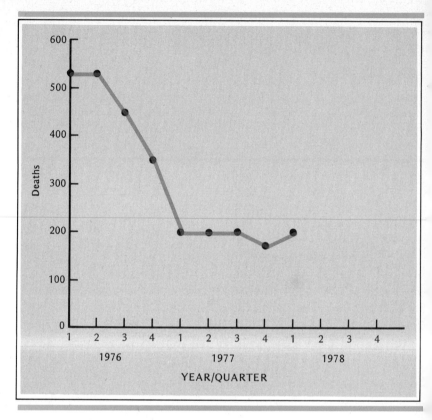

Figure 4-1. Heroin-related Deaths, 1976–1978.
Source: DAWN Quarterly Report, April/June 1978 *(Rockville, Maryland: National Institute on Drug Abuse, 1979).*

cently the federal government has placed restrictions on its sale, but physicians can still prescribe it.

Narcotics as a group are among the most dangerous of all drugs. Their greatest danger is the way they decrease the heartbeat and the breathing rate—and these can lead to death from an overdose. Since narcotics are highly addictive, users who cannot get hold of them when they need them or who attempt to stop using them may get severe withdrawal symptoms: chills and tremors, cramps, twitching, vomiting, diarrhea, and sleeplessness. The attempt to avoid these symptoms and the high that the narcotic brings account for the compulsion to continue their use. This compulsion is a major source of urban crime, since narcotics are expensive and addicts often must steal to support their habit.

Preventing Drug Abuse

The key to preventing drug abuse is to understand its causes. And the cause, more often than not, is stress and the desire to remove it—quickly and without effort. As you saw in Chapter 3, in the long run some ways of trying to remove stress simply create more stresses, and a drug habit, prolonged drug taking, is one of those ways. That doesn't mean, of course, that the first drink will make you a drunkard or the first joint will make you a drug fiend; in fact, some people do manage to use drugs without losing their heads over them. But others do not. They get some relief and some pleasure from the drug, but in the long run they pay for it since they do not solve the problems that made them turn to drugs in the first place—and the use of drugs adds more and more stress to their lives.

Before using any drug, think about why you are using it. If you are seeking relief from minor frustration, this may mean, simply, that you are human, with common human weaknesses. But if you attempt to solve long-standing or long-term problems through drug taking, or if you take drugs because you are pressured into it by your friends, you may have a drug problem—and right now.

Mimi Forsyth/Monkmeyer

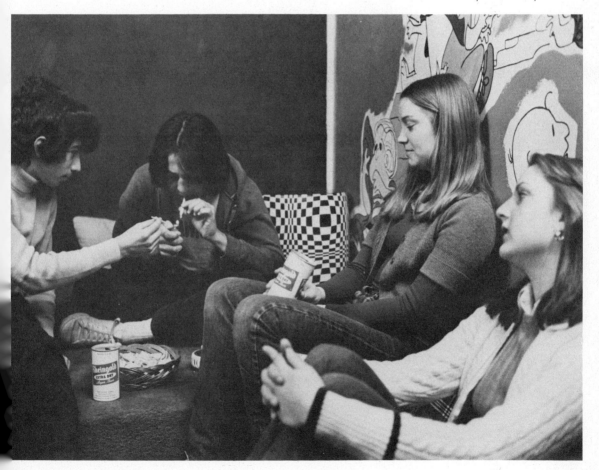

Rehabilitation

Drug-treatment programs make use of two methods. First, the *drug therapy* approach tries to satisfy the addict's craving for drugs in a less destructive way, before attempts are made to change behavior. In the United States the best-known method of drug therapy is the use of Methadone to wean addicts away from Heroin and other narcotics. Although Methadone is itself a narcotic, it can be given by physicians so that it does not produce a high but does stave off withdrawal symptoms. At this stage the addict remains an addict but may learn to live without drug-induced pleasure. If the treatment is a success the addict leaves the "drug subculture"—the company of other addicts—and sets up a life that is not built around the getting and taking of drugs. If all goes well, the addict's need for drugs will taper off, and then the use of Methadone can be decreased and finally ended.

Some researchers think that taking the addict off drugs should be the *first* step in treatment, not the last. Such treatments seek to change the addict's personality by breaking down the defenses, rationalizations, and evasions (see Chapter 1) used to justify and prolong the drug addiction. In some programs, the addicts are removed from their day-to-day world and placed in a *therapeutic community*, a group residence mainly run by the addicts themselves. By forcing addicts to run their daily lives, these communities attempt to make them self-controlled, trustworthy, and self-sufficient.

SUMMARY

Drugs affect the body and the mind. Psychoactive drugs (those affecting the mind) are used for many reasons, but the most important of them is that they help people cope with stress. And the use of drugs can be a very harmful form of coping.

Caffeine, tobacco, and alcohol are the most widely used psychoactive drugs in our country. But many people have used illicit drugs—drugs that are illegal or are used illegally—marijuana, amphetamines, cocaine, barbiturates, psychedelics, tranquilizers, and narcotics. Of these, marijuana is the most widely used, cocaine the most fashionable at present, and Heroin and the barbiturates the most dangerous.

Some drugs are legal, others illegal. The use of many legal drugs is controlled, so that they cannot be used without a prescription or by people under a certain age. Some substances are commonly called drugs, but others—tobacco, alcohol, and caffeine—are not. The distinctions between legal and illegal drugs, controlled and uncontrolled drugs, and recognized and unrecognized drugs are not always based on the real dangers of each drug. Drugs in all these groups are psychoactive—and they can undermine health.

Our society insists on the distinction between these groups, so it is a social reality. And it is based, in part, on another: the fact that certain legal drugs, though quite dangerous, are also quite popular and respectable. In the next two chapters we shall take a look at two of these drugs: alcohol and tobacco.

Suggested Readings

Benjamin, Fred B. *Alcohol, Drugs, and Traffic Safety.* Springfield, Ill.: Charles C. Thomas, 1980. This book discusses government programs on drugs and alcohol and the effect they have had on traffic safety. Thus far, the results of these programs have been largely negative. The focus is on what is not known and how we can get the required data—what was wrong in other programs and how these mistakes can be avoided in the future.

Dusek, Dorothy, and Girdano, Daniel A. *Drugs; A Factual Account,* 3rd ed. Reading, Mass.: Addison-Wesley, 1980. A factual overview of the total drug scene that, while general, zeroes in on topics based on current research. It depicts the historical, social, and legal impact of drugs on our society.

Eisenman, Russell, Grossman, Jan Carl, and Goldstein, Ronald. "Undergraduate Marijuana Use as Related to Internal Sensation Novelty Seeking and Openness to Experience." *Journal of Clinical Psychology*

36 (1980): 1013–1019. This study expanded on previous findings in marijuana personality research. It was found that the greater the self-reported use of marijuana, the higher were the scores on creativity and adventuresomeness tests and the lower the scores on authoritarianism. A new factor, internal sensation novelty seeking, was found to be correlated with self-reported frequency of marijuana use.

Vourakis, Christine, and Bennett, Gerald. "Angel Dust: Not Heaven Sent." *American Journal of Nursing* 79 (1979): 649–653. The article discusses the pharmacology and patterns of use of PCP. It is of concern as a drug of abuse in the United States because of its high potential for physical and mental harm after as little as one dose.

Ward, Nicholas G., and Schuckit, Marc A. "Factors Associated with Suicidal Behavior in Polydrug Abusers." *Journal of Clinical Psychiatry* 41 (1980): 379–385. Drug abuse goes with a high rate of fatal and nonfatal suicide attempts. This study examines demographic, diagnostic, familial, and drug-use factors and past history of suicide attempts.

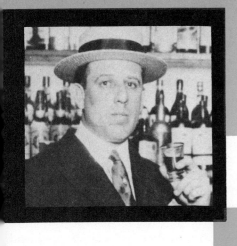

5

Alcohol

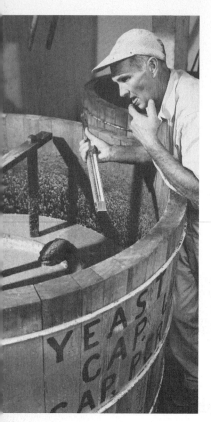

Fermentation.

Joe Monroe/Photo Researchers

Alcohol—CH₃CH₂OH, the active agent in wine, whiskey, and beer—is really a drug with several faces. Many people drink it for its taste, and a drink helps some people to relax. Most people use it for those reasons, and they manage not to misuse it. But not everyone is that lucky—since alcohol is a powerful drug, known and used since ancient times for its mood-altering effects. Unlike the drugs discussed in Chapter 4, alcohol is socially respected—it is served at the White House. It can also be found on Skid Row. In fact, alcohol is our country's most popular drug—it accounts for our leading drug problem.

"Drinking" is a firmly established fact of American behavior—among men and women; rich and poor; city people, country people, and even people in the suburbs. Although a large minority of Americans do not "drink," ours *is* a "drinking" society. Almost 70 percent of all American adults, and more than 87 percent of all college students, drink alcohol in one form or another.

Why is alcohol so respectable? In part, because of its long use in Western society; we are so familiar with it that it does not frighten us. Partly, too, because it is advertised widely as a refreshment, not a drug. These advertisements show a drink as the well-earned reward for a hard day's work ("This beer's for you!") and encourage its use by the status-conscious ("Here's to your first million"). They suggest that it is the normal complement to friendship ("Here's to good friends") and a symbol of manhood ("Who is the ale man?").

What We Drink

Alcohol is a natural substance formed when sugar or starch (carbohydrates) ferments in the presence of yeast. Different kinds of alcoholic drinks are produced by different means using different raw materials. Beer (from malted barley and grains) and wine (from grapes and berries) are made by the *fermentation* process. Fermented drinks have an alcohol content of no more than about 12 percent, because after that the alcohol simply kills the yeast and ends the process. Whiskey (from whole grains), vodka (from grains or potatoes), and rum (from molasses) are made by the process called *distillation*, in which the fermented alcohol is treated to extract pure alcohol.

Alcoholic Content.   Most American beers have 3 to 6 percent alcohol by volume, while dinner (or table) wines, such as Chablis and Burgundy, have about 12 percent. Most distilled spirits have between 40 percent and 50 percent alcohol by volume. The common measure of the amount of alcohol in a product is called *proof*. Proof equals twice the volume (or content) of alcohol in a beverage—so, a distilled spirit that is 50 percent alcohol by volume is called 100 proof.

Don't let the seemingly low alcoholic content of beer fool you. A 12-

In the 70's the 3 top beer-drinking countries were Czechoslovakia, West Germany, and Australia, in that order. The United States ranks only 13th.

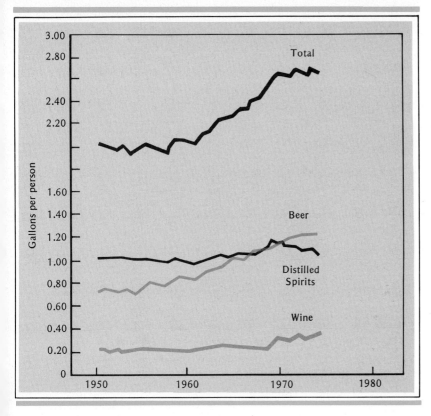

Figure 5-1. This graph shows how much beer, wine, and distilled spirits Americans have been consuming.

Source: Third Special Report to the U.S. Congress on Alcohol and Health. Secretary of HEW, Government Printing Office, June 1978.

ounce can of beer has about the same amount of alcohol in it as a cocktail with one ounce of 100-proof (50%) alcohol. In beer, the alcohol is just more dilute than in a vodka gimlet. Even if you never touch the hard stuff, it doesn't mean that you can't get just as drunk!

Preferences. While more than 50 percent of those who drink in this country use distilled spirits, only about 37 percent claim to use them exclusively or almost so. About 40 percent of those who drink report that they do not use distilled spirits at all; about 4 percent drink only wine, while about 15 percent drink only beer. Although the absolute amount of alcohol used by American drinkers has not changed much recently, we report drinking less distilled spirits but more wine.

The Effects of Alcohol

Mood. Most people think of alcohol as a stimulant. In fact, it is a depressant, but it does have a "stimulating" effect at first. Under the in-

What Can Happen If You Drink and Take Drugs

The effects of mixing alcohol with other drugs fall into three categories:

- Antagonistic—the effect of either (or both) drugs is blocked or reduced.
- Additive—the total effect of the combination of two or more drugs equals the combined effects of each individual drug.
- Synergistic (potentiating)—the total effect of the combination of two or more drugs is *greater than* the combined effect of each individual drug.

The chart below indicates the range of unpleasant and dangerous reactions caused by the use of alcohol with other drugs.

Drug	Effect When Mixed with Alcohol
Analgesics (Narcotic) (Demerol, Darvon, etc.)	Depresses central nervous system; can cause respiratory failure and death
Analgesics (non-Narcotic, such as Aspirin)	Irritates stomach; can cause bleeding in stomach and intestines
Antidepressants (Tofranil, Triavil, etc.)	Reduces even further the functioning of the central nervous system; taken with red wine, may cause high blood pressure crisis
Antihistamines (Actifed, Coricidin, etc.)	Increases sleep-inducing effect; driving extremely hazardous with this combination
Antihypertensive Agents (Serpasil, Aldomet, etc.)	Lowers blood pressure further, causing dizziness; depresses central nervous system
Barbiturates (Amytal, Nembutal, Seconal, Quaalude, etc.)	Increases tolerance to dosage prescribed or taken; can cause anxiety, loss of memory, and slurred speech
Diuretics	Reduces blood pressure, causing dizziness
Psychotropics (Tindal, Mellaril, Thorazine, etc.)	Depresses central nervous system; can cause respiratory failure and death
Tranquilizers (Valium, Librium, etc.)	Decreases motor control and mental functions; diminishes control over emotions; increases danger of car and household accidents

Drug	Effect When Mixed with Alcohol
Amphetamines (Dexedrine, Benzedrine, etc.)	Reverses effect of alcohol; gives drunk person sense of control—but not actual control—over movements; can provoke symptoms such as paranoia
Antidiabetic Agents (Insulin, Diabenese, Orinase, etc.)	Can produce severe and unpredictable reactions
Antibiotics (Seromycin, Cloromycetin, etc.)	Can cause nausea, headaches, and (possibly) convulsions, especially when mixed with drugs prescribed for urinary-tract infections.
Cocaine	Has effects similar to those of combining amphetamines and alcohol, but also produces mental distortions.
Vitamins	Keeps vitamins from entering bloodstream and thereby from taking effect
Marijuana	In small amounts, produces no ill effect; may cause emotional problems and depression when used excessively with alcohol.

fluence of this effect drinkers lose their restraint—they talk more freely at parties, they tell secrets, they make passes, they dance, and so on. To feel this freedom from restraint—a freedom that, within limits, serves many useful functions—is why most people begin to drink.

Alcohol's stimulating effect wears off quite soon. Then, if more and more is consumed it begins to slow the neural actions in the brain, those which control perception and motor function. Soon the drinker begins to feel sluggish, tired, heavy, even numb. The true, the depressant, nature of alcohol has begun to make itself felt.

Perception.　One drink can measurably interfere with sight and hearing, as well as impair both judgment and mental performance. Another drink or two may impair brain function, so that the sharpness of visual images is lost and double vision may set in. Once the brain is dulled by alcohol, the drinker's perception of the world and even of the self becomes distorted.

Motor Control.　One drink affects the motor nerves and relaxes muscles that normally are slightly tensed. Further drinks make the nervous system carry signals ever more slowly to the muscles, which respond with movements that are not precise and slowed reflexes. Even more drinks produce slurred speech, an unsteady walk, and the glassy-eyed stare of the heavy drinker.

Taste. The effects of alcohol on judgment, perception, and motor function can be measured without bias. Alcohol's taste cannot. People prefer one taste to another and are willing to spend large amounts of money on status labels of wines, brandies, whiskeys, and so forth. And many people were taught that certain wines and beers enhance the taste of certain food. This gourmet approach leads to many sales, and to many drinks, and it may lead to too many drinks.

Measuring the Effects. The blood alcohol level (BAL) is a way of measuring the amount of alcohol that concentrates in the bloodstream. It is simply the proportion of the total weight (in milligrams) of 100 units of blood (in milliliters) made up by alcohol. Different concentrations of alcohol—that is, different BALs—produce different effects.

One mixed drink or one can of beer commonly yields a BAL between .02 and .03 percent. Based on the size and the stomach contents of the drinkers, and what has been drunk and how quickly, two or three drinks yield a reading of about .05 percent. At this level, alcohol can be the cause of an auto accident. In almost all states a BAL of .10 percent puts the driver in the loser's circle when the highway patrol demands a breath or urine test. At .10 percent, even if you feel great, you are legally drunk.

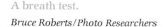

A breath test.

Bruce Roberts/Photo Researchers

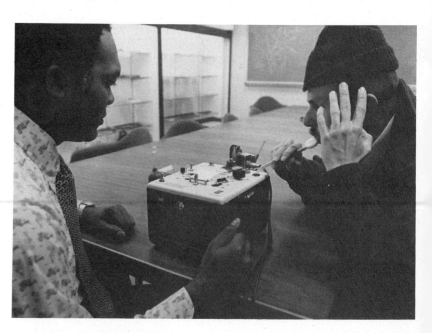

Blood Alcohol Level*

Number of Drinks†	Blood Alcohol Concentration	Mental and Physical Effects
1	.02–.03%	No overt effects, slight feeling of muscle relaxation, slight mood elevation.
2	.05–.06%	No intoxication, but feeling of relaxation, warmth. Slight increase in reaction time, slight decrease in fine muscle coordination.
3	.08–.09%	Balance, speech, vision, and hearing slightly impaired. Feelings of euphoria. Increased loss of motor coordination.
4	.11–.12%	Coordination and balance becoming difficult. Distinct impairment of mental faculties, judgment, etc.
5	.14–.15%	Major impairment of mental and physical control. Slurred speech, blurred vision, lack of motor skill. Legal intoxication in all states (.15%).
7	.20%	Loss of motor control—must have assistance in moving about. Mental confusion.
10	.30%	Severe intoxication. Minimum conscious control of mind and body.
14	.40%	Unconsciousness, threshold of coma.
17	.50%	Deep coma.
20	.60%	Death from respiratory failure.

*For each one-hour time lapse, subtract .015% blood alcohol concentration, or approximately one drink.
†One drink = one beer (4.0% alcohol, 12 oz.) or one highball (1 oz. whiskey, 4 oz. ginger ale).

Source: Adapted from Daniel A. Girdano and Dorothy D. Girdano, *Drug Education: Content and Methods,* 2nd ed. (Reading, Mass.: Addison-Wesley, 1976), Table 3.2. © 1976. Reprinted with permission.

The Costs of Alcohol

Alcohol is big business, one that clears about $11 billion a year. It is also a big source of tax money for governments—about $5 billion a year, in all.

The misuse of alcohol also produces some big figures: its toll in 1975 was $43 billion, according to the National Institute on Alcohol Abuse and Alcoholism (NIAAA). This cost included $19.64 billion in lost production of goods and services, as well as $17.97 billion spent for the goods and services needed to deal with the results of alcohol misuse. Those included health care, police protection, and social welfare payments. Then, in 1977, motor vehicle accidents caused by drunk drivers cost $5.14 billion.

According to one estimate about half of the arrests made in the United States have some connection with alcohol.

Human Costs of Alcohol Use.   Not only is the cost of alcohol counted in days lost from work, health care, and money spent, but it is also counted in human costs. Data from the National Institute on Alcohol Abuse and Alcoholism shows that in 1975, drinking was indirectly involved in between 30 and 50 percent of all motor vehicle deaths; 44 percent of deaths from falls; 52 percent of deaths from fire; and 11 percent of deaths in other accidents. Alcohol use was also indirectly involved in 49 to 70 percent of all homicides and in up to 80 percent of all suicides.

The Rise, Fall, and Rise of Drink

Alcohol was used and misused in all those countries from which men and women came to people the United States. The history of alcohol use in this country began in 1607, when the first settlers in what is now Virginia arrived bearing (among other things) distilled spirits. America's history of alcohol control began only 12 years later, when the first law against drunkenness was passed.

By the 19th century, the goal of the temperance (antialcohol) movement had shifted from moderate use to non-use (abstinence). In the mid-19th century, Maine and 13 other states tried to prohibit the use or sale of alcohol. They failed in their state-wide efforts, but in 1919 they got what they wanted: an amendment to the Constitution (the 18th) to prohibit the possession and sale of alcohol. However, the 18th Amendment ushered in the chaotic and violent era known as Prohibition.

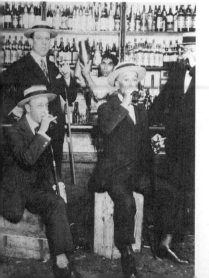

A "speakeasy."

The Bettmann Archive, Inc.

Prohibition.   The "Drys" could not know how hard it would be to enforce Prohibition. Boats and trucks were loaded with "bootleg" liquor from abroad, while uncounted millions of gallons of black-market booze were turned out in this country. The police counted 32,000 "speakeasies"—places where liquor was sold—in New York City alone. Instead of changing or ending the country's drinking habits, Prohibition gave birth to a multitude of large-scale criminal gangs that supplied drinks to a more and more thirsty nation.

After 13 years, it was seen that Prohibition had failed and in 1933 it was brought to an end. Today, while many state and local laws seek to end public drunkenness, disorderly conduct, drinking in public, and driving while drunk, the use of alcohol remains, for the most part, uncontrolled for adults.

Kinds of Drinkers

Prohibition's failure to end the use, misuse, and abuse of alcohol points up how popular alcohol is and the many reasons for this: It can reduce restraint and lessen stress, and people like its taste. Drinkers drink at different times and for different reasons—and in different amounts. They even behave in different ways. *Light drinkers* drink only for medicinal purposes or, in moderation, during social events. *Moderate drinkers* drink to relax and be sociable at parties and at other social events. They may also believe (as many do) that beer and wine enhance the taste of food. Their drinking is always under control. By contrast, *heavy drinkers* drink in large amounts, daily, or whenever possible. Unlike moderate drinkers, they drink to relieve tension, anxiety, and self-doubt, not just to break the ice. They manage to fulfill their duties to job and family, but they are ever more dependent on alcohol to dull feelings of inferiority, frustration, or failure. Heavy drinkers are problem drinkers. They have trouble limiting their intake and controlling their behavior while drinking. Some, but not all, become *alcoholics*. An alcoholic has regular or periodic "drunks" and can no longer control the use of alcohol. Alcoholics most often want to be continually drunk because they are always deeply troubled by or dissatisfied with their families, jobs, or schools. To say the same thing in a different way, their self-images are defective. Ultimately the cells of their bodies become dependent on alcohol for fuel. They are addicted. Alcoholism is a serious disease—and an addiction that only medical treatment can reverse.

Alcohol Abuse

The number of Americans who are heavy drinkers is on the increase. Just how bad is the problem?

In an effort to answer that question, the National Institute on Alcohol Abuse and Alcoholism did a survey in 1979. The NIAAA concluded that about 10 million Americans—or 7 percent of those over the age of 18—have a serious drinking problem, and that many are truly addicted to alcohol. An even larger number of drinkers have less serious symptoms of alcohol dependency—like gulping or sneaking drinks, trouble in stopping, drinking in the morning or drinking to get rid of a hangover, and loss of memory. Such symptoms are on the increase in both sexes and are quite high for men—20 percent of drinkers—compared with 10 percent for women.

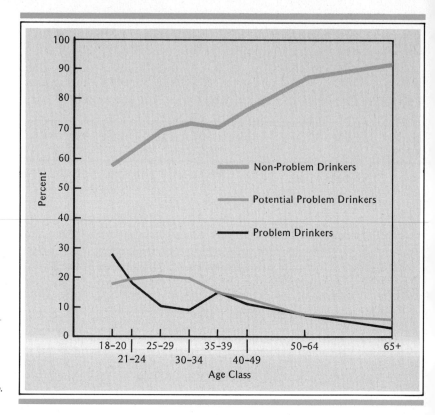

Figure 5–2. Drinkers, Problem Drinkers, and Potential Problem Drinkers.

Source: U.S. Department of HEW, Alcohol and Health. Rockville, Md.: Public Health Service, 1974, p. 27.

Dynamics of Alcohol Dependence

For most problem drinkers, dependence on alcohol develops gradually, going through a series of well-defined stages, each with specific symptoms and changes in behavior.

Warning.   At the outset, someone who is heading toward a drinking problem simply uses alcohol to relieve stress, tensions, or frustrations, as many people do. The relief expressed by "Thank God it's Friday," may be pursued all week.

At this warning stage, the use of alcohol becomes frequent, then regular, and then daily. The drinker may enter a sort of "drinking culture," a circle of friends who are heavy drinkers. But the drinker still manages to cope with the job, school, and family.

The warning stage may last for some time. From all outward appearances, the drinker still seems to be using alcohol in a social way, but may be using it more and more often.

Dependence.   After a while, the development of a tolerance for alcohol (see Chapter 4) forces the drinker to consume steadily increasing amounts to achieve the desired effect. Looking forward to the pleasant change of mood that will follow the first drink takes over the drinker's thoughts. The drinker's way of life is now shifting to fit in some daily drinking and, perhaps, some daily drunkenness as well—followed by some daily hangovers!

Rationalization.   The drinker must now devote much mental energy to the defense of drinking: "I have a tough job . . . big test . . . cold romance . . . crazy boss . . . boring life," or perhaps even "I only drink at the happy hour" or "I only drink beer and wine." The drinker's thoughts, in short, become filled with self, self-indulgence, and lies to support the drinking.

Since the drinker's mind is filled with the effort it takes to deny the alcohol dependency, the problems that led to it in the first place are ignored. Guilt over personal faults causes the drinker's self-image to plummet. Alcohol no longer produces a sense of ease; it is now required to stave off real depression.

Franklin Wing/Stock, Boston

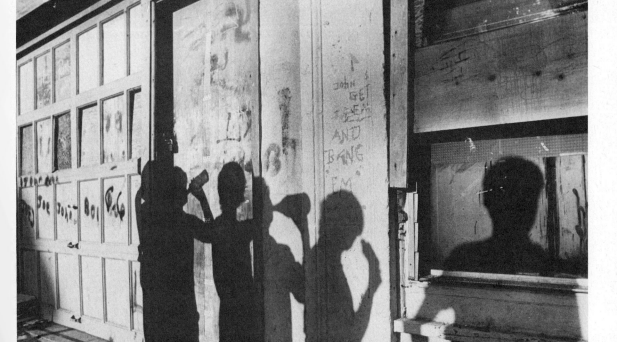

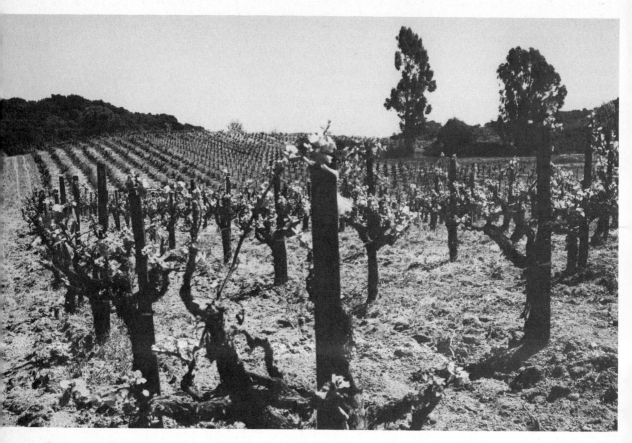

Grapes growing in a vineyard. They will later be picked, pressed into grape juice, and fermented into wine.

Dick Davis/Photo Researchers

Rigidity.   In the long run, the drinker's need for alcohol becomes so great that daily behavior centers on getting some and drinking it. Any break in the drinking routine provokes anxiety or hostility. Because the duties of a job, schoolwork, or a family interfere with these rigid routines, duties are abandoned. Money, human relations, and acceptance of authority (that of a boss, for instance) become real hassles. A student who reached this stage would probably have a long record of absences, incompletes, and failures and would likely be asked to leave school.

Alcoholism.   People who have lost control over drinking usually drink to the point where they are drunk. Drinking becomes less and less comfortable, more and more harmful to the drinker's physical health. But the drinking goes on, despite the physical discomfort that goes with it and follows it. The compulsion to drink gives way to an actual physical addiction. The drinker must now have alcohol, or withdrawal symptoms appear. The drinker is so dependent—physically dependent—on the drug that its sudden withdrawal can kill.

Why People Misuse Alcohol

The picture is not a pretty one, but people misuse alcohol anyway. Why? The search for the underlying causes of alcohol misuse has inspired three kinds of theories.

Physiological. One theory states that alcoholism results from a physical craving, a craving due (according to various theorists) to genetic predisposition (see Chapter 10), nutritional deficiencies, malfunctions of the glands, and allergic reactions.

While it is true that the rate of alcoholism may appear to be higher among some ethnic groups than others, this by itself does not suggest that genetic rather than social factors are to blame. Then too, the metabolic abnormalities often found among alcoholics are probably not solely responsible for the misuse of alcohol. Also, it cannot be proved that certain physical malfunctions point some people toward alcoholism.

Psychological. Many people use alcohol in some way to solve problems, yet very few who do so become dependent on it. All those who depend on it, though, use it to solve or to escape from problems, and they had poor self-images before they became alcoholics. That is why they drink their problems away instead of facing them. And alcoholism, of course, goes on to depress their self-images even more, so that they end up with no way to do something about their problems at all.

Sociological. There is good reason to think that social attitudes, values, and drinking customs are linked to rates of alcoholism. Alcoholism seems to be worst in cultures that regard drinking as pleasureful but sinful, those that reject problem drinkers and isolate them socially. Where drinking is taken for granted, as within the framework of the family, problem drinking tends to be avoided and rates of alcoholism are low.

Diseases Connected with Alcoholism

Alcohol pervades the body, and the more of it you drink the worse is the effect on your health. Heavy drinking can lead, for example, to cancer (see Chapter 10) of the tongue, mouth, esophagus, larynx, and liver. Smoking and drinking at the same time greatly increases the risk of mouth and throat cancer and cancer of the esophagus. Heavy drinking is also associated with *cardiomyopathy* (a disease of the heart muscle), and it increases the incidence (occurrence) of *coronary artery diseases* (see Chapter 10). Recent data, by the way, suggest that total abstainers run a slightly higher risk of coronary artery diseases than do light drinkers.

Cirrhosis of the Liver.   At least 95 percent of the incidence of this disease is related to alcohol use along with its resulting poor nutrition, states the NIAAA. Cirrhosis (scarring) of the liver is caused by the replacement of active liver cells by scar or connective tissue. Early signs of the disease include abdominal tenderness and weight loss. As the disease gets worse, severe jaundice may develop along with a wasting away of the body's flesh. As the liver becomes stiff, the blood does not circulate well, resulting in high blood pressure and bleeding within the digestive tract. Pressure from the enlarged liver may cause breaks in the blood vessels of the esophagus.

Alcohol and Pregnancy.   Recent studies show that a pregnant woman may endanger herself and her unborn child by drinking alcohol. The greater the amount of alcohol drunk by the mother, the greater becomes the risk to both. Mothers who drink suffer more miscarriages and difficult births than those who do not drink (see Chapter 13). Their infants are much more likely to have birth defects (of varying kinds and degrees) that stem from problems of fetal development.

Paul Conklin/Monkmeyer

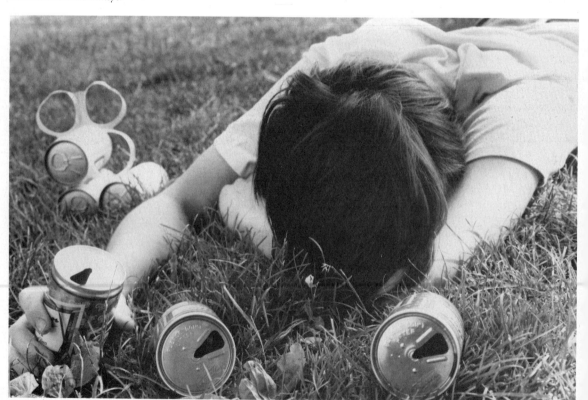

A serious problem goes with the use of alcohol by pregnant women. The *Fetal Alcohol Syndrome (FAS)* is a set of abnormal signs that appears in infants born to mothers who have used alcohol (generally heavily) during their pregnancies. These signs most frequently include smaller-than-normal size at birth, small head size, failure to grow normally after birth, a delay in mental development, poor coordination, and even mental deficiency. There are other minor problems in the face, joints, and genitals. Animal studies indicate that pregnant women who drink three ounces of alcohol—about six drinks—daily greatly increase the risk that their children will be born with FAS. The exact dose and the spacing of the doses are not known. A rule of thumb for expectant mothers is this: Do not drink at all during pregnancy and you will not have to be concerned at all about FAS.

The Impact of Alcoholism on Family Life

Alcoholism is sometimes called the family illness because it affects the whole family, and mainly the children. In 1974, about 27 million children lived in households in which at least one parent was an alcoholic.

The dynamics of the way a family relates to an alcoholic parent parallels the dynamics of the disease itself. In other words, the fabric of family life often unravels in roughly the same stages as the drinker does, since the drinker's spouse and children, too, are subject to the social and emotional stresses of the dependency.

First comes denial, as the members of the family try to convince themselves that no problem exists. They make excuses and cover up for the drinker. Then, after it is clear that alcohol is a real problem, the promises come, and the threats, and the lectures. The members of the family—even the children—believe themselves to be in some way a cause of the condition. Guilt and shame cut the whole family off from social events. Then, in many cases, the drinker admits defeat and the members of the family resign themselves to some very destructive behavior. Often, the family thinks that if it had loved the drinker more or better, then the problem might have been solved. The home may become tense and lose its sense of order; and this takes its toll on both the physical and the emotional health of all the other family members.

Reorganization/Recovery.   The choices that the family has are now hard to make. It may continue as a family by closing ranks and trying to keep the alcoholic out of its life. Or the other parent may decide to leave the alcoholic. (Far more husbands leave wives in these cases than the reverse.) Sometimes the breakup of the family (or the threat of a breakup) pushes the victim toward a treatment program—with or without the aid of other family members. Sometimes the family does break up, and the alcoholic may then go on to skid some more or, at the end, commit suicide.

Even if the person recovers and stops drinking, there may be no happy ending for the family. Families are fragile and some suffer such damage that once broken they stay broken. In fact, unless the other family members get treatment too, they may also bear emotional scars, and negative and self-destructive feelings, throughout their lives.

Among the long-term effects that alcoholic parents have on their children is the fact that 40 to 60 percent of these children become alcoholics too, bringing the legacy of alcohol misuse into a second generation—and, often, the child of an alcoholic marries an alcoholic!

Treatments for Alcoholism

There are almost as many treatments for alcoholism as there are reasons for its misuse in the first place. All the thousands of programs now in operation use one or more of a few basic techniques, however. These include the following:

- *Psychotherapy* deals with the attempts of problem drinkers to hide repressed feelings, like self-hatred, inadequacy, hostility, anxiety, and alienation.
- *Behavior modification* conditions the drinker's behavior through aversion therapy, making use of hypnosis or one of a number of drugs, including *disulfiram.* This drug works by producing severe symptoms of nausea in anyone who drinks alcohol within 12 hours of taking it.
- Biofeedback devices, exercise programs, and group therapy are also used to treat alcoholics.
- The best-known, and perhaps most successful, treatment program is run by Alcoholics Anonymous (AA). The heart of the AA technique consists of informal meetings, run by and for alcoholics. At these meetings (and by other means, as well), they work out and pinpoint problems and, perhaps for the first time in their lives, achieve status and prestige by devoting themselves to helping others remain sober. AA also helps the other family members through Alanon (for husbands and wives of drinkers) and Alateen (for children of drinkers).

Student Drinkers

Ours is a drinking culture. Most adults drink, and so do most teenagers, since it lets them feel "adult."

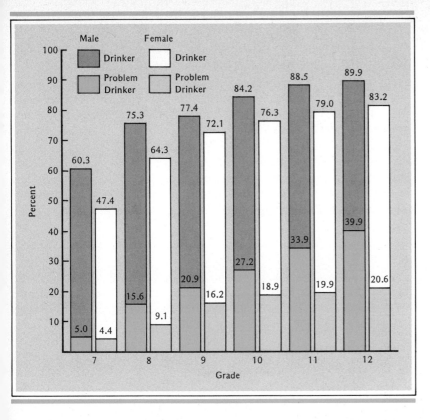

Figure 5–3. This 1978 report on young drinkers was based on answers given by people who are now college students or of college age.

Source: Ernest P. Noble, ed., Alcohol and Health: Third Special Report to the United States Congress *(Rockville, Md.: U.S. Public Health Service, June 1978), p. 24.*

Teenage Drinking. A 1980 survey conducted for the NIAAA found that 8 out of 10 high school students drank moderately to heavily.

Young people pick up most of their attitudes toward drinking from their parents and the other adults in their lives. Children of heavy drinkers are more likely to become problem drinkers, early on or later in life; children of regular or moderate drinkers also imitate their parents' behavior. Urban children, like urban adults, tend to drink more than do rural ones; and children from families of low social status drink more than the children of doctors, lawyers, and others with jobs that have prestige. Finally, young people who drink heavily seem to be less satisfied with themselves than young people are in general, and at the same time more removed from society and, indeed, from life.

College Students. You have probably seen with your own eyes that the great majority of college students drink—88 percent of them did in a 1979 survey.

Other highlights of the survey include: Most college drinkers (56 percent) had never or had rarely been drunk, but about 22 percent reported being drunk from 3 to 8 times a month, and 4 percent admitted being drunk even more regularly! Most college drinkers (60 percent) had never had a blackout from drinking, but 30 percent had. (Ten percent did not answer the question.) Since blackouts are regarded as a symptom of serious alcohol abuse, a third of college drinkers can be regarded as potential alcoholics.

An Epidemic among Students.   At the moment, problem drinking seems to be an epidemic among teens and young adults. A problem drinker in this age group is someone who drinks frequently, drinks to get drunk, and as a result gets into trouble at work or in school.

SELF-ASSESSMENT DEVICE 5-1: CHECK UP ON YOUR BOOZE USE

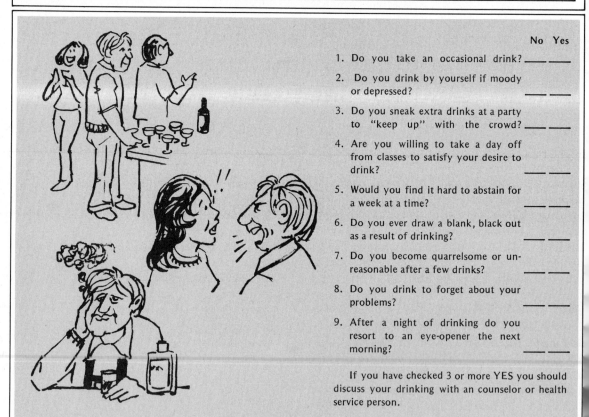

	No	Yes
1. Do you take an occasional drink?		
2. Do you drink by yourself if moody or depressed?		
3. Do you sneak extra drinks at a party to "keep up" with the crowd?		
4. Are you willing to take a day off from classes to satisfy your desire to drink?		
5. Would you find it hard to abstain for a week at a time?		
6. Do you ever draw a blank, black out as a result of drinking?		
7. Do you become quarrelsome or unreasonable after a few drinks?		
8. Do you drink to forget about your problems?		
9. After a night of drinking do you resort to an eye-opener the next morning?		

If you have checked 3 or more YES you should discuss your drinking with an counselor or health service person.

Source: Adapted from *Am I a Problem Drinker.* Commonwealth of Pennsylvania, Department of Health, Division of Behavioral Problems and Drug Control, Alcohol Studies and Rehabilitation Section.

Myths about Drinking

- I ONLY DRINK BEER. Beer has long been touted as the "beverage of moderation." But a 12-ounce can of beer packs the same punch as one ounce of 100-proof vodka, gin, rum, or whiskey. It's not what you drink that makes you drunk, but how much and how quickly you put it away.
- I CAN HOLD MY LIQUOR. You might think having a "hollow leg" is a social asset, but, in fact, developing a tolerance for alcohol is one sign of a dependence on it.
- I ALWAYS HAVE A CUP OF COFFEE BEFORE I HIT THE ROAD. Only time and the normal processes of the body can remove alcohol from your system. Coffee, cold showers, fresh air, and exercise will not sober you up, but a good long sleep will.
- I'M MORE FUN WHEN I'M DRUNK. But are your friends laughing with you or at you? Drunkenness is a form of overdosing, a quite serious condition. It should be avoided, not treated as funny.
- I FEEL UP WHEN I DRINK. Alcohol is not a stimulant but a depressant. The mild euphoria after one or two drinks quickly wears off, and then you start slowing down and getting numb.
- I'M A BETTER LOVER AFTER A FEW DRINKS. Ask your date or your mate. Alcohol may lessen your restraint, but too much drink usually leads to sleep, not sex.
- I'M FRIENDLIER WHEN I'M DRUNK. Maybe, but you may also end up feeling blue, hostile, homicidal, or suicidal, if these feelings are part of your life. Research has linked the use of alcohol to dangerous and criminal behavior.

What are the reasons for this epidemic of problem drinking among students? One reason might be that the nation's attention was focused on illicit drug use in the 1960s and 1970s, mainly on Heroin and marijuana. This let students regard alcohol as a better, legal, easy way to get high. Yet even at the height of the nation's obsession with illegal drugs, the drug used and misused most often, and with the greatest impact, was none other than alcohol. A second reason may be that as the number of adult problem drinkers climbs, so too does the number of young people exposed to them and influenced by them.

Responsible Drinking

Alcohol has somewhat different effects on different people, and different effects on the same people at different times. Since its effects cannot be predicted, the amount of it that can be drunk without harm cannot be set for all drinkers at all times. Responsible drinking is not a matter of setting fixed limits for maximum use; rather, it is an attitude.

To be responsible for something is to recognize that you yourself have some degree of control over it. Responsible drinkers do not say things like: "I didn't know the punch was loaded," or "My stomach was empty—that's why I got so bombed." You know that you are drinking responsibly if alcohol does not interfere with your duties.

Drinking Precautions

Think before you drink. You can reduce your chances of having a problem with drinking if you follow some simple rules:

1. Never drink on an empty stomach. Eat along with your drink.
2. Don't gulp your drinks. Take your time, pace yourself, enjoy the flavor.
3. At a party, talk, dance, eat, and join the fun to help pace your alcohol intake.
4. Don't drink before facing a demanding or unpleasant task.
5. Don't mix alcohol with *any* other drug.
6. Set a limit for drinking, and stick to it—a time limit or a number of drinks.
7. Don't be pressured into drinking if you don't want a drink.
8. Dilute distilled spirits (whiskey, rum, and gin, for example) with a mixer. Water or juice are better mixers than soda, so choose the best mixer for the drink.
9. Let someone else drive you home if booze is making you feel numb or spacy.
10. If you're giving a party, provide nibbling food, lots of mixers, and lots of ice to keep drinks cool and dilute. Arrange a place to sleep or a way to get home for friends who are too drunk to drive.

Bill Anderson/Monkmeyer

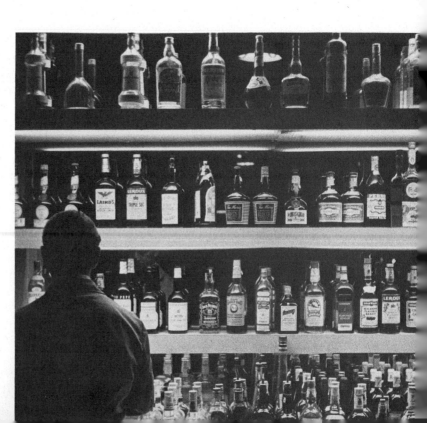

Recognize Irresponsible Drinking

You ought to know when you are not drinking responsibly—that is, when you are drinking so much that you cannot do all the things that need to get done. But just as alcohol sometimes interferes with getting things done, it likewise interferes with the way you recognize that you are not doing them. Here are some signs that you or your friends might have an alcohol problem:

1. Gulping drinks to get a quick effect—a pick up or to relax fast.
2. Drinking alone when bored, lonely, or frustrated.
3. Starting the day with a drink.
4. Overdosing often on alcohol (that is, getting drunk).
5. Losing friends as a result of drinking behavior.
6. Having blackouts (alcohol-induced amnesia).
7. Experiencing a sweeping personality change after drinking.
8. Drinking to relieve a hangover.
9. Rationalizing drinking behavior with a defense like, "I only drink beer" or "I only drink on weekends."
10. Needing medical help for minor accidents or the physical complaints that result from drinking—sprained ankles, scraped knees, body bruises, broken limbs, or the multiple problems that result from an auto wreck.

Barbara Alper/Stock, Boston

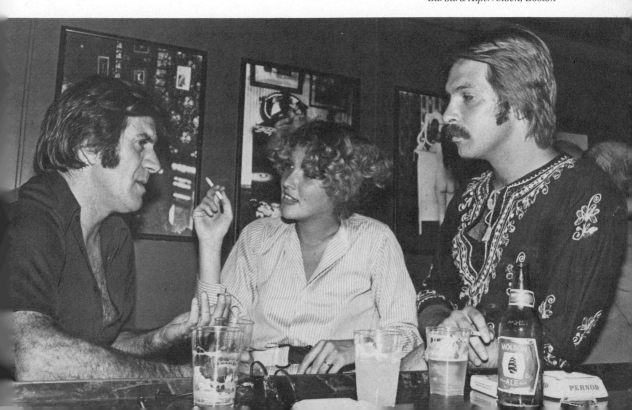

SUMMARY

Alcohol is a legal drug that enjoys widespread social respect in the United States. It is also the drug misused the most.

The majority of Americans drink, and many Americans drink too much. Alcohol misuse leads to mental and physical problems for the offspring of alcoholics as well as to mental illness and heart and liver diseases for the drinkers themselves.

People drink mainly because, like many other drugs, alcohol is thought to relieve stress. It can reduce anxiety and social restraint, so that people can be relaxed and sociable—perhaps, in some cases, even a little more human. This is not to be denied, but too much drinking can destroy these good effects. Knowledge of yourself and the drug you are using is the key to control. Thereby we can enjoy its benefits, while avoiding its dangers.

Suggested Readings

Chafetz, Morris E. "Alcohol and Alcoholism." *American Scientist* 67 (1979): 293–299. A general overview of alcohol abuse and the many research approaches toward effective treatment and prevention.

Dusek, Dorothy, and Girdano, Daniel A. *Drugs: A Factual Account,* 3rd ed. Reading, Mass. Addison-Wesley, 1980, pp. 36–70. Although most adults and teenagers have used alcohol and are familiar with its general effects, use alone does not give one a complete understanding of the drug. In this chapter a number of the common misconceptions and important considerations about the use of alcohol are offered.

Lavin, Thomas J., III, "The Alcohol Problem—More of the Same?" *Journal of the American College Health Association* 29 (1980): 96–99. In view of recent prevalence and other data on alcohol use by college students, this article considers whether alcohol represents a problem or a changeable problem for these students and/or their colleges.

Mendelson, Jack H., and Mello, Nancy K. eds. *The Diagnosis and Treatment of Alcoholism.* New York: McGraw-Hill, 1979. The knowledge that alcohol abuse exists when alcohol use leads to impairment of health and social functioning is the thesis of this work. It covers diagnosis, physical complications, genetic determinants, and treatments for the alcohol abuser.

Noel, Nora E., and Lisman, Stephen A. "Alcohol Consumption by College Women Following Exposure to Unsolvable Problems: Learned Helplessness or Stress-induced Drinking?" *Behavior Research and Therapy* 18 (1980): 429–440. The three experiments in this study were to examine the relationship between alcohol, depression, and learned helplessness. Specific questions were raised regarding the boundary conditions of learned helplessness, while factors bearing on stress-related alcohol use are discussed.

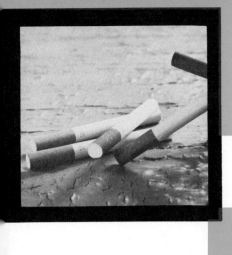

6

Tobacco

chapter objectives

When you have finished reading this chapter you should be able to:

1. Discuss the trends of smoking and of smokers in the United States
2. Understand the health hazards of smoking and be able to discuss the effect of tobacco smoke on the body
3. Offer practical advice to anyone who is trying to quit smoking
4. Discuss the federal government's policy of subsidy for the tobacco industry, along with hazard warnings to the consumer

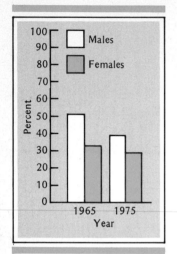

Figure 6–1.   Cigarette smoking has been on the decline since 1965.

Source: National Clearinghouse for Smoking and Health, *Adult Use of Tobacco—1975.* U.S. Public Health Service.

The tobacco plant.
Daniel S. Brody/Stock, Boston

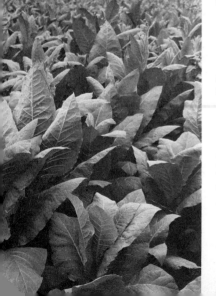

Bad habits can mean big business, as we have seen, and tobacco is one of the biggest businesses, formed from one of the worst habits. Tobacco is native to the New World and was used, in many ways and for many reasons, by the Indians of North, Central, and South America. Columbus brought tobacco use to Europe, and it soon spread to the Near East and Asia. As it caught on, tobacco growing became one of the most important businesses in Europe's New World colonies.

The dangers of tobacco smoking were noted soon after the habit's arrival in Europe (so many people took to using snuff). But in our country and most others, alcohol, not tobacco, roused the fury of reformers. The use of tobacco did not become an important public issue here until 1964, when the U.S. Surgeon General issued a report describing tobacco as a danger to health. A notice to that effect was then ordered to be placed on every pack, carton, and cigarette ad. The report persuaded millions of people to quit smoking. But not everyone—not by a long shot: Among people of college age, for instance, 34 percent were smoking in 1977. In fact, during the 1970s tobacco use among young people was on the increase, and mainly among girls.

Table 6–1.   Tobacco Products—Production and Consumption: 1960 to 1979

Item	Unit	1960	1965	1970	1972	1973	1974	1975	1976	1977	1978	1979
Production:												
Cigarettes.....	Billions ..	506	562	562	593	616	652	627	688	673	688	707
Cigars...........	Billions ..	6.9	8.9	8.0	8.0	11.4	8.7	8.3	6.7	5.8	5.6	5.1
Tobacco	Mil. lb	176	169	164	157	149	152	155	153	155	156	159
Per Capita Consumption:												
All products .	Lb...........	11.8	11.5	9.6	9.7	9.5	9.4	9.1	8.6	8.5	8.1	7.9
Cigarettes.....	1,000	4.2	4.3	4.0	4.0	4.1	4.1	4.1	4.1	4.1	4.0	3.9
Cigars...........	Number .	61	70	62	52	49	44	39	36	33	47	43
Tobacco	Lb...........	.99	.88	.83	.79	.75	.75	.72	.73	.70	.81	.79

Source: U.S. Bureau of the Census, *Statistical Abstract of the United States, 1980* (101s ed.), table 1458, p. 824.

The use of tobacco by girls is now leveling off; and the proportion of smokers in the total U.S. population is smaller now than it was in 1970. But our population has continued to grow and so has the number of cigarettes sold and consumed. Despite the heated debate over tobacco and its ill effects, its use remains, like alcohol's, a part of our culture.

Anatomy of a Habit

Why Do People Smoke?

A writer of social satire, Russell Baker, once noted that people smoke although the act itself—burning a stick under their noses—seems like a silly one. But many people do burn sticks under their noses. Why?

One reason is that each generation of smokers raises and shapes the next one. Teenagers whose parents or whose older brothers or sisters smoke are four times more likely to do so than are those with no smokers in their families. Cigarettes are available; they are sold almost everywhere, even in hospitals. Free packs are given away on street corners as a promotion gimmick. Although cigarettes are not supposed to be sold to minors, almost any child who tries can buy them—in shops or from vending machines. Social custom, too, tolerates smoking, whether in private or public places.

About 75 percent of all smokers pick up the habit before the age of 20. And for young people, mainly those in their teens, smoking is a form of rebellion. Sometimes, too, young people are trying to imitate someone special who smokes—a parent, a rock star, a movie star, a glamorous stranger, or even an older friend they see as a leader. They (and adults too) may start smoking because they think cigarettes look glamorous, witty and wise, sophisticated, tough, or liberated ("You've come a long way, baby!"). They may start smoking to help lose weight so that they may look even more like that idol.

Kinds of Smokers

Smoking satisfies a number of needs and supposed needs, and so people smoke for several reasons. Sometimes they smoke for only one of the reasons listed below—sometimes for more than one.

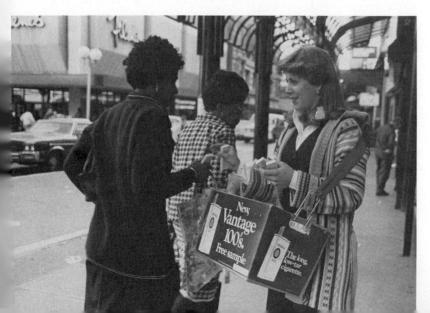

Barbara Alper/Stock, Boston

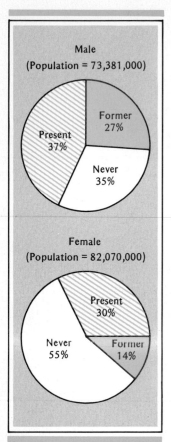

Male
(Population = 73,381,000)

Former
27%

Present
37%

Never
35%

Female
(Population = 82,070,000)

Present
30%

Never
55%

Former
14%

Figure 6–2.   Male and female smokers and nonsmokers, aged 17 and over.

Source: U.S. Bureau of the Census, *Statistical Abstract of The United States,* 1980 (101st ed.), table 209, p. 130.

Pleasure.   Over the ages, humans have searched for natural products that satisfy the senses—things to eat, drink, smoke, chew, swallow, and sniff. Tobacco is simply one among these, and cigarettes are one form of tobacco—people also smoke pipes, cigars, and cigarillos; they sniff snuff, and they chew tobacco, too. They even used to drink a brew made from tobacco leaves or ash.

People who smoke for pleasure may use cigarettes either as a stimulant or a relaxant. In the first group, many people get out of bed in the morning and light up to wake up. Then they drink their coffee to get the stimulant effect of caffeine. In the second group are people who use cigarettes as a relaxant, often in the first moments after dinner, for a work break, or while having a cocktail. Cigarette ads promote the notion of smoking with relaxing, by using photos that show smokers holding hands on a sunny beach or cuddled up next to roaring fires. Needless to say, many smokers just smoke all day—about once every 10 minutes—and for both reasons. In fact, the nicotine in smoke is a stimulant, not a relaxant.

Coping with Stress.   *Negative-affect smokers* smoke to relieve their negative feelings. We have all sat and talked with an upset or angry friend who chain-smokes and lights up end to end. We know people who have quit and who have then started up again because of some upset. These smokers are trying to reduce their feelings of anxiety, anger, and disappointment.

Habit.   Some smokers simply smoke out of force of habit, although they might have started smoking for pleasure or to relax. At times, they may smoke without even being aware of it. Habit smokers sometimes go to light up, not realizing that they already have a smoke in their mouths.

Addicted Smokers.   Have you ever had friends who had to have a smoke? Have you seen them scramble through their pockets, purses, or glove compartments desperate—in search of a "weed"?

These are the addicted smokers. In part, they are addicted because certain chemicals, or drugs, in cigarette smoke, like nicotine, are physically habit-forming. But there is also a strong mental aspect to cigarette addiction. Addicted smokers are always "aware" of a lack of cigarettes. They become anxious and think that only a smoke can help them. When they do get that smoke, the anxiety is relieved. Smoking cigarettes like this amounts to reinforced learning (see the section called Behaviorism in Chapter 1).

Reversing an addiction of this sort is harder than breaking any other kind of smoking habit.

SELF-ASSESSMENT DEVICE 6-1: WHAT KIND OF A SMOKER ARE YOU?

Here are statements made by some people to describe what they get out of cigarettes. How often do you feel this way when you are smoking them? (Circle one answer for each statement.)

	Always	Frequently	Occasionally	Seldom	Never
1. I smoke cigarettes to stimulate me, to perk myself up.	X	X	X	X	X
2. Part of the enjoyment of smoking a cigarette comes from the steps I take to light up.	X	X	X	X	X
3. I find cigarettes pleasurable	X	X	X	X	X
4. When I feel "blue" or want to take my mind off cares and worries, I smoke cigarettes	X	X	X	X	X
5. I am very much aware of the fact when I am not smoking a cigarette	X	X	X	X	X
6. I've found a cigarette in my mouth and didn't remember putting it there	X	X	X	X	X
7. I smoke cigarettes to give me a "lift"	X	X	X	X	X
8. Handling a cigarette is part of the enjoyment of smoking it	X	X	X	X	X
9. Smoking cigarettes is pleasant and relaxing	X	X	X	X	X
10. When I feel uncomfortable or upset about something, I light up a cigarette	X	X	X	X	X
11. I get a real gnawing hunger for a cigarette when I haven't smoked for a while	X	X	X	X	X
12. I smoke cigarettes automatically without even being aware of it	X	X	X	X	X
13. I light up a cigarette when I feel angry about something	X	X	X	X	X
14. When I have run out of cigarettes I find it almost unbearable until I get them	X	X	X	X	X
15. I light up a cigarette without realizing I still have one burning in the ashtray	X	X	X	X	X

Type:	Stimulation	Manipulation	Relaxation	Reduction of Negative Feelings	Pscyhological Addiction	Habituation
Items summed	1 + 7	2 + 8	3 + 9	4 + 10 + 13	5 + 11 + 14	6 + 12

Source: Edgar F. Borgatta and Robert Evans, eds., *Smoking, Health, and Behavior* (Chicago: Aldine, 1968), pp. 20-21.

Effects of Smoking

It is hard for some people to understand why simply drawing cigarette smoke into the body should be dangerous. After all, "It's just hot air, isn't it?" Or is it?

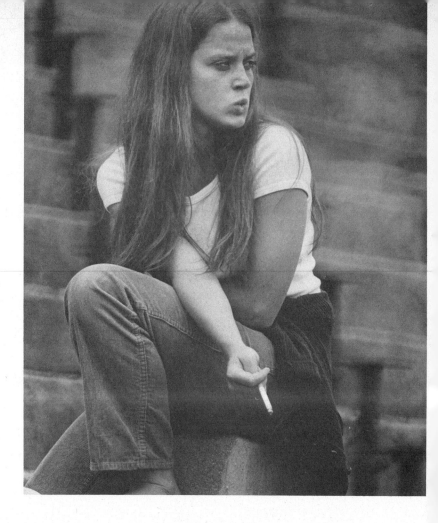

Ellis Herwig/Stock, Boston

The Strange Case of Sigmund Freud

The points made against smoking are very good ones. Yet they failed to move some of our most brilliant thinkers, among them Sigmund Freud.

Freud routinely smoked 20 cigars a day. When he developed heart problems, at the age of 38, his best friend and personal physician told him to quit. Freud tried many times, but found not smoking painful.

Freud then tried getting his habit down to one cigar a week, and finally stopped smoking for more than a year. But he could not endure the suffering and went back to cigars. He continued to smoke even after he developed mouth cancer. The initial cancer was cured, since Freud had no recurrence for 8 years. He continued to smoke. But over the next 16 years he underwent 33 operations for removal of cancerous jaw tissue. Still he continued to smoke. By then, his entire jaw had been removed. Still he continued to smoke. He suffered constant pain and had difficulty eating and swallowing. Still he continued to smoke. Freud died at age 83.

Why not find out for yourself. Take a clean handkerchief and blow cigarette smoke through it. *Warning*: This experiment will ruin it. And the tarry black substance that messes it up is evidence of the many harmful components in cigarette smoke.

What Is the Smoke?

What exactly are you doing to your body when you take a deep drag? Although you see nothing but a gray-blue cloud, you are taking in hundreds of separate components, of both gases and particles.

Gases.   Cigarette smoke contains many gases, but we can only discuss a few of them. One is *carbon monoxide,* a gas which makes it difficult for the red blood cells to absorb oxygen and, thus, reduces the body's supply of it. *Hydrogen cyanide,* a poisonous gas in the smoke, is one of the reasons why a hacking cough often develops.

Particulates.   Besides gases, the smoke also contains liquid substances called *particulates.* One of them, *nicotine,* is thought to be the chief cause of physical dependence as well as the cause of tobacco's stimulant effect. Nicotine constricts the blood vessels and raises the blood pressure; it also triggers some other diseases that are often found in smokers. *Tar,* another of the particulates in the smoke, contains all the particulate matter plus the material condensed from the gases. As the cigarette is smoked, tar is formed by the burning of tobacco dust. The tar, rich in hydrocarbons, is the primary cancer-causing (carcinogenic) agent in the smoke.

Diseases Associated with Smoking

Since 1964 hundreds of studies have been made to confirm that inhaled tobacco smoke causes lung cancer. The conclusion is that smokers do have ten times more lung cancer than nonsmokers do. This does not really prove that smoking *causes* lung cancer, but since those first studies many researchers have become convinced that smoking and lung cancer *are* causally (and not just statistically) related. As for other kinds of cancer, cigarette smoking has been statistically linked with cancer of the gastro-intestinal system and cancer of the urinary tract.

Respiratory Diseases.   Many substances in cigarette smoke deplete the body's oxygen supply. Others cause many smokers to cough through the day. One of the diseases of the respiratory system that goes with smoking is *emphysema,* in which the air sacs in the lungs break as the tissues lose elasticity. This eventually makes its victims depend on oxygen tanks. Chronic bronchitis, a disease in which the bronchi are blocked with mucous, is also found in cigarette smokers.

Cigarette smoke alters the action of drugs in a few ways. Smoke sometimes increases the harmful effects of a drug. For instance, women who take birth control pills run a higher than normal risk of heart attack, as do women who smoke. Women who both smoke and also take birth control pills have heart attacks at a rate much higher than the "smoker rate" and "pill taker rate" *combined.*

Tobacco smoke may also hasten the rate at which the body metabolizes a drug (see Chapters 4 and 8), so that smokers come to think they need greater doses or doses more often, when in fact they need to stop smoking. For instance, nicotine and other factors in the smoke speed up the body's use of Darvon, a common painkiller.

The problem of combining tobacco smoke with drugs is compounded by the fact that smokers use far more drugs than do nonsmokers. Smoking, too, is often part and parcel of an unhealthy lifestyle that includes high stress, the use of drugs, and little exercise.

Cardiovascular Diseases. When cigarette smoking depletes the supply of oxygen in the blood and constricts the small arteries, the brain signals the heart to pump more quickly, to try to get more oxygen into the system. The heart does so, and this raises the level of pressure in the blood vessels (see Chapter 10), which can itself be a serious health problem. Smoking also seems to encourage the buildup of plaque on the walls of the arteries; this, in turn, causes blockage that often results in heart attacks and strokes (see Chapter 10).

Figure 6–3. The effect of smoking on the lining of the bronchial tubes.

Source: Adapted from U.S. Department of Health, Education, and Welfare, *Progress against Cancer 1970,* p. 48.

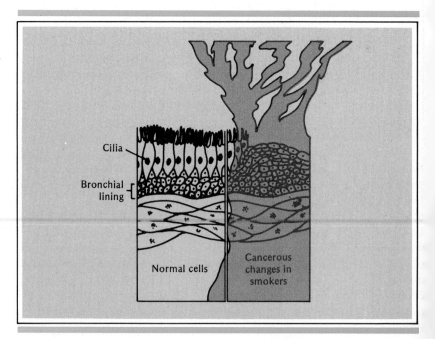

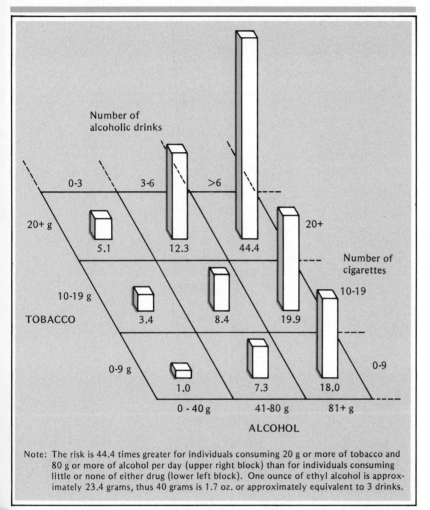

Number of
alcoholic drinks

0-3   3-6   >6

20+ g   20+

5.1   12.3   44.4

Number of
cigarettes

10-19 g   10-19

TOBACCO   3.4   8.4   19.9

0-9 g   0-9

1.0   7.3   18.0

0 - 40 g   41-80 g   81+ g

ALCOHOL

Note: The risk is 44.4 times greater for individuals consuming 20 g or more of tobacco and
80 g or more of alcohol per day (upper right block) than for individuals consuming
little or none of either drug (lower left block). One ounce of ethyl alcohol is approximately 23.4 grams, thus 40 grams is 1.7 oz. or approximately equivalent to 3 drinks.

Figure 6-4. Relative risks of
esophageal cancer in relation
to the daily consumption of
alcohol and tobacco.
Source: Third Special Report to the
U.S. Congress on Alcohol and
Health. *Secretary of HEW, Government Printing Office, June 1978.*

Smoking during Pregnancy. Women who smoke while they are
pregnant expose their unborn children to many dangers. For starters,
heavy smoking during this time raises the risk of a miscarriage or a
stillbirth (see Chapter 13) by at least 30 percent. If the infant is indeed
born, and born alive, it will probably weigh less than it would have
weighed if the mother had not smoked. Records show that by 11 years
of age, children of mothers who smoked during pregnancy are, on the
average, smaller than those of nonsmoking mothers. In fact, the children of *fathers* who smoke more than 10 cigarettes a day are more
prone to death in infancy than those of nonsmoking fathers. Also, more
hyperactive children are born in families were the mother smoked a

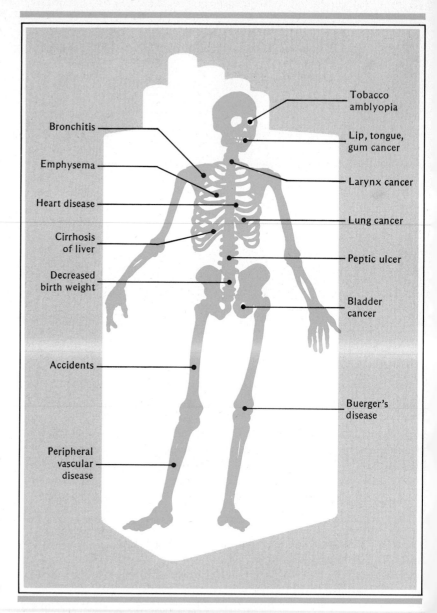

Bronchitis

Emphysema

Heart disease

Cirrhosis
of liver

Decreased
birth weight

Accidents

Peripheral
vascular
disease

Tobacco
amblyopia

Lip, tongue,
gum cancer

Larynx cancer

Lung cancer

Peptic ulcer

Bladder
cancer

Buerger's
disease

Figure 6–5. Many diseases and conditions go with smoking. Only some are causally related. Accident rates are higher for smokers than nonsmokers; this includes fires in the home caused by the smoker.

Source: National Clearinghouse for Smoking and Health, *Adult Use of Tobacco—1975.* U.S. Public Health Service.

good deal during pregnancy. (The cause of this relationship is not yet explained, but the relationship is clear.)

Newborn infants and growing children exposed to cigarette smoke are more likely than other children to suffer from health problems, mainly in the respiratory tract. Finally, parents who smoke often pass along the habit to their children, who are twice as likely to smoke than the children of nonsmokers.

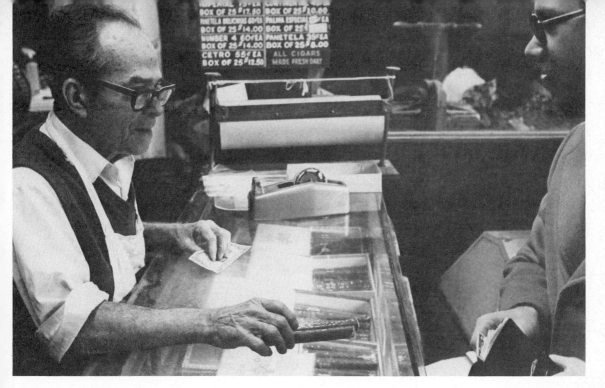

Pipes and Cigars

So far we have mostly been looking at the dangers of cigarette smoke, since cigarettes are now the most often sold form of tobacco. They are followed by pipes and cigars, and these too are dangerous to your health. In fact, the tobacco used in pipes and cigars contains *higher* levels of cancer-causing agents than cigarettes do. And the hot smoke of pipes and cigars, as it lingers in the mouth, promotes cancer of the mouth, lips, throat, and stomach.

The big difference between smoking cigarettes as opposed to other tobacco products is that cigarette smoke is inhaled, while the smoke of the other tobacco products is not. They therefore expose the lungs less to the gases and particles, since the smoke was not inhaled. But cigarette smokers who switch to pipes and cigars often keep the habit—they inhale—and this *increases* their chances of serious heart and lung disease.

Quitting

There are many ways to quit smoking. But they all suffer from a common defect: motivation. Smokers can only quit if they want to quit. They have to quit for themselves, not for others. They have to believe—in their hearts, not just in their minds—that they have a personal stake in quitting. Finally, they must believe that they have the power to quit.

And they *do* have the power to quit; *millions* of people have done so.

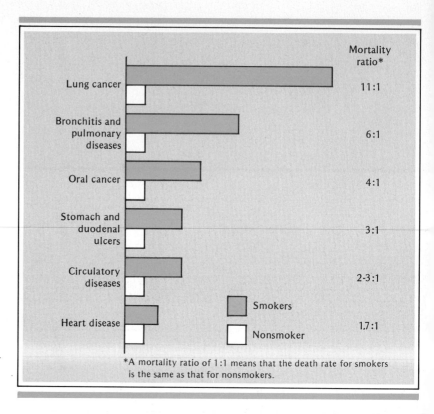

Figure 6-6. Death ratio of smokers to nonsmokers for selected diseases.

Source: Adapted from U.S. Department of Health, Education, and Welfare, *Progress against Cancer 1970*, p. 41.

Why Quit?

The most obvious reason to quit smoking—although many people ignore it—is one's health, pure and simple. Cigarettes are destructive to your health; and that message is constantly spread in newspapers, on billboards and posters, and on radio and TV, by family, friends, and fellow students and workers, and wherever cigarettes are shown or sold—*"Warning: The Surgeon General Has Determined That Smoking Is Harmful To Your Health."*

Yet concern for your health is not the only reason to quit. Pregnant women often quit because they are afraid—and quite rightly—that their smoking will damage the health of their unborn children. Others quit to set an example—like parents who would not like to see their children smoking or doctors who want their patients to stop. Some smokers quit because smoking is costly (at 75¢ a pack, it costs $273.75 a year to buy a pack a day, $547.50 to buy two packs a day). Some are tired of being reminded that many people find their habit offensive, awful, even loathsome. One antismoking ad points out that for a nonsmoker kissing a

Quitting is easy. I've done it a hundred times—Mark Twain (a cigar smoker).

smoker is like kissing a tray full of butts. On the positive side, many people quit smoking to restore their sense of smell or taste. Finally, certain smokers are more frightened by their lack of control over their habit than by the threat of disease or death. These smokers quit simply to prove to themselves that they can.

A fire at one end, a fool at the other, and a bit of tobacco in-between—Anon.

How to Quit

Like smoking itself, quitting is a process that takes some time, not a one-moment-in-a-lifetime event. Like smoking, quitting has to be worked into the normal pattern of life. And although some people simply make a resolve not to smoke any more and then stick to it, others find that they have to approach quitting bit by bit, just as they built up their cigarette habits. What follows are step-by-step bits of advice for quitters. They are suggestions, not rules.

Before you quit. Pick a target date for quitting, one that is important to you, like your birthday. Mark the day in red on all your calendars, and let nothing change it.

Start getting into shape a few weeks before the target date. Drink at least eight glasses a day of liquids, get plenty of rest, and avoid as much stress as you can.

Reduce the number of cigarettes you smoke day by day. Try to smoke only half of each cigarette. Each day, try to postpone lighting up your first smoke by one hour. Set a daily limit.

Don't carry any extra packs in your pockets or handbags. If you go to school or work, leave your extra pack at home. If you are at home, put it in a hard-to-reach place.

Don't smoke for the sake of smoking. Smoke only when you really want to.

The Day You Quit. Is this the long-awaited day of liberation? Throw away your cigarettes, matches, lighters, and ashtrays; you are now forever free of them. Visit the dentist and have the tobacco stains cleaned from your teeth. Above all, indulge yourself. Buy yourself a record or a pair of jogging shoes, go to the movies, visit a friend. Fool around. Celebrate your liberation from smoking throughout the whole day.

After You Quit. Spend time in places like theaters or libraries where smoking is not allowed. Drink lots of fluids—juices, mineral water, tea—up to eight glasses a day. If you long to hold a cigarette in your hand, play with something else: Worry beads, pencils, and rosary beads are quite effective. If you miss the feeling of a cigarette in your mouth, try chewing gum or a plastic cigarette holder. If you miss lighting up, carry a pack of matches and light one as you feel the need.

When You Get the "Crazies." Keep raisins, carrots, apples, nuts, and gum handy. Try taking deep breaths. Imitate inhaling. Above all, don't light up "just one."

Marking Progress. Make a 90-day calendar; as you progress, cross off each day. Add up how much money you have saved to date. Spend the money you have saved on something very special.

Gaining Weight. Most people who quit do not gain weight. Besides, you would have to gain upwards of 75 pounds to offset the health benefits of quitting. Still, some people who quit do gain weight, so weigh yourself carefully each day, exercise each day, and stock up on low-calorie drinks and snacks. Be sure not to substitute food for tobacco; food tastes good and if you gain weight you may use this as an excuse to go back to smoking.

If You Are Not Ready to Quit. Quitting is hard. Many people want to bring their habits under control but are not ready to quit. Here are some things you can do to reduce the risks of smoking while you are building up the resolve to quit.

Mimi Forsyth / Monkmeyer

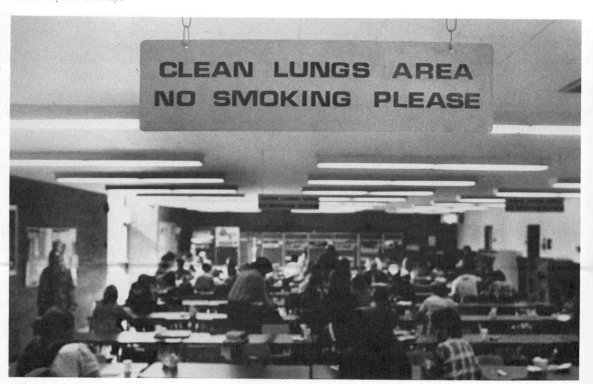

"Safer" Cigarettes. Cigarettes that are rated low in tar and nicotine are less harmful than the others, since these substances are carcinogens. Filter-tipped cigarettes filter out some of the carcinogens, so they somewhat reduce the dangers of smoking. But not all filter-tipped cigarettes are low in tar and nicotine, and some filters are not effective. You must therefore do some research to find out which are the "safest" brands. Remember, by the way, that the benefits of smoking a "safer" cigarette are lost if you smoke more of them than you did of your other brand—as many smokers report doing.

Pipes and Cigars. Most of the damage from cigarettes comes from inhaling the smoke, so there is some benefit from smoking "little cigars" (the size of cigarettes but made from cigar tobacco), cigars, or pipes, at least if you do not inhale the smoke. But if you do inhale pipe or cigar smoke, the risks become greater than when you inhaled cigarette smoke.

Changes in Smoking Patterns. Take fewer puffs. Smoke only the first half of a cigarette. Switch to a pipe or cigars. All lessen the dangers of smoking.

Smoking and Society

In the 19th century and in the early part of the 20th, the movement to end the use of alcohol played an important role in U.S. politics. Alcohol was prohibited, but only by law; the people who wanted it went on using it. After the end of Prohibition, in 1933, the trend was toward *less* regulation of the respectable drugs—alcohol and tobacco—not more.

Then, in 1964, the government (through the Surgeon General's Report on Smoking) declared that tobacco was a danger to health. The first product of that report was the message printed on each pack of cigarettes, warning of smoking's dangers. Soon, however, it began to appear that those dangers were not limited to the smokers themselves. In 1972 the American College of Chest Physicians stated that *second-hand* smoke (first inhaled, then exhaled) is harmful to nonsmokers who breathe it in. A 14-year study done in Japan shows that nonsmoking wives of men who smoke are twice as likely to die of lung cancer as the nonsmoking wives of nonsmokers. Those and later findings have led many people to fight for laws that restrict the right to smoke in public and enclosed places. Some cities passed such laws, but they were and are contested and hard to enforce.

Smoking imposes financial as well as health costs on nonsmokers, because smokers have high rates of illness and death. The cost of those high rates is largely borne by all of us in the form of insurance and welfare payments. Also all of us pay the price for the many fires (over

Smoking and the Third World

Tobacco use has grown quickly in the Third World: in Africa, Asia, and Latin America. Label and ad restrictions are rare there, so tobacco firms now focus on the Third World, where smoking is thought to go with social status and industrial progress. Since tobacco firms "dump" substandard tobacco in this market, the cigarettes sold there may have as much as twice the cancer-causing agents of those sold elsewhere under the same brand name.

100,000 a year) that smokers start—the costs of insurance, repairs, large fire departments, and the replanting of the nation's forests and wilderness areas.

The Government's Role

The federal government now tries to discourage the sale of tobacco products in several ways: high taxes, health warnings, and restrictions in the way tobacco can be advertised. But it also subsidizes the farmers who grow tobacco. Let's examine the history of what seems to be a contradiction.

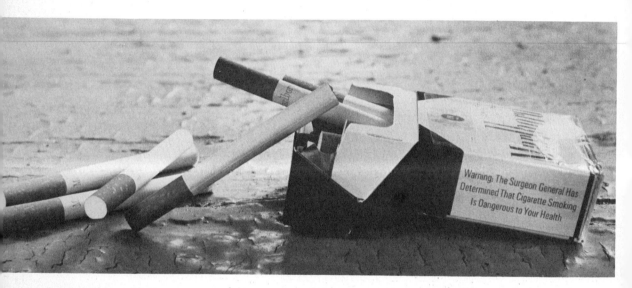

Richard Hutchings / Photo Researchers

The Surgeon General's 1964 Report. The medical profession's concern about the hazards of smoking is not new. Research on how tobacco affects health began in earnest in the late 1940s. Statistics showed a possible connection between smoking and lung and heart disease, and more and more evidence showing this was gathered over the years. But the government did not act on these findings. Then in 1964 the Surgeon General of the United States, a high-ranking government official, issued a report that stressed the dangers of smoking. The publication of this report was a milestone in the antismoking struggle. The first result was the warning label on cigarette packages and ads. Then, in 1971, cigarette ads were banned from TV.

Cigarette Advertising and the Law. The 1971 ban did not put an end to cigarette ads. In fact, today, most of the money—about $1 billion a year—now goes into magazines and newspapers. The huge profits of

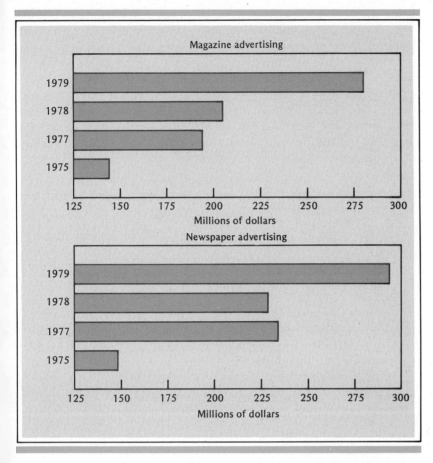

Magazine advertising

Newspaper advertising

Figure 6–7. Expenditures for national advertising for tobacco products and smoking materials (in millions of dollars).

Source: Adapted from U.S. Bureau of the Census, *Statistical Abstract of the United States, 1980* (101st ed.), tables 1023; 1024, p. 599.

the tobacco industry prevail over doubts about whether it is morally right to promote an unhealthy habit. Publications that carry ads indeed have a moral responsibility in this matter, and they are ignoring it.

Tobacco Subsidies.   The worst thing that anyone can say about the federal government and its policy toward tobacco ads is that not enough is done *against* smoking. But in one respect the government is *helping* the tobacco industry. In fact, the government is subsidizing it. This means that tax money is used to promote tobacco production in several ways: through a price-support program for tobacco (a program that requires the government to pay the difference if the price of tobacco falls below a certain minimum), also through crop inspection, grading, tobacco research (to develop a hardier leaf), export promotion, and market research. The opponents of smoking have tried to halt all those subsidies, and so far they have failed.

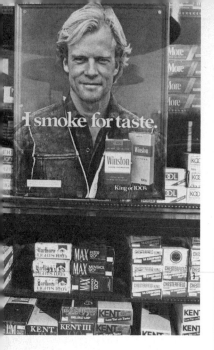

Barbara Alper/Stock, Boston

Ending the tobacco price-support program would not have much effect on the number of cigarettes that people smoke; and under some conditions, the end of the program might even allow tobacco firms to sell their products at a lower and, therefore, more attractive price. The tobacco price-support program involves an interesting sociological problem. Tobacco is one of the few crops still grown on small family farms. The end of price supports for tobacco would probably force many or most of these small farmers to change their crop or sell their lands. Supporters of this program claim that the subsidy is a part of the price that Americans have to pay in order to keep small family farms.

SUMMARY

The seeming contradiction in the actions taken by the federal government shows very well the conflict between the major forces of the debate over tobacco: industry, government officials, smokers, and nonsmokers. The tobacco industry gets huge subsidies from the federal government; government officials seek through regulation to protect the public from known hazards; smokers demand the right to buy and use tobacco; nonsmokers form groups to protect their rights. Despite the debate, tobacco remains socially acceptable. Its use is declining somewhat, but it still remains a part of our culture.

Tobacco is a danger to health mainly because inhaling the smoke damages the respiratory and circulatory systems. Quitting is hard, but millions of people have done so. No one method of quitting is effective for all smokers; the approach must be tailored to the person.

Tobacco smoke is dangerous to nonsmokers as well as to smokers. More and more, nonsmokers are asserting their claim to smoke-free air. That claim is rejected by most smokers, but smoking is at last a political issue.

Suggested Readings

Cooreman, J., and Perdrizet, S. "Smoking in Teenagers: Some Psychological Aspects." *Adolescence* 15 (1980): 581–588. The object of this study, conducted among teenage smokers in France, was to determine what factors related school, family, and smoking habits.

Dusek, Dorothy, and Girdano, David A. *Drugs: A Factual Account*, 3rd ed. Reading, Mass. Addison-Wesley, 1980, pp. 136–154. The health hazards of smoking, the psychological and social forces for and against smoking, and the personal rights versus public safety debate are the issues of this chapter.

Haworth, J. C., et al. "Relation of Maternal Cigarette Smoking, Obesity, and Energy Consumption to Infant Size." *American Journal of Obstetrics and Gynecology* 138 (1980): 1185–1190. In this study birth weight and crown-heel length of offspring were related to maternal size (weight for height) and smoking habits. In all weight categories, infants of smokers were lighter and shorter than those of nonsmokers. Maternal obesity and cigarette smoking are independent of each other and maternal overweight does not protect the fetus against the growth-retarding effect of smoking.

Johnston-Early, Anita, et al. "Smoking Abstinence and Small Cell Lung Cancer Survival." *Journal of the American Medical Association* 244 (1980): 2175–2179. Continuation of smoking during the treatment of small cell lung cancer was associated with a poor prognosis; not continuing to smoke, even at diagnosis, may have beneficial effects for survival.

Physical Health

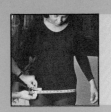

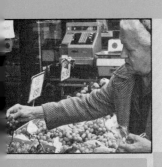

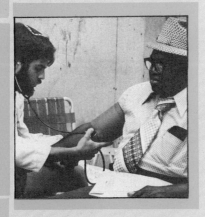

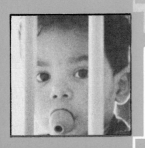

UNIT THREE

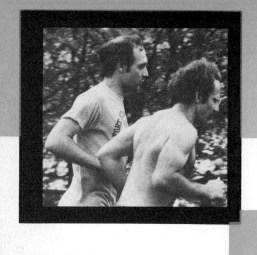

7

Exercise

chapter objectives:

When you have finished reading this chapter you should be able to:

1. Describe the advantages of exercise
2. Design a program that will build strength, cardiorespiratory fitness, flexibility, and muscular endurance
3. Discuss the principles of aerobics
4. Explain how exercise may aid weight reduction
5. Discuss how sleep and relaxation relate to personal fitness

Most of the games played today are ballgames, and most of these ballgames were invented at the same time and in the same place: 19th-century England. In the early part of that century students at many English public schools began to play games whose object was to push a ball past a goal. Since all these schools had invented their own games, there could be little competition among them. In the 1840s, representatives of many schools met at Cambridge University to devise common rules. As the century continued, two schools of thought emerged: the "kickers" and the "throwers." At Cambridge the kickers were in the majority, and they created the rules of the game now called soccer (or, in Europe, football). The throwers went off to another place, where they formulated the rules of Rugby, a game (still played today) that a few years later was modified by Americans into what we know as football.

Many other games were invented and formalized at about this time, including tennis and baseball. Why so many at one time? The answer is that these games answered a great human need that was no longer being met by work—the need for physical exertion. Before the 19th century, physical exertion could hardly be avoided, for until then there were few mechanical sources of power; physical exertion was a way of life. Until then, most people did not need more physical exertion in the form of games; they needed relief from back-breaking physical labor.

As machines came to do more and more of the work formerly done by human muscles, the need for substitute forms of physical activity became more and more acute. Games answered this need. But games are not always convenient, and their effect on the body, though good, is usually diffuse and short-term. Research showed that particular muscles and muscle groups could be worked out more efficiently through the use of certain bodily movements called exercises.

Advantages of Exercise

We have noted that the body needs physical exertion. But why? The answer is that when the body is used, its physical capacities are developed; when it is not used, those capacities waste away. Also, without physical exertion humans have a tendency to become fat. For the body to be "used," it needs energy. We get energy from food. Food, in other words, is our input, our source of energy. If there is not an equal energy output, in the form of physical exertion, the body must gain weight (see Chapter 9 for further details). Carrying around an excess weight of 20 pounds is like carrying around a knapsack of that weight. It tires you and puts greater stress on the heart and the circulatory system.

Food cannot be used in the body's cells without oxygen. The food and the oxygen have to be delivered to the cells, and the more efficiently they are delivered—by the heart and the lungs—the more efficiently the body works. There are many kinds of fitness, but the most important

Calories Used per Mile of Running

Weight (lbs.)	Pace Per Mile			Weight (lbs.)	Pace Per Mile		
	6:00 min.	8:00 min.	10:00 min.		6:00 min.	8:00 min.	10:00 min.
120	83	79	76	190	128	123	118
130	89	85	82	200	135	129	124
140	95	92	88	210	141	136	130
150	102	98	94	220	148	142	136
160	109	104	100				
170	115	111	106				
180	121	117	112				

Source: *The Aerobic Way* by Kenneth H. Cooper, M.D. © 1977 by the author and reprinted by permission of M. Evans & Co., Inc., New York.

kind is *cardiorespiratory fitness,* the fitness of the heart and lungs, on which all the body's systems rely for their supply of energy. Certain kinds of exercise, called *aerobics* (see below), are very good for simulating such fitness. These exercises increase the amount of oxygen that the lungs take in with each breath, and they make the heart muscle stronger, so that it pushes more oxygen and energy-rich blood to the

Rafael Macia/Photo Researchers

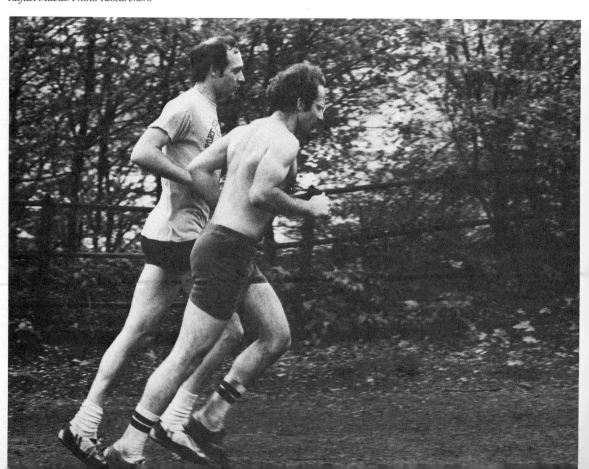

working tissues. Cardiorespiratory fitness gives you endurance, or "wind," the ability to work and play over a long period while resisting fatigue. That is why it is the key to fitness in general, and why most experts think that aerobic exercises are the most important of all. In addition, these exercises help prevent cardiorespiratory disease (see Chapter 10), today the chief cause of death in the United States. The fact that this disease now kills so many people reflects, in part, the lack of physical exertion that has become much of this country's way of life.

The benefits of exercise are not only physical. Exercise not only makes you feel better but also makes you feel better *about yourself,* and it reduces the effects of stress by helping you work out your anxieties. Modern research confirms these insights, but it did not discover them; even in ancient times, philosophers knew that a sound mind is more often than not perched atop a sound body.

The First Steps

Your body is unique—not only in structure, but also in its level of fitness—and that is why your exercise program should be designed just for you, not for humanity in general. First of all, that means finding out how fit you are right now. It also means deciding how fit you want to be, for although everyone ought to be fit, everyone does not have to be equally fit. Once you have fixed your goals you must embody them in a program of specific exercises and sports. The program should start at your present level of fitness, and it should become more and more demanding until you reach your goal.

Let us take a look at the different stages of putting together and starting up an exercise program.

Measuring Your Fitness

Like most other human attributes and qualities, fitness is not a single thing but the sum of many things, and you can be fit in one way without being fit in another. These different ways of being fit are called the "dimensions" of fitness. The most important of these dimensions are cardiorespiratory fitness, muscular strength, flexibility, and muscular endurance. Each of them can be measured in several ways, so the discussion below is not complete.

Cardiorespiratory Fitness.   The Kasch Test: We saw earlier that cardiorespiratory fitness, the fitness of the heart and lungs, is the most important kind. The Kasch Test is one standard way of measuring cardiorespiratory fitness. To take it, you need a bench or step 12 inches high (two 6-inch steps will do), a watch with a sweep hand, and a friend. There is one further requirement: Avoid physical exertion and tobacco for 2 hours before taking the test.

Table 7–1.   Fitness Level as Measured by Kasch Test

	18–26 years	
	Pulse Count for Men	*Pulse Count for Women*
Excellent	69–75	76–84
Good	76–83	85–94
Average	84–92	95–105
Fair	93–99	106–116
Poor	100–106	117–127

Now for the test itself. First, go up and down the stairs (or bench) for 3 minutes, at the rate of 24 times a minute. Each time you get to the top you must keep both feet there, and each time you get to the bottom you must do the same. After you have gone up and down for 3 minutes, sit down for 5 seconds without talking. Then take your pulse. You do this by placing your three middle fingers on the side of the opposite wrist, which is held palm up, and counting the throbs. (Do not use your thumb; it has a pulse of its own.) You can also take your pulse by placing the same three fingers on either side of the throat, just below the joint in the jaw. (By the way, it's a good idea to locate your pulse before taking the test.) To get a total, you can count your pulse for 30 seconds

Figure 7–1. The Kasch Test: try this test of your cardiorespiratory fitness—the fitness of your heart and lungs.

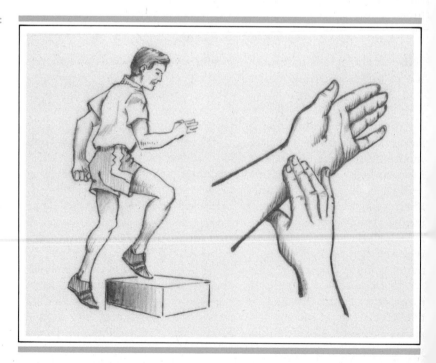

and multiply by two, or for 15 seconds and multiply by four. The significant figure is the number of pulse throbs each minute.

To find your level of cardiorespiratory fitness, by pulse count per minute, check the results against Table 7–1.

The Cooper Field Test: Another way of measuring cardiorespiratory fitness is called the Cooper Field Test. It is more vigorous than the Kasch Test, so do not try taking it unless you have been involved in a fitness program for at least 6 weeks.

The Cooper Field Test simply requires you to run or walk on a level surface for 12 minutes. Check the results against the table below (which is valid only for people under 30).

Table 7–2.   Fitness Level by Distance Covered in 12 Minutes

	Excellent	Good	Fair	Poor	Very Poor
Men	1.75 miles	1.50–1.74 miles	1.25–1.49 miles	1.0–1.24 miles	1.0 mile or less
Women	1.65 + miles	1.35–1.64 miles	1.15–1.34 miles	.95–1.14 miles	.95 mile or less

Since most college campuses have tracks, the Cooper Field Test should be a convenient way to measure your cardiorespiratory fitness. Most tracks are a quarter of a mile long, so you have to go around 4 times (or 4 laps) to complete 1 mile. On your first try, remember that the important thing is to do the laps; do not exhaust yourself.

Muscular Strength.   Muscular strength is the force exerted in one movement of a muscle. Since there are many muscles, there are many tests of muscular strength. To test the strength of the biceps of your arms, for example, you measure the amount of weight you can lift. But the most common test of muscular strength measures the force of the subject's grip, which correlates well with overall body strength. A dynamometer, an apparatus that measures force or power, may be available in the physical education department of your school.

Flexibility.   Flexibility is the range of motion that can be made by muscles and joints. Since there are many muscles and joints, there are many tests of flexibility. A useful one is called the "sitting toe touch," which measures the flexibility of the lower back and the back of the thigh.

The test is conducted as its name would suggest. Warm up by toe touches. (Lock knees, bend at the waist, and gently reach toward the toes as far as possible. Straighten up and repeat the bend-and-stretch in a slow rhythm.) Then sit on the floor with your legs straight out and your heels about 5 inches apart. Put a mark (with adhesive tape) at the

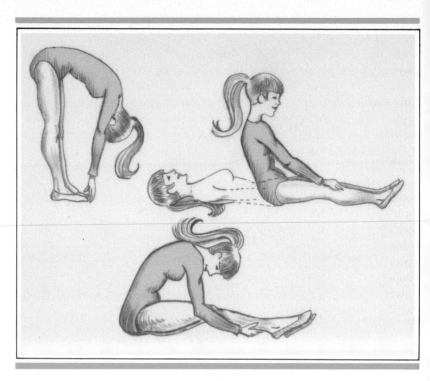

Figure 7–2. To test your flexibility, try the standing toe touch, the sit-up, and the sitting toe touch.

bottom of each heel. Then put a yardstick between your legs and parallel to them, so that the 15-inch mark touches the adhesive tape and the beginning of the yardstick points in the direction of your crotch. The idea of the test is to see how far along the yardstick you can touch your fingers without bending your knees.

Women tend to be more flexible than men and therefore do better on this test. A stretch no further than the 12-inch mark is poor for both men and women. A stretch to 22 inches is excellent for men, but women must stretch to least 24 inches to get that rating.

Muscular Endurance.   Muscular endurance is the ability to work for a long period of time before fatigue forces you to rest. It differs somewhat from general endurance, although the two are related. Muscular endurance refers to specific muscles or muscle groups that work for an extended period of time (as in arm wrestling). Local muscle endurance is reflected by the overall strength of the muscle and the blood vessels within it. General endurance is associated with the use of the whole body and involves many muscle groups (as in the butterfly stroke, in swimming). General endurance is the most important single measure of fitness, because it reflects the constitution of the cardiovascular and respiratory systems, and the general condition of the muscles.

One of the tests for muscular endurance is the familiar sit-up. Lie on your back and flex your knees. Have a friend hold your ankles, or slip your toes under some heavy furniture, to keep yourself from sliding around. Place your hands on your thighs and raise your head and shoulders from the floor, sliding your hands over your knees. Repeat until fatigue keeps you from sitting up. Count each sit-up as one. A poor level of fitness is fewer than 14 sit-ups for men and fewer than 12 for women. Fifty or more is an excellent score for both sexes.

Goals

If you have taken the tests just described, you ought to know how fit you are. Next question: How fit do you want to be? If you want to cut a figure on the beach, go disco dancing, and avoid heart disease, you can probably get by with 30 minutes of swimming or running, 5 times a week. Champion athletes have to do more—a lot more. The fitness programs in this book were designed to make you fit, but they will not get you into the final four at Wimbledon.

You must also decide what kind of fitness interests you. No single exercise is going to develop all the dimensions of fitness; you have to choose an exercise for each goal. Jogging and running, for example, are good for building up cardiorespiratory fitness, but they do little for the muscles of the upper body. Push-ups (see below) will do that but will do little for cardiovascular fitness.

Kinds of Exercise

We saw earlier that cardiorespiratory fitness is the most important kind of fitness because it develops the body's energy resources and helps prevent heart disease. Exercises that develop this kind of fitness have both immediate effects and effects that are slower in appearing. The immediate effects include an increase in the output of the heart; in blood levels of carbon dioxide, fatty acids, and cholesterol; and in blood flow back to the heart. Eventually, the size and strength of the heart increase, permitting it to pump more slowly yet provide more blood to the tissues. The heart can then rest longer between contractions, more blood flows through the heart, and it has a faster recovery rate, even from heavy workloads. A network of efficient small blood vessels (collateral vessels) is generated within the heart, and these small vessels deliver blood within the heart if larger ones shut down (as in the case of heart attack).

The immediate effects of exercise on the respiratory system are obvious: You breathe faster and deeper. In time the respiratory muscles become stronger, so that they allow an increased amount of air into the lungs with each breath. The number of blood vessels in the lungs also increases; this allows more oxygen to be absorbed faster, so that breathing becomes more efficient. Deeper, more efficient breathing means that less effort is needed; you save energy and recover rapidly from exertion. Muscles get oxygen more efficiently, so they contract with more force, and wastes are removed more rapidly from them. This, in turn, increases the efficiency and endurance of the muscles. The long-term effect of exercise is called the "training effect."

Not all exercises produce an equal training effect, and some exercises do not produce any training effect at all. The reason is that, although all exercises use up some oxygen, not all exercises require large amounts of oxygen over a sustained period of time. Exercises that *do* make such requirements, like swimming and jogging, increase the body's ability to take in and use oxygen and fuel. The building up of this capacity is the training effect.

Dr. Kenneth Cooper, who has studied the way that various exercises develop (and fail to develop) the training effect, divides them into four categories.

- *Isometrics:* Exercises that tense muscles but produce no movement and require little or no oxygen beyond what is consumed ordinarily—for example, pushing against a doorjamb.
- *Isotonics:* Exercises that tense muscles to produce movement but, like those in the first group, require little or no extra oxygen—for example, weight lifting.
- *Anaerobics:* Exercises that demand a lot of oxygen, but do not last long enough to produce a real training effect—for example, running the 100-yard dash.
- *Aerobics:* Exercises that demand a lot of oxygen and *do* last long enough to produce a training effect—for example, long-distance swimming and running.

Aerobic exercises are the most valuable of all for developing general fitness, that is, for achieving the training effect.

Isometrics

You can try an isometric right now by pulling up on your chair seat. In isometrics, one set of muscles is tensed against another or against an immovable object (like a chair when you are sitting on it). These exercises were first promoted by one Charles Atlas, who promised to turn 90-pound weaklings into "he-men" in 15 minutes a day. In the 1950s, some experts claimed that people could stay fit with just 60 seconds of isometrics each day and they became a fad. Research later showed that they can and do increase the size and strength of skeletal muscles (those in the arms, legs, and chest). But that is about all they can do: They produce little or no training effect, but they are convenient, can be

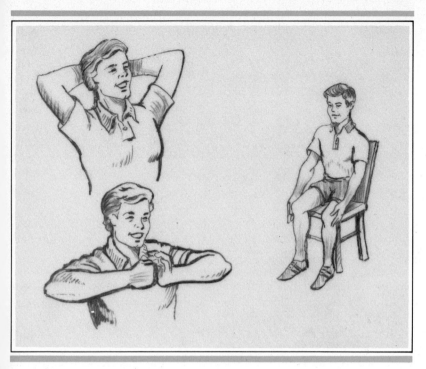

Figure 7–3. Isometrics: to increase the size and strength of your muscles, try these arm, shoulder, and chest presses.

done nearly any place and in any kind of clothing, and cause little fatigue or sweating. Before each exercise take a deep breath and hold it until the contraction is finished and then exhale. Each exercise must last 8 to 10 seconds.

One isometric exercise that makes the chest stronger is to clasp your hands on the back of your head and push backwards with the head while resisting with the hands.

An isometric that strengthens the arms and shoulders is placing the fist of one hand into the palm of the other, at shoulder level, with elbows extended. Press with the fist, while resisting with the other hand. Reverse hands and repeat.

An isometric for the arms is to sit in a chair and spread your knees about a foot apart. Then place your hands at the outsides of your knees. Press out with your knees while pushing in with your hands.

Isotonics

Isotonics are the exercises that we all do in school, in camp, and in exercise clubs, salons, and classes: push-ups, sit-ups, and leg lifts, for example. They strengthen selected muscle groups through *movement*, so they are better for fitness than isometrics; but they do not promote

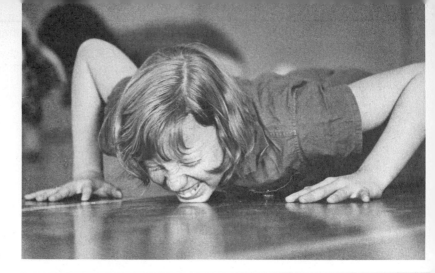

"Ugh!"
Richard Frear/Photo Researchers

the training effect very much, because they make little demand for extra oxygen.

The most popular kinds of isotonics are called calisthenics. We have already described one of these: the sit-up. Another is the push-up, which has versions for men and women. Push-ups strengthen the upper body—the arms and shoulders.

Figure 7–4. Isotonics: try some calisthenics, like the push-up or the trunk raise, to increase your muscle tone and flexibility.

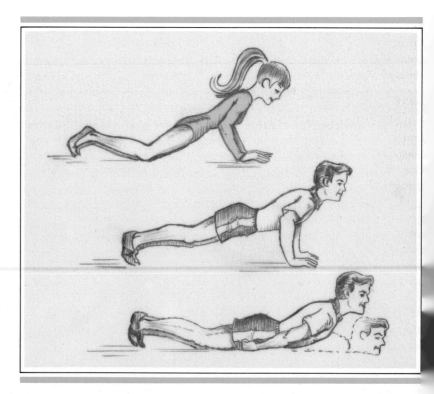

- Men: Lie on the floor with hands directly under the shoulder joints, facing down. Extend the arms to lift yourself fully from the floor, supporting your weight on your hands and toes. There should be a straight line between head and heels (no sag in the middle). Lower yourself until your chest just touches the floor or within an inch of it. Repeat in a slow rhythm (5-20 times).
- Women: The same as for men, except that the knees remain in contact with the floor throughout the exercise.

Here is an exercise that will help strengthen the lower back muscles and the abdominal ones—but if you have low back problems, do not do this exercise.

- Trunk Raise: Lie on the floor, face down, with hands under your thighs. Keep your legs together and straight. Keeping legs in contact with the floor, raise your head. At the same time, pull your shoulders back and lift your trunk as high as you can. Return to the starting position, then repeat in a slow rhythm (5–10 times).

Anaerobics

Isometrics and isotonics do not require much extra oxygen. Anaerobic exercises do—but still they do not produce a substantial training effect. These exercises—sprinting, or running very quickly, is typical—use up more oxygen than the body can take in during the exercise itself, creating an "oxygen debt." Waste products (lactic acids) accumulate in the muscles, and the exercise ends in sheer exhaustion.

Aerobics

In the 1940s young people swallowed goldfish. In the 1950s they crammed into telephone booths. Today they go jogging. And here, at least, times have changed for the better, for jogging is not only an exercise, but an *aerobic* exercise, the most useful kind. What does this mean?

You will remember that isometrics and isotonics demand little oxygen beyond what people commonly use. Anaerobic exercises require a lot of oxygen, but only for a short period; they require more oxygen than the body can supply, so they create an "oxygen debt." Aerobic exercises, like anaerobic ones, require extra oxygen. But because they are less vigorous, they require less oxygen at any one time. For this reason, they can be carried on for a long time, and they use (over the whole course of the exercise) a greater total amount of oxygen than any other form of exercise. There is no "oxygen debt": On the contrary, aerobic exercises produce the training effect.

The trick is to do the right kind of exercise for the right amount of time or, to put it another way, to do an exercise that is vigorous enough

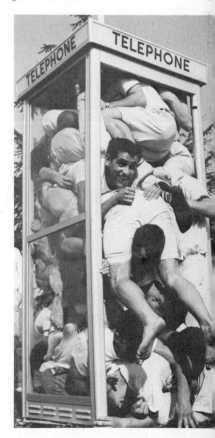
"Maybe we'd be better off swallowing a few goldfish!"
Joe Munroe/Photo Researchers

Today, jogging and running are very popular exercises among Americans. Below are some of the advantages of jogging and some suggestions should you decide to take it up.

Advantages:

- Dr. Cooper rates jogging as an excellent aerobic exercise. It greatly increases oxygen consumption and helps you to lose weight and release frustration.
- Thanks to Dr. Cooper and his point system, people can determine their needs and individualize their programs.
- It is cheap (although a good pair of shoes is necessary) and it is convenient: jogging can be done nearly anywhere, under nearly all conditions.
- It is popular—if you like to have a companion to jog with, start jogging and you will likely find one.

Precautions and Suggestions:

- "The stitch in the side"—caused by temporary interruption in the oxygen supply to the diaphragm and breathing muscles. If this happens just slow down and allow the oxygen to get moving again.
- Chest pain—a sharp pain in the chest is a signal to stop and rest. Get a medical checkup before starting exercise again.
- Shin splints—due to tearing of connective tissue from the shin bone. Often due to running on hard surfaces. Immediate care: sit down, and rotate and stretch the foot. When you resume, jog, and vary the terrain between dirt, grass, and hard surfaces.
- Cramps—due to temporary interruption of blood supply to muscles. Immediate care: stop, and stretch the muscles. You might try putting your index finger under your nose, then push in and up.
- Blisters—due to friction "burns" from shoes that do not fit or are not broken in. Blisters need to be cleaned with antiseptic solution if they have been broken; or they should be drained carefully, cleaned with an antiseptic, and covered with light gauze. Blister control: Tape gauze over areas of the foot that are irritated, or adjust the fit of your shoes with heavier socks to help prevent blisters from forming.

Suggestions:

- Get a *good pair of shoes* before you start. Many brands are available at a variety of costs (mostly high). Quality shoes will pay for themselves by helping to spare you from blisters, sore feet, and fallen arches, and knee and hip pain.
- *Heat and humidity* is a dangerous combination, causing a higher heart rate. In addition, cold showers taken to cool off can have a "shock" effect on the heart (especially for those who have a history of heart disease). The best shower temperature is about 70°F.
- *Neither alcohol nor cigarette smoking* mix well with exercise. Alcohol interferes with oxygen exchange in the tissues. Smoking causes increased airway resistance and interferes with the oxygen-carrying ability of red blood cells.
- Finally, *be reasonable* about your jogging program, vary it and do not think you must jog no matter what—getting upset about a broken routine defeats your purpose. Do not run if your feet are bloody or if shin splints are causing great pain. If your feet and knees ache after running, take up swimming or walking.

to require extra oxygen, but not vigorous enough to create "oxygen debt." The right kind of exercises (among others) are swimming, jogging, running, handball, and basketball. But what is the right amount of time? Dr. Cooper (whose work on the training effect has already been mentioned) says that, to be aerobic, an exercise has to produce a sustained heart rate of at least 150 beats a minute, and it has to be carried on (at this level) for at least 5 minutes. If an exercise demands extra oxygen, but produces a heart rate of fewer than 150 beats a minute, it has to be done for more than 5 minutes. How much longer depends on how much oxygen is consumed.

Cooper's Point System.   Since it would be difficult for most of us to make these calculations, Cooper devised what he calls a "point system," which tells you how to get the training effect. He believes that the best exercises for aerobic fitness are running and jogging, followed (in that order) by swimming, bicycling, walking, stationary running, handball, basketball, and squash. Cooper determined the amount of each activity that would produce the same training effect. Every time you do this

SELF-ASSESSMENT DEVICE 7-1: AEROBICS FOR YOUR HEALTH AND WELFARE

To help you decide whether aerobic exercise has any application to you personally from the physiological standpoint, here's a group of ten yes-no questions.

	Yes	No
1. My physician is satisfied with my weight.		
2. I have adequate control over my eating, smoking and drinking habits.		
3. I can run a few blocks or climb a few flights of stairs without becoming short of breath.		
4. My resting heart rate is usually in the efficient 55-to-70 beats per minute range. (As a test, sit and relax for five minutes, then check your pulse for a minute against a watch or clock with a second hand.)		
5. My doctor says my blood pressure is normal.		
6. My heredity gives me nothing to worry about in terms of heart or lung disease or diabetes.		
7. My blood vessels seem to be healthy enough—for example, I don't have a problem with varicose veins.		
8. I rarely have trouble with acid stomach, heartburn, indigestion and the like.		
9. I'm seldom if ever constipated.		
10. I have nice firm muscle tone—no flabs or sags.		

If your answer to any one of the above questions is "no," you ought to think seriously about an aerobics exercise program.

Source: From *Aerobics for Women* by Mildred Cooper and Kenneth H. Cooper, M.D. © 1972 by the authors and reprinted by permission of the publisher, M. Evans & Co., Inc.

888888888888888888888888888888888888

amount of exercise, in any activity, you get 5 points. A man should get 30 points a week (6 sessions), a woman 24 points.

Each of the following activities constitutes 1 exercise session and is worth 5 points:

- Running 1 mile in less than 8 minutes
- Swimming 600 yards in less than 15 minutes
- Bicycling 5 miles in less than 20 minutes
- Running in place for a total of 12½ minutes
- Playing handball for 35 minutes

Some words of caution: Do not try to achieve the full 24 or 30 points in the first week; work up to them over 6 weeks. Also, in the beginning you do not have to do the exercises nonstop; run a bit and then rest, then continue running and resting until you have covered the distance. Soon enough, you should be able to run a mile without stopping.

One of the advantages of Cooper's point system is that it lets you get your points in a variety of ways—by running, swimming, and bicycling, and by playing several games. Remember that if you mix your activities you are less likely to become bored.

A Way of Life

It may seem odd, but exercise, like smoking, can be dangerous for your health. If you know people who exercise a lot, you know that such people constantly talk about their injuries. It pays to avoid the strains and sprains that beset people who exercise, not only because these injuries are painful but also because they often force people to stop exercising. And to derive real benefits from exercise, you have to make it a way of life, not something you start one month and stop the next.

Warm-Up

The most common cause of athletic injuries is simply rushing right into exercise, without preparing for it. The way to avoid them is to prepare your muscles with "stretch exercises," and then to begin your workout slowly, so that your heart and lungs can adjust to the increased demands you are making on them. This slow increase of activity is called a warm-up. The amount of time that should be spent on the warm-up varies from person to person, but a good general rule is to spend 10 minutes. It takes longer to warm up on a cold day than on a warm one.

The main danger in starting up with vigorous exercises is the possibility of tearing or pulling a muscle, so stretching and flexibility exercises, which loosen the muscles, are very good for warming up.

Average Amount of Calories Expended for Various Activities

These are approximate average values for someone weighing 140–150 lbs. They include the energy needed for basal metabolism.

Activity			Calories Per: Hour	Half-hour	Minute
Sleeping (for comparison)			75	38	1.25
Recreation and Exercise					
Walking on Level	2.0	mph	180	90	3.00
	3.0	mph	260	130	4.33
	3.5	mph	300	150	5.00
	4.0	mph	350	175	5.83
	4.5	mph	480	240	8.00
	5.3	mph	620	310	10.33
Walking upstairs	1.0	mph	195	98	3.25
	2.0	mph	640	320	10.67
Walking downstairs	2.0	mph	215	108	3.58
Running on level	5.5	mph	660	330	11.00
	7.2	mph	720	360	12.00
	8.0	mph	825	413	13.75
	10.0	mph	1140	570	19.00
	11.4	mph	1390	695	23.17
Hiking (20-lb. pack)	2.5	mph	300	150	5.00
	3.0	mph	312	156	5.20
	3.5	mph	380	190	6.33
	4.0	mph	450	225	7.50
Hiking (40-lb. pack)	1.0	mph	210	105	3.50
	2.0	mph	270	135	4.50
	3.0	mph	348	174	5.80
	4.0	mph	540	270	9.00
Swimming					
Crawl stroke	0.7	mph	300	150	5.00
	1.0	mph	420	210	7.00
	1.6	mph	700	350	11.67
	1.9	mph	850	425	14.17
	2.2	mph	1600	800	26.67
Breast stroke	0.7	mph	300	150	5.00
	1.0	mph	410	205	6.83
	1.3	mph	600	300	10.00
Side stroke	1.0	mph	550	275	9.17
	1.6	mph	1200	600	20.00

Average Amount of Calories Expended for Various Activities

Activity			Calories Per:		
			Hour	Half-hour	Minute
Swimming (cont'd)					
Back stroke	0.8	mph	300	150	5.00
	1.0	mph	450	225	7.50
	1.2	mph	540	270	9.00
	1.33	mph	660	330	11.00
	1.6	mph	800	400	13.33
Bicycling	5.5	mph	240	120	4.00
	9.0	mph	415	208	6.92
	13.0	mph	660	330	11.00
Skiing					
on level	3.0	mph	540	270	9.00
	5.0	mph	720	360	12.00
Downhill	Various		300–500	150–250	5.0–8.33
Skating	Leisurely		350	175	5.83
	9.0	mph	470	235	7.83
	11.0	mph	640	320	10.67
	13.0	mph	780	390	13.00
Snowshoeing	2.5	mph	620	310	10.33
Rowing	2.5	mph	300	150	5.00
	3.5	mph	660	330	11.0
	11.0	mph	970	485	16.17
Canoeing	Leisurely		230	115	3.83
	4.0	mph	420	210	7.00
Baseball					
(Except pitcher)			300	150	5.00
Pitcher			400	200	6.67
Volleyball					
Recreational			350	175	5.83
Competitive			600	300	10.00
Basketball			608	304	10.13
Tennis					
Recreational			450	225	7.50
Competitive and Singles			600	300	10.00
Golf (no carts)			300	150	5.00
Bowling			270	135	4.50
Squash			600–800	300–400	10.00–13.33
Fencing			630	315	10.50
Horseback riding (trot)			415	208	6.92

Average Amount of Calories Expended for Various Activities

Activity	Calories Per: Hour	Half-hour	Minute
Badminton			
Recreational	350	175	5.83
Competitive	600	300	10.00
Mountain climbing	600	300	10.00
Table tennis	360	180	6.00
General Fitness Exercises			
Basic level	200	100	3.33
Intermediate and advanced			
levels	400	200	6.67
General			
Lying down	*85*	*43*	*1.42*
Watching TV in chair	*107*	*54*	*1.78*
Mental work (seated)	*110*	*55*	*1.83*
Sewing, handwork	*115*	*58*	*1.92*
Dressing and undressing	*140*	*70*	*2.33*
Driving a car	*150*	*75*	*2.50*
Office work	*155*	*78*	*2.58*
Light housework	*165*	*83*	*2.75*
Ironing	*150*	*75*	*2.50*
Sweeping, vacuuming	*180*	*90*	*3.00*
Cleaning windows	*195*	*98*	*3.25*
Polishing	*210*	*105*	*3.50*
Laundry work	*240*	*120*	*4.00*
Making beds	*270*	*135*	*4.50*
Mopping	*300*	*150*	*5.00*
Gardening	*250*	*125*	*4.17*
House painting	*225*	*113*	*3.75*
Chopping wood	*480*	*240*	*8.00*
Sawing wood	*515*	*258*	*8.58*
Stacking firewood	*370*	*185*	*6.17*
Carpentry work	*230*	*115*	*3.83*
Shoveling dirt	*425*	*213*	*7.08*
Stone masonry	*420*	*210*	*7.00*
Machinist work (light)	*180*	*90*	*3.00*
Printing work	*150*	*75*	*2.50*

Source: Reprinted from *Keep Your Heart Running*, Paul J. Kiell, M.D., and Joseph Freylinghuysen, published by Winchester Press, P.O. Box 1260, Tulsa, OK 74101.

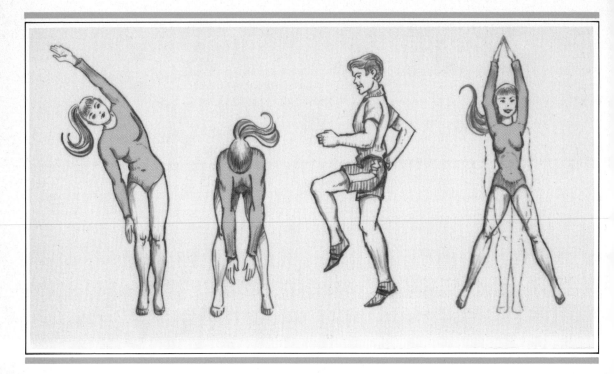

Figure 7–5. Warm-ups help you get ready for exercise by slowly preparing your body for increasing demands. Try the side bender, the forward bend, the slow jog, and the jumping jack.

- *Side bender.* Stand with feet together, one arm stretched straight upward and the other at your side. Slowly bend to the arm-down side as far as you can, bob gently (which means, start the return movement but bend quickly again), then come up, switch arm positions and repeat (5 or 10 times).

- *Forward bend.* Stand with feet apart and hands on hips. Bend the knees slightly, and curl the head and trunk down. Extend your arms between your legs and gently touch the ground at heel level. Bob once and reach farther back, then return to standing position and thrust your shoulders back (5 to 10 times).

- *Slow jog.* Stand in place, with arms in running position, and slowly run in place, counting each time the left foot strikes the ground. Pick up your pace at each count of 10, until you are running in place at full speed, with the knees thrust up high.

- *Jumping jack.* Stand with arms at your sides and jump, spreading your feet to each side while at the same time swinging your arms over head. Then jump your feet together while at the same time lowering your arms to your sides (15–20 times at a moderate speed).

Cool-Down

Cool-downs are the opposite of warm-ups: Instead of getting your body ready to exercise, they get it ready for normal activity. Exercise speeds blood to the working muscles. Without a cool-down, blood builds up in these muscles and in nearby veins, sometimes causing light-headedness or chills. The best cool-down is a brisk walk of 5 or 10 minutes; slow your speed gradually. Follow this by stretching.

- *Toe Touch.* With feet comfortably apart and knees locked, bend forward, extending your hands toward your toes. (You need not touch them.) Bob gently and straighten up (5–10 times).
- *Side twists.* Stand comfortably with feet apart and extend your arms out at each side, with your palms down. Slowly twist to the side as far as you can, bob gently, and twist to the other side. Repeat.

Overload

As we saw earlier, you do not get a training effect from exercise unless you exercise for a sufficiently long time. And you cannot increase your level of fitness without increasing the demands that you make on your body. This is called the principle of adaption, or "overload." That is why your exercise program should force you to increase the demands you make on your body until you reach your fitness goal. Then you can

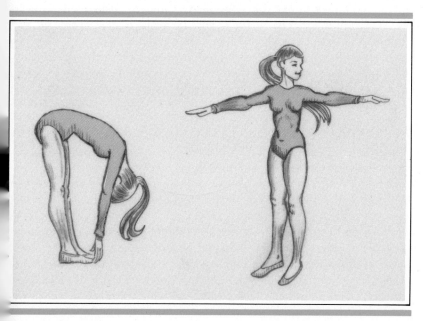

Figure 7–6. Cool-downs help your body get ready for normal activity. Slow down and cool down with a brisk-to-slowed walk, the toe touch, and the side twist.

stop increasing your level of activity and just maintain the one that you have achieved. This might mean less exercise and more sports.

How Much?

We have seen that you have to do a certain amount of exercise to benefit from it, and that you have to increase this amount to benefit even more. But there is still such a thing as *too much* exercise. How much is enough? Dr. Lenore Zohman, an authority on exercise, says that all people have a "target" zone that will make them fit but will not strain their capacities. This target zone is the amount of exercise that uses between 60 and 80 percent of your maximum aerobic power—maximum oxygen intake, that is—or that stimulates a heart rate of between 70 and 85 percent of your maximum rate.

Since you cannot measure your aerobic power, you will have to estimate your maximum heart rate, with the Karvonen formula. For a man under 30, just subtract your age from the number 220. (If you are 20, your maximum heart rate is: $220 - 20 = 200$.) For a woman under 30, subtract your age from the number 227. Immediately after exercising at a steady pace for 3 to 5 minutes, take your pulse. At the age of 20, this ought to be within 140 to 170 beats per minute. Let us say that it is 150 and that your maximum heart rate is 200. Exercise therefore stimulates a heart rate that is 75 percent of your maximum rate. You are fit!

Fatigue

Since you have to exercise vigorously to get real benefits from exercise, a certain amount of fatigue cannot be avoided. But chronic fatigue, fatigue that lasts more than 2 hours, is avoidable. If fatigue does last longer than that you are working too hard—reduce your level of activity. In any case, exercise hard only for short periods; be sure to warm up and cool down; progress from easier to harder exercise; and do not use drugs to reduce fatigue.

Sustaining Interest

Boredom is really more of a problem for most exercisers than fatigue. It is not enough merely to choose a program that will develop your body; you also have to choose one that interests you, so that you will stick with it. Often, that means picking several activities, not just one. And it means avoiding any exercise that does not fit your life style, interests, and convenience. Do not decide to play tennis, for example, if there are no courts nearby, or if you have no way to learn the skills. Avoid competitive sports if you are not a competitive person. Some people, however, enjoy competition and are spurred by it to exercise regularly. Even in this case, the best exercise program is one that forces you to achieve your goals because you want to, not so that you can beat someone else.

When?

Injuries, fatigue, and boredom are not the only things that can end an exercise program. There is also the problem of timing. To sustain an exercise program you have to fit it into your schedule—into your life, in fact. Be sure to pick a time that is convenient, a time when you will not be interrupted or tempted by something else. Two bad times to exercise are just after eating and just before going to bed.

Another point about scheduling exercise: Many short workouts are better than a single long one. Exercise 4 times a week for half an hour each instead of once for 2 hours. But it is always better to exercise at a lower level of intensity for a longer period, than at a higher level of intensity for a shorter one.

Exercise Logs

A truth of human nature is that many people enjoy the feeling that they are *making progress* more than they enjoy achievement itself. That is why keeping records of your exercise program is so important. These records do not have to be complex; simply jotting down the day's accomplishments in a notebook will do. The precise type of records you keep depends on the type of exercises you decide to do, but your records might include your speed and distance (for a runner) or the number of times you repeat a calisthenic. You might also record your progress in approaching your target heart rate.

Sleep: The Complement of Exercise

In the long run, exercise, sports, and vigorous activity will add to your energy, but in the short run they use it up. The body's way of restoring energy is rest and sleep. In this sense, sleep is the complement of exercise.

When you first lose awareness after going to sleep, you enter what is called Stage 1 sleep, which is light and easily aroused. Your sleep then becomes more and more profound, moving through Stages 2 and 3, and eventually reaching Stage 4—deep, or delta, sleep. The next stage is called REM (rapid eye movement) sleep; the lids of your eyes are now closed, but the eyes themselves move rapidly from side to side. Dreaming occurs in REM sleep, which is also called D (for dreaming) sleep; Stages 1 to 4 (non-REM sleep) are also called S sleep. Through the night you move back and forth between REM and non-REM sleep, but as morning approaches deep sleep becomes less frequent and REM sleep more so.

Much remains to be learned about the role of sleep, but researchers generally agree that sleep serves more than one function. Ernest Hartmann, foremost among sleep researchers, theorized that S sleep, espe-

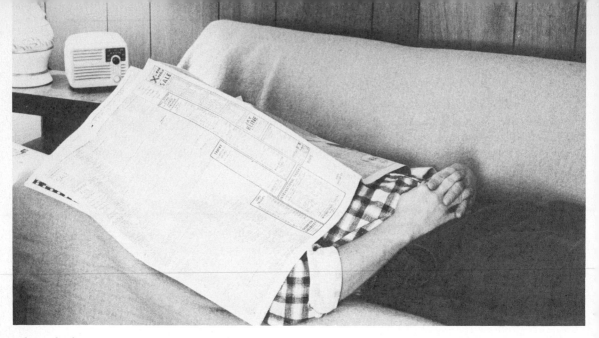

cially the delta phase, helps to restore physical strength after periods of exertion and to prepare the mind for D sleep. D sleep appears to restore the ability to concentrate and to maintain optimism and self-confidence. It also seems to help consolidate memory for long-term storage.

Sleep lowers the body's temperature and its demand for oxygen, and it slows the heart rate. These, too, would conserve the body's stores of energy.

How Much Do Students Sleep?

If asked how long people usually sleep, most of us would say about 8 hours. This is generally true, but it is not true of everyone—and certainly not of college students. College students are less dominated than most people by regular work hours, and they are buffeted more often by variations in schedule.

For 2 weeks, a group of 89 students (47 men and 42 women) at the University of Florida kept a sleep log in which they carefully recorded when they went to bed and when they got up. The average amount of sleep each night was 7 hours and 40 minutes, although there was great individual variation. The average amount of sleep during each 24-hour period, including naps, was 8 hours and 5 minutes. On weekdays, the average amount of sleep was 7 hours and 25 minutes; on weekends, 8 hours and 20 minutes.

The researchers were surprised by the large amount of napping. During the two-week period, 16 percent took no naps, 26 percent took 1 to 2 naps, 16 percent took 3 to 4 naps, and 42 percent took 5 or more naps. The last figure—the whopping 42 percent—made the researchers wonder how natural it is to concentrate most of our sleeping at night.

SUMMARY

Exercise does wonders for the body. It helps you to reduce weight, lessen the effects of stress, prevent many diseases, and build up general endurance. Overall fitness has four major elements: muscular strength, cardiorespiratory fitness, flexibility, and muscular endurance. To decide which exercise program is right for you, you must find out how fit you are now and choose your goals, then design an exercise program to help you achieve them.

For most people cardiorespiratory fitness is the most important kind of fitness because it builds up energy and helps prevent heart disease, the leading cause of death in the United States. Cardiorespiratory fitness helps the heart get more oxygen and nutrients to the tissues with each beat. The increase in the heart's pumping power and the lungs' breathing efficiency as a result of exercise is called the training effect.

Not all exercises promote the training effect equally. The exercises that do most to promote it are those that improve the body's ability to absorb more and more oxygen, which is then sent by the heart to the tissues. Isometrics have little training effect, but do help build up muscle strength. Anaerobic exercises also have relatively little training effect. The exercises that really promote the training effect are called aerobics: swimming, running, bicycling, stationary running, handball, basketball, and squash, among others.

Exercises should start at your present level of ability and increase in difficulty as you go along. Once you start exercising, make sure that you are working out enough to promote the training effect and to progress, but not so much as to suffer chronic fatigue. To avoid strains and sprains, warm up before every workout and cool down afterward. Doing more than one kind of activity will help keep you interested in your program—and so will measuring your progress frequently.

Sleep is important in restoring the body's energy and in that sense is the complement of exercise.

Suggested Readings

Cooper, Kenneth H. *The Aerobic Way.* New York: Evans, 1977. Highlights include "Your Personal Coronary Risk Profile," how to begin an aerobics program, plus exercise charts for self-evaluation.

Cooper, Mildred, and Cooper, Kenneth. *Aerobics for Women.* New York: Evans, 1972. Presents the concept of aerobics from a woman's perspective.

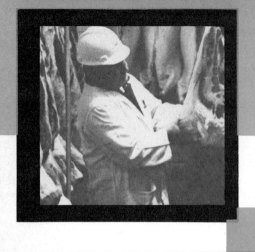

8

Nutrition

chapter objectives

When you have finished reading this chapter you should be able to:

1. Recognize that diet and exercise are the fundamental building blocks for health
2. Apply your knowledge of the nutrients to your daily diet practices, and use this knowledge to evaluate diets
3. Discuss nutritional goals and deficiencies of the American diet
4. Define food sources of vitamins and minerals
5. Recognize nutritional fallacies

Eating food is a universal human activity. Yet ideas about *what* things should be eaten and *how* to eat them vary from one culture to the next. In Taiwan, dogs are regarded as a great delicacy. But to an American, the idea of eating a dog seems horrible. And in some places belching after a meal is supposed to be a polite way of indicating that you enjoyed it, but in the United States belching is merely boorish. Other social attitudes help to determine how much we eat, what we eat, and when we eat.

Like other social attitudes, attitudes toward food change. About 100 years ago, most Americans ate much more fruit, vegetables, and whole grains than they eat today; they ate fewer fatty foods, then, and fewer foods containing refined sugar. Their total consumption was less than it now is, too.

One fact about food is universal and unchanging, however: People eat it to end their hunger. This hunger, despite its sometimes dreadful consequences, is useful, for it forces people to eat and thereby to give their bodies the food they need. But the body cannot use food without breaking it down (digesting it) into its component parts. Almost all foods have more than one component. Some of these components, such as cellulose in plants, are not used by the body directly. Those components that are used are called *nutrients.*

Nutrients

The basic nutrients are carbohydrates, fats, minerals, proteins, vitamins, and water. The body needs varying amounts of these nutrients, and no single food contains all of them. A balanced diet is a diet that contains all the nutrients that we need. Since each of us needs differing amounts of each nutrient, one person's "balanced" diet may not be the same as another's.

Nutrients are divided into two fundamental categories: those that provide the body's basic need for energy and those that do not. The energy contained in food is measured in *calories.* Foods that are high in calories are therefore high in energy potential, but they are more fattening than foods that are lower in calories, too (see Chapter 9 for further details).

Nutrients That Provide Energy

Carbohydrates.   When you eat a bar of candy, a grapefruit, or a piece of bread, you are taking into your body its most important source of energy, carbohydrates. When carbohydrates are broken down in the body, they produce a sugar called glucose, which is the first substance the body uses for energy. (When there is no glucose available, other substances are converted to glucose.) Carbohydrates should make up about half of the calories in the diets of most Americans. Unit for unit they are lower in calories than fat is.

Carbohydrates are divided into two great classes—the simple and the complex. Simple carbohydrates are sometimes called "the sugars," such as sucrose (table sugar), lactose (milk sugar), and fructose (fruit sugar). Simple carbohydrates come from such foods as refined sugar, fruit, milk, and the host of sugar-sweetened products: soda pop, candy bars, cookies, cake, and frosting. Complex carbohydrates include such substances as starch, glycogen (a variety of starch the body stores), and cellulose (a plant substance indigestible by humans). These substances (except cellulose) contribute glucose, and thus energy, to the diet. Complex carbohydrates are found in such foods as rice, pasta, beans, peas, potatoes, wheat, barley, and corn.

Proteins.   The organic compounds used to repair and build body tissues are called proteins. Most people know that animal meat is a good source of protein. But proteins are also available in fish, poultry, milk, grains, nuts, peas, and beans. Proteins make up about 10 to 15 percent of our diet, but extremely active people and pregnant women may need a higher proportion. Protein is essential to building body tissues. As we age, we grow less active and therefore our daily caloric requirements go down. But the amount of protein that we need remains relatively constant throughout our lives.

Protein is composed of carbon, hydrogen, oxygen, and nitrogen. These atoms are combined into substances called amino acids, which in turn are linked together to form proteins. Proteins (like carbohydrates) are divided into two large classes: proteins that contain the eight "essential" amino acids (those the body requires but cannot produce in sufficient quantity to meet its needs) and proteins that do not contain all eight. After proteins are eaten, digestive enzymes unravel the complex chains of amino acids and chemically reduce them into smaller, less complex compounds. Some of these compounds are used to repair the body or help it grow, and some are used for energy. Per unit, proteins are less rich in calories than are carbohydrates or fats.

Fats.   Of all the fuels used by the body, fats (or lipids) are the richest in energy—for each unit of weight they produce more than twice the calories of carbohydrates and proteins. There are three basic varieties of lipids in the diet: triglycerides (which make up 95 percent of the total); phospholipids, and sterols (which together make up the other 5 percent). Three kinds of triglycerides are the *saturated* fats, the *polyunsaturated* fats, and the *monosaturated* fats, whose hydrogen atoms are arranged somewhat differently. Saturated fats are found in beef, lamb, pork, whole milk products, some vegetable shortenings, coconut oil, cocoa butter, and palm oil. Generally speaking, the more saturated

Table 8–1.   Principal Sources and Functions of Nutrients

Nutrients	Functions	Principal Sources	
Proteins	Build and repair the body	Beef	Fish
		Veal	Milk
		Pork	Cheese
	Regulate body processes	Lamb	Eggs
		Liver	Dried beans
		Poultry	Peas
Carbohydrates	Furnish energy*	Sugars	Crackers
		Syrups	Cereal
		Molasses	Potatoes
		Flour	Rice
		Flour products	Noodles
		Bread	Other starchy vegetables
Fats	Furnish energy*	Butter	Bacon
		Lard	Oils
		Vegetable oils	Nuts
		Shortening	Cheese
		Margarine	Cream
		Salad dressings	Meat fats
Minerals	Build and repair the body	(See Mineral Table 8–3)	
	Regulate body processes		
Vitamins	Regulate body processes	(See Vitamin Table 8–2)	

*Although carbohydrates and fats are the principal sources of energy, protein also provides energy. This, however, is not the major function of protein.
Source: Adapted from National Live Stock and Meat Board (Washington, D.C.: Government Printing Office, 1964).

a fat may be, the harder it is at room temperature; for example, soft margerine is less saturated than butter.

Equal weights of all fats have the same number of calories, but meats that are rich in saturated fats, such as beef and pork, are also rich both in triglycerides and in a substance called *cholesterol*. Both are necessary for some physiological processes, but they are also linked to a condition called atherosclerosis, hardening of the arteries (Chapter 10).

Unsaturated (or polyunsaturated) fats are found in such liquid vegetable oils as those made from corn, soybeans, cotton seeds, safflower seeds, sunflower seeds, and sesame seeds. Monosaturated fats are found in such foods as olive oil.

Fats have a reputation that is not altogether deserved. The body requires a certain amount of fat, and for a number of reasons. Fats help create a sense of "fullness" during the digestion process, since, of all the nutrients, they take the longest to digest. Fats improve the taste of many foods. Certain vitamins—A, D, E, and K—are provided in part by foods that contain fats. And fats help to support and protect vital organs, to insulate the body against the environment, and to store certain vitamins.

Most experts still believe that Americans consume too much fat. And they think so for good reason, too. During this century, the percentage of fat in our diet has, on average, risen from 33 percent to about 45 percent. Many nutritionists believe that 35 percent or so is a much healthier proportion, and they believe that at least one-half to two-thirds of this 35 percent should be in the form of unsaturated fats. To put it more concretely, you ought to be eating less "red" meat than poultry, fruits, vegetables, and fish. And to keep your total intake of cholesterol low, you should be eating no more than three or four eggs a week. It is also a good idea to eat very little fried food and to use unsaturated vegetable oils for cooking and baking.

Figure 8–1. Current Diet versus Dietary Goals.
Sources for current diet: "Changes in Nutrients in the U.S. Diet Caused by Alterations in Food Intake Patterns." B. Friend. Agricultural Research Service. U.S. Department of Agriculture, 1974. Proportions of saturated versus unsaturated fats based on unpublished Agricultural Research Service data.

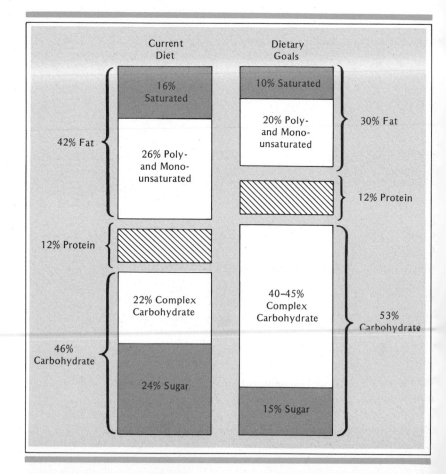

Nutrients That Do Not Provide Energy

Vitamins.   Although *vitamins* themselves do not provide energy, they make possible many of the body's chemical reactions, including those that set energy free from other nutrients. The body requires only a minute amount of each vitamin, but since it cannot make them itself, it has to get a steady supply through food. "Fat-soluble" vitamins—A, D, E, and K—are those that, when absorbed through digestion, are transported to the tissues and stored in body fat. They are found in foods that contain fats. Normally, they are not excreted in the urine, an important point because it means they can be stored in the body, which therefore does not have to take in a supply of them each day. The "water-soluble" vitamins—including the B-complex and vitamin C—are those that are excreted in the urine when they are in excess of body needs. That means that they are not stored in the body, which *does* have to take them in each day. Vitamin pills (multivitamins) usually contain both fat- and water-soluble vitamins.

Minerals.   *Minerals* are similar in function to vitamins, but unlike vitamins (and all the other nutrients except water), they are elements, not compounds, and they are inorganic—they do not contain carbon. Seven minerals are required by the body in amounts of 1/10th of a gram or more each day; these include calcium and phosphorus. Other minerals are needed in amounts of 1/100 of a gram or less, or in trace amounts; these include iodine and zinc. The list of the trace elements required in the diet seems to grow each year as nutritional research continues to discover uses for them.

   Minerals are vital to many body functions. Two of them, calcium and phosphorus—found in milk and in leafy green vegetables, like collard greens and spinach—form most of the structure of bones and teeth. Calcium is important in nerve activity, blood clotting, and metabolic functions (see Chapter 9). Iron, from red meats, oysters, lima beans, berries, and green vegetables, helps the red blood cells to carry oxygen.

   Among the other major required minerals are potassium, sodium, and chlorine. Other trace elements include flourine, cobalt, and copper. Some minerals, such as sodium and potassium, may be lost through the sweat during exercise, but you should get all you need (of these and other minerals) from your normal diet.

Water.   Just about everything that lives in this world is made up mostly of water, including things that appear to be quite solid—your body, for instance, is about 60 to 70 percent water. Water not only plays a vital role in the chemical reactions within the body but also helps it to absorb other nutrients and to remove wastes. You can live without the other nutrients much longer than you can live without water. Average

Table 8–2.   Vitamins: Where You Get Them and What They Do

Best Sources	Main Roles	Deficiency Symptoms	Risks of Megadoses
Fat Soluble			
A			
Liver; eggs; cheese; butter; fortified margarine and milk; yellow, orange, and dark-green vegetables and fruits (e.g., carrots, broccoli, spinach, cantaloupe). Vitamin A is preformed in animal foods. In plants the yellow-orange "provitamin," called carotene, is converted to an active vitamin in the body.	Assists in the formation and maintenance of healthy skin, hair, and mucous membranes; aids in the ability to see in dim light (night vision); needed for proper bone growth, teeth development, and reproduction.	Night blindness; rough skin and mucous membranes; infection of mucous membranes; drying of the eyes; impaired bone growth and tooth enamel.	Blurred vision, loss of appetite, headaches, skin rashes, nausea, diarrhea, hair loss, menstrual irregularities, extreme fatigue, joint pain, liver damage, insomnia, abnormal bone growth, injury to brain and nervous system. Excessive consumption of carotene-containing foods, while not poisonous, can cause yellowing of skin.
D			
Fortified milk; egg yolk; liver; tuna; salmon; cod liver oil. Made on skin in sunlight, but required in diet by dark-skinned persons in cold climates, babies, and those confined indoors.	Aids in the formation and maintenance of bones and teeth; assists in the absorption and use of calcium and phosphorus.	In children, rickets: stunted bone growth, bowed legs, malformed teeth, protruding abdomen. In adults, osteomalacia: softening of the bones leading to shortening and fractures, muscle spasms, and twitching.	In infants, calcium deposits in kidneys and excessive calcium in blood; in adults, calcium deposits throughout body (may be mistaken for cancer), deafness, nausea, loss of appetite, kidney stones, fragile bones, high blood pressure, high blood cholesterol, increased lead absorption.
E (alpha tocopherol)			
Vegetable oils; margarine; wheat germ; whole-grain cereals and bread; liver; dried beans; green leafy vegetables.	Aids in the formation of red blood cells, muscles, and other tissues; protects vitamin A and essential fatty acids from oxidation.	Not seen in human beings except after prolonged impairment of fat absorption. Deficiency symptoms in laboratory animals (e.g., reproductive failure, liver degeneration, heart damage, muscular dystrophy) not seen in people, not even those getting very little vitamin E for six years.	None definitely known. Reports of headache, blurred vision, extreme fatigue, muscle weakness. Can destroy some vitamin K made in the gut.
K			
Green leafy vegetables; cabbage; cauliflower; peas; potatoes; liver; cereals. Except in newborns, made by bacteria in human intestine.	Aids in the synthesis of substances needed for the blood to clot; helps maintain normal bone metabolism.	Hemorrhage, especially in newborn infants. In adults, loss of calcium from bones (however, this deficiency is extremely rare). Extra K needed by persons on prolonged antibiotic therapy and those with impaired fat absorption, cancer, or kidney disease.	Jaundice in babies; anemia in laboratory animals.

Table 8–2.   Vitamins: Where You Get Them and What They Do

Best Sources	Main Roles	Deficiency Symptoms	Risks of Megadoses
		Water Soluble	

Thiamin (B_1)

Best Sources	Main Roles	Deficiency Symptoms	Risks of Megadoses
Pork (especially ham); liver; oysters; whole-grain and enriched cereals, pasta, and bread; wheat germ; oatmeal; peas; lima beans. May also be made by intestinal microbes.	Helps release energy from carbohydrates; aids in the synthesis of an important nervous-system chemical.	Beriberi: mental confusion, muscular weakness, swelling of the heart, leg cramps. Need for thiamin is increased if calories consumed increase.	None known. However, since B vitamins are interdependent, excess of one may produce deficiency of others.

Riboflavin (B_2)

Best Sources	Main Roles	Deficiency Symptoms	Risks of Megadoses
Liver; milk; meat; dark-green vegetables; eggs; whole-grain and enriched cereals, pasta, and bread; mushrooms; dried beans and peas.	Helps release energy from carbohydrates, proteins, and fats; aids in the maintenance of mucous membranes.	Skin disorders, especially around nose and lips; cracks at corners of mouth; sensitivity of eyes to light.	None known. See thiamin.

Niacin (B_3, nicotinamide, nicotinic acid)

Best Sources	Main Roles	Deficiency Symptoms	Risks of Megadoses
Liver; poultry; meat; tuna; eggs; whole-grain and enriched cereals, pasta, and bread; nuts; dried peas and beans. Body can convert tryptophan in protein into niacin.	Participates with thiamin and riboflavin in facilitating energy production in cells.	Pellagra: skin disorders (especially on parts of body exposed to sun), diarrhea, mental confusion, irritability, mouth swelling, smooth tongue.	Duodenal ulcer, abnormal liver function, elevated blood sugar, excessive uric acid in blood, possibly leading to gout. See thiamin.

B_6 (includes pyridoxine, pyridoxal, and pyridoxamine)

Best Sources	Main Roles	Deficiency Symptoms	Risks of Megadoses
Whole-grain (but not enriched) cereals and bread; liver; avocados; spinach; green beans; bananas; fish; poultry; meats; nuts; potatoes; green leafy vegetables.	Aids in the absorption and metabolism of proteins; helps the body use fats; assists in the formation of red blood cells.	Skin disorders; cracks at corners of mouth; smooth tongue; convulsions; dizziness; nausea; anemia; kidney stones. Mild deficiency caused by oral contraceptives may cause depression. Otherwise, deficiencies rare. Need for B_6 is increased by increased protein in diet.	Dependency on high dose, leading to deficiency symptoms when one returns to normal amounts.

B_{12} (cobalamin)

Best Sources	Main Roles	Deficiency Symptoms	Risks of Megadoses
Only in animal foods: liver; kidneys; meat; fish; eggs; milk; oysters; nutritional yeast.	Aids in the formation of red blood cells; assists in the building of genetic material; helps the functioning of the nervous system.	Pernicious anemia: anemia, pale skin and mucous membranes, numbness and tingling in fingers and toes that may progress to loss of balance and weakness and pain in arms and legs. At risk: strict vegetarians who eat no animal foods; persons who have had part of their stomach removed; those with a genetic inability to absorb B_{12}.	None known. See thiamin.

Table 8-2.   Vitamins: Where You Get Them and What They Do

Best Sources	Main Roles	Deficiency Symptoms	Risks of Megadoses
		Water Soluble (cont'd)	
		Folacin (folic acid)	
Liver; kidneys; dark-green leafy vegetables; wheat germ; dried beans and peas. Stored in the body so that daily consumption is not crucial.	Acts with B_{12} in synthesizing genetic material; aids in the formation of hemoglobin in red blood cells.	Megaloblastic anemia: enlarged red blood cells, smooth tongue, diarrhea; during pregnancy, deficiency may cause loss of the fetus or fetal abnormalities. Women on oral contraceptives may need extra folacin.	None identified. But body stores it, so it is potentially hazardous. Can mask a B_{12} deficiency.
		Pantothenic acid	
In all plants and animals, especially liver; kidneys; whole-grain cereal and bread; nuts; eggs; dark-green vegetables. Also made by intestinal bacteria. Lost in refined and heavily processed foods.	Helps in the metabolism of carbohydrates, proteins, and fats; aids in the formation of hormones and nerve-regulating substances.	Not known except experimentally in human beings: severe abdominal cramps, vomiting, fatigue, difficulty sleeping, tingling in hands and feet.	Increased need for thiamin, possibly causing thiamin deficiency symptoms.
		Biotin	
Egg yolk; liver; kidneys; dark-green vegetables; green beans. Made by microorganisms in the intestinal tract.	Aids in the formation of fatty acids; helps release energy from carbohydrates.	Not known under natural circumstances. Large amounts of raw egg white can destroy biotin, causing loss of appetite, nausea, vomiting, pallor, depression, fatigue, and muscle pain. (Cooked egg white has no harmful effect.)	None known. See thiamin.
		C (ascorbic acid)	
Citrus fruits; tomatoes; strawberries; melon; green peppers; potatoes; dark-green vegetables.	Aids in the formation of collagen; helps maintain capillaries, bones, and teeth; helps protect other vitamins from oxidation; may block formation of cancer-causing nitrosamines.	Scurvy: bleeding gums, degenerating muscles, wounds that don't heal, loose teeth, brown, dry, rough skin. Early symptoms include loss of appetite, irritability, weight loss.	Dependency on high doses, possibly precipitating symptoms of scurvy when withdrawn (especially in infants if megadoses taken during pregnancy); kidney and bladder stones; diarrhea; urinary-tract irritation; increased tendency for blood to clot; breakdown of red blood cells in persons with certain common genetic disorders (such as glucose-6-phosphate dehydrogenase deficiency, common in blacks); may induce B_{12} deficiency.

Source: Jane Brody, *Jane Brody's Nutrition Book* (New York: Norton, 1981), pp 159–164.

Table 8–3.   Minerals: Where You Get Them and What They Do

Best Sources	Main Roles	Deficiency Symptoms	Risks of Megadoses
Macromineral			
Calcium			
Milk and milk products; sardines; canned salmon eaten with bones; dark-green, leafy vegetables; citrus fruits; dried beans and peas.	Building bones and teeth and maintaining bone strength; muscle contraction; maintaining cell membranes; blood clotting; absorption of B_{12}, activation of enzymes.	Children: distorted bone growth (rickets). Adults: loss of bone (osteoporosis) and increased susceptibility to fractures.	Drowsiness; extreme lethargy; impaired absorption of iron, zinc, and manganese; calcium deposits in tissues throughout body, mimicking cancer on X-ray.
Phosphorus			
Meat; poultry; fish; eggs; dried beans and peas; milk and milk products; phosphates in processed foods, especially soft drinks.	Building bones and teeth; release of energy from carbohydrates, proteins, and fats; formation of genetic material, cell membranes, and many enzymes.	Weakness, loss of appetite, malaise, bone pain. Dietary shortages uncommon, but prolonged use of antacids can cause deficiency.	Distortion of calcium-to-phosphorus ratio, creating relative deficiency of calcium.
Magnesium			
Leafy, green vegetables (eaten raw); nuts (especially almonds and cashews); soybeans; seeds; whole grains.	Building bones; manufacture of proteins; release of energy from muscle glycogen; conduction of nerve impulse to muscles; adjustment to cold.	Muscular twitching and tremors; irregular heart beat; insomnia; muscle weakness; leg and foot cramps; shaky hands. Deficiency may occur in persons with prolonged diarrhea, kidney disease, diabetes, epilepsy, or alcoholism, and in those who take diuretics.	Disturbed nervous-system function because the calcium-to-magnesium ratio is unbalanced; catharsis; hazard to persons with poor kidney function.
Potassium			
Orange juice; bananas; dried fruits; meats; bran; peanut butter; dried beans and peas; potatoes; coffee; tea; cocoa.	Muscle contraction; maintenance of fluid and electrolyte balance in cells; transmission of nerve impulses; release of energy from carbohydrates, proteins, and fats.	Abnormal heart rhythm; muscular weakness; lethargy; kidney and lung failure. Deficiency may occur among heavy laborers and athletes who work hard in heat, persons taking diuretics and purgatives, and those with prolonged diarrhea.	Excessive potassium in blood, causing muscular paralysis and abnormal heart rhythms.
Sulfur			
Beef; wheat germ; dried beans and peas; peanuts; clams.	In every cell as part of sulfur-containing amino acids; forms bridges between molecules to create firm proteins of hair, nails, and skin.	Not known in humans.	Unknown.
Chloride			
Table salt and other naturally occurring salts.	Regulates balance of body fluids and acids and bases; activates enzyme in saliva; part of stomach acid.	Disturbed acid-base balance in body fluids (very rare).	Disturbed acid-base balance.

Table 8–3.   Minerals: Where You Get Them and What They Do

Best Sources	Main Roles	Deficiency Symptoms	Risks of Megadoses
Trace Minerals (cont'd)			
Iron			
Liver (especially pork, followed by calf, beef, and chicken); kidneys; red meats; egg yolk; green leafy vegetables; dried fruits (raisins, apricots, and prunes); dried beans and peas; potatoes; blackstrap molasses; enriched and whole-grain cereals.	Formation of hemoglobin in blood and myoglobin in muscles, which supply oxygen to cells; part of several enzymes and proteins.	Anemia, with fatigue, weakness, pallor, and shortness of breath.	Toxic build-up in liver, pancreas, and heart.
Copper			
Oysters; nuts; cocoa powder; beef and pork liver; kidneys; dried beans; corn-oil margarine.	Formation of red blood cells; part of several respiratory enzymes.	Animals: anemia; faulty development of bone and nervous tissue; loss of elasticity in tendons and major arteries; abnormal lung development; abnormal structure and pigmentation of hair.	Violent vomiting and diarrhea. Cooking acid foods in unlined copper pots can lead to toxic accumulation of copper.
Zinc			
Meat; liver; eggs; poultry; seafood; followed by milk and whole grains.	Constituent of about 100 enzymes.	Delayed wound healing; diminished taste sensation; loss of appetite. In children: failure to grow and mature sexually. Prenatally: abnormal brain development.	Nausea, vomiting; anemia; bleeding in stomach; premature birth and stillbirth; abdominal pain; fever. Can aggravate marginal copper deficiency. May produce atherosclerosis.
Iodine			
Seafood; saltwater fish; seaweed; iodized salt; sea salt.	Part of thyroid hormones; essential for normal reproduction.	Goiter (enlarged thyroid with low hormone production). Newborns: cretinism, with retarded growth, protruding abdomen, swollen-looking features, thick lips, enlarged tongue. Persons living far from sea coast should use iodized salt to prevent deficiency.	Not known to be a problem, but could cause iodine poisoning or sensitivity reaction.
Fluorine			
Fish; tea; most animal foods; fluoridated water; foods grown with or cooked in fluoridated water.	Formation of strong, decay-resistant teeth; maintenance of bone strength.	Excessive dental decay; possibly osteoporosis.	Mottling of teeth and bones; in larger doses, a deadly poison.
Chromium			
Meat; cheese; whole-grain breads and cereals; dried beans; peanuts; brewer's yeast.	Metabolism of glucose.	Possibly, abnormal sugar metabolism (chemical diabetes) and adult-onset diabetes.	Not known.

Table 8–3. Minerals: Where You Get Them and What They Do

Best Sources	Main Roles	Deficiency Symptoms	Risks of Megadoses
Trace Minerals (cont'd)			
Selenium			
Seafood; whole-grain cereals; meat; egg yolk; chicken; milk; garlic.	Antioxidant, preventing breakdown of fats and other body chemicals; interacts with vitamin E.	Not known in human beings. Animals: degeneration of pancreas. Parts of country where selenium is low have higher cancer rates and more deaths from high blood pressure.	Animals: "blind staggers"—stiffness, lameness, hair loss, blindness, death.
Manganese			
Nuts; whole grains; vegetables and fruits; tea; instant coffee; cocoa powder.	Functioning of central nervous system; normal bone structure; reproduction; part of important enzymes.	Not known in human beings. Animals: poor reproduction; retarded growth; birth defects; abnormal bone development.	Masklike facial expression; blurred speech; involuntary laughing; spastic gait; hand tremors.
Molybdenum			
Legumes; cereal grains; liver; kidney; some dark-green vegetables.	Part of the enzyme xanthine oxidase.	Not known in human beings. Animals: decreased weight gain; shortened life span.	Goutlike syndrome; loss of copper.

Source: Jane Brody, *Jane Brody's Nutrition Book* (New York: Norton, 1981), pp. 184–188.

people need about 2 to 3 quarts of water each day and perhaps more, depending on how active they are and on conditions in the environment (heat, for example).

Essential Nutrients

Many nutrients are required by the body, but essential nutrients are those that must be supplied by food; the body cannot make them. We have already seen that the diet must provide the eight essential amino acids. Other dietary essentials include water, certain fats, vitamins, and minerals.

Non-Nutrients

Some of the components of food are not nutrients, since they do not take part in any of the body's chemical reactions. Nonetheless, they play an important role in the body's workings. The most important of these non-nutrients is *fiber,* the general term for the indigestible parts of food. Fiber forms the greater part of the roughage (the indigestible portion of plants, mostly cellulose) that passes through our intestinal tracts. Certain animals are able to break down cellulose (and other fibers) and get energy from them, but humans cannot.

Although indigestible, fiber is important to human digestion. Statis-

Table 8–4. Approximate Fiber Content of Selected Foods

Product	Serving Size	Dietary Fiber g/serving
Cereals, Breads, and Flours		
Bran	1 oz	14.40
Whole grain flour	½ c	13.20
White flour	½ c	4.00
All bran	½ c	—
Bran flakes	¾ c	—
Raisin bran	½ c	—
Oatmeal, cooked	1 c	—
Cornflakes	1 c	3.08
Cream of wheat, cooked	1 c	—
Bread, "high fiber" type	1 slice	—
Bread, whole wheat	1 slice	2.00
Bread, pumpernickel	1 slice	—
Bread, white, enriched	1 slice	0.60
Fruits and Vegetables		
Peas, green	⅔ c	7.20
Pear	1 medium	3.90
Carrots	⅔ c	3.80
Banana	1 medium	3.10
Cabbage, cooked	⅔ c	2.80
Apple with skin	1 medium	2.60
Strawberries	½ c	1.60
Tomato, raw	1 medium	1.40
Plum	1 medium	1.10
Potato	3¼″ diam.	—
Orange	3″ diam.	—
Corn, canned	½ c	—
Raisins, dried, seedless	½ c	—
Beans, fresh green	½ c	—
Spinach	½ c	—
Celery, stalk	1 large	—
Grapes, green seedless	18–20	—
Fruit juice	1 c	—
Legumes		
Chick peas	½ c	—
Beans, navy	½ c	—
Lentils	½ c	—
Meat and Dairy Products	—	
Nuts and Seeds		
Sunflower seeds	3½ oz	—
Sesame seeds	3½ oz	
Walnuts, English	½ c	—
Peanuts, roasted, with skin	1 tbs	1.40
Pistachio nuts	30	—
Cashews, roasted	6–8	—

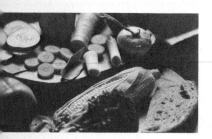

Fiber foods.

Jan Halaska/Photo Researchers

Source: D. A. T. Southgate, B. Bailey, E. Collinson et al., "A Guide to Calculating Intakes of Dietary Fiber," *Journal of Human Nutrition* 30 (1976): 303.

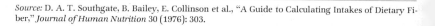

tics show that in places where diets are high in fiber content the incidence of colon cancer (see Chapter 10) is low. The reason seems to be that high-fiber diets help the feces pass through the colon rapidly, thus keeping harmful substances from making much contact. Fiber also helps to prevent constipation. So it is important to get enough fiber in your diet; eat fresh fruit, leafy vegetables, and whole-grain breads and cereals.

Additives

Manufacturers of processed food conduct market-research surveys to find out what the public wants. These surveys show, among other things, that people want their chickens to look yellow, and their meat to be red and "raw," and their bread to be so doughy "fresh" that it often sticks to the roofs of their mouths. Additives are put into food to cater to these and other fancies. Some of them contain nutrients, and some do not.

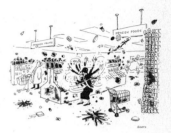

"Artificial coloring, artificial flavoring, artificial glop, artificial slop, artificial this, artificial that . . ."

Drawing by Booth; © 1972 The New Yorker Magazine, Inc.

Flavor and Color

One class of additives simply makes foods more appealing: colors, flavors, flavor enhancers, and sweeteners. Almost all processed foods contain food colors, which add little or nothing to any product's nutritional value. About half the 35 colors now permitted for use in the United States are synthetic, and many are derived from petroleum. More than 1,700 natural and synthetic—mostly synthetic—substances are used to flavor foods. These flavors, although artificial, are less artificial than the flavor enhancers, which change our perception of flavor, rather than give flavor. Some do so by temporarily deadening certain nerves or by enhancing the nerve impulses that allow us to perceive flavor.

One flavor enhancer, monosodium glutamate (MSG), used commonly in restaurants and in prepared foods, was banned from baby foods because it produced deformities in experimental animals. It is still widely used in prepared soups, gravies, cold cuts, breadings, and other convenience foods. In restaurants, so much may be used that MSG has been linked to the so-called Chinese Restaurant Syndrome—headaches, a tightness in the chest, difficulty in breathing, and a burning sensation in the neck and forearms.

Food Processing

Another class of additives helps process and prepare foods that need a long shelf life in the supermarket. Emulsifiers, for instance, are used in salad dressings to keep the oil mixed with vinegar. Without emulsifiers, peanut butter and mayonnaise would separate and form an oily top layer. Thickeners and stabilizers help to give food a uniform tex-

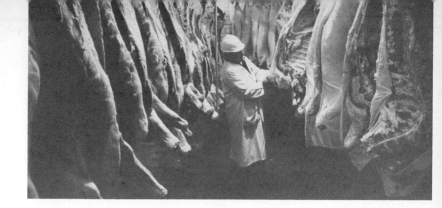

ture. Certain compounds keep powdered products free-flowing by absorbing moisture. Glycerine is used in certain foods to retain moisture.

Preservatives protect natural color and flavor, prevent fats and oils from tasting rancid, and stop the spoilage caused in foods by molds, bacteria, fungi, and yeasts.

Nutrition

Some things are actually put into foods to improve their nutritional value. The processing of foods may destroy nutrients, and these may be added back later: Vitamin A to margarine, for example, Vitamin C to fruit drinks, and the B vitamins to breads and cereals. All this seems well and good, and sometimes it is. But sometimes a manufacturer adds vitamins and minerals that most people are probably getting in sufficient amounts from other sources. Since your body only uses what it needs, some extra vitamins are stored, but most are excreted.

The Basic Four

Humans need about 50 nutrients. Not all these nutrients are available in any one food, but you do not have to eat all foods to get all the nutrients you need. The reason is that all foods, despite their great variety, can be divided among four basic food groups: meats, fruits and vegetables, grains, and milk. If you include in your daily diet enough foods from each of these four groups, you will get all the nutrients you need.

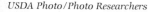

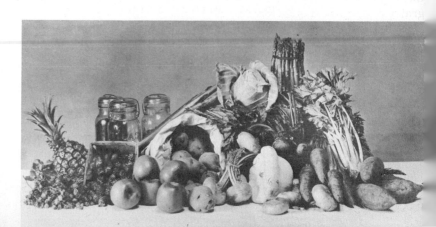

Meats

Besides red meats, the meat group includes poultry, fish, eggs, and such rich sources of protein as dried beans, peas, and nuts. In fact, the meat group as a whole is a good source of protein, and also of iron and the fat soluble and B-complex vitamins (thiamine, riboflavin, niacin, B_6, and B_{12}). Alas, however, the meat group also abounds in calories, fats, and cholesterol. You only need about 5 ounces of these foods each day. Most of us eat much more of them than we need.

Fruit and Vegetables

The fruit and vegetable group contributes 90 percent of the vitamin C in the average diet, and 60 percent of the vitamin A. These are the vitamins in which the average diet is most often deficient. Fruits and vegetables also give us important amounts of minerals, folic acid, fiber, and carbohydrates. Nutritionists recommend four servings of fruits or vegetables daily. A typical serving might include either 1 cup of raw salad; ½ cup of cooked fruit or vegetables; ½ medium banana or grapefruit; or 1 medium peach, pear, or apple. Most of us do not eat enough fruits and vegetables.

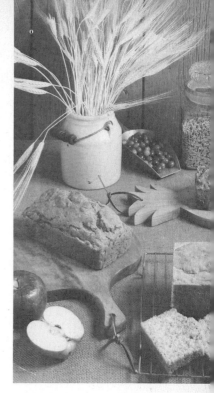

Sara Watts/Photo Researchers

American Dairy Association and Dairy Council, Inc.

Grains

Many people think that the group of foods made from grains like wheat, corn, rice, and barley are more fattening than other foods, so grains are too often avoided. But they are really less fattening than people think. And grains provide carbohydrates and protein, and such vitamins and minerals as riboflavin, niacin, thiamine, and iron. In about half of the states the nutritional value of bread, the most important food product made with grain, has been regulated by "enrichment laws" that require bread manufacturers to add important vitamins and minerals back to the bread if they are lost in baking. Nutritionists recommend 4 servings each day from this group. A typical serving might include either 1 slice of bread, ½ cup of cooked cereal, 1 roll or biscuit, 1 ounce of ready-to-eat cereal, or ½ cup of cooked pasta. When you eat these kinds of foods try to be sure that they are made from whole grains or enriched flour.

Milk

You have been told, no doubt, that milk is the "perfect food." But nothing is perfect, and certainly milk is not. First, whole milk has many calories (about 170 calories in a single cup) because of the fat it contains. Second, some people (especially adults) are allergic to milk and have digestive problems when they drink it. Third, milk does not con-

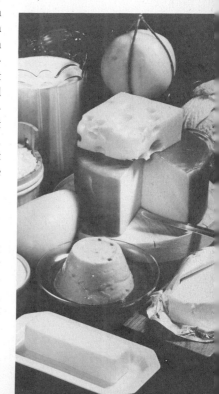

tain each and every nutrient. But it does have some solid virtues: For each unit it supplies more calcium than the foods in any other group; and it is a source of protein, riboflavin, vitamin A, and (if fortified) vitamin D. Nutritionists recommend 2 servings a day from this group for adults and 3 for children. One serving might include either 1 cup of whole, skim, or reconstituted milk; 1 slice of cheese; 1 cup of yogurt; or 1 cup of baked custard.

Table 8–5.   The Basic Four Food Groups: What's "A Serving"?

Food	Amount per Serving*	Servings per Day
Milk Group		
Milk	8 ounces (1 cup)	Children 0–9 years: 2 to 3
Yogurt, plain	1 cup	Children 9–12 years: 3
Hard cheese	1¼ ounces	Teens: 4
Cheese spread	2 ounces	Adults: 2
Ice cream	1½ cups	Pregnant women: 3
Cottage cheese	2 cups	Nursing mothers: 4
Meat Group		
Meat, lean	2 to 3 ounces cooked	2 (can be eaten as mixtures of ani-
Poultry	2 to 3 ounces	mal and vegetable foods; if only
Fish	2 to 3 ounces	vegetable protein is consumed, it
Hard cheese	2 to 3 ounces	must be balanced)
Eggs	2 to 3	
Cottage cheese	½ cup	
Dry beans and peas	1 to 1½ cups cooked	
Nuts and seeds	½ to ¾ cup	
Peanut butter	4 tablespoons	
Vegetable and Fruit Group		
Vegetables, cut up	½ cup	4, including one good vitamin C
Fruits, cut up	½ cup	source like oranges or orange juice
Grapefruit	½ medium	and one deep-yellow or dark-
Melon	½ medium	green vegetable
Orange	1	
Potato	1 medium	
Salad	1 bowl	
Lettuce	1 wedge	
Bread and Cereal Group		
Bread	1 slice	4, whole grain or enriched only,
Cooked cereal	½ to ¾ cup	including at least one serving of
Pasta	½ to ¾ cup	whole grain
Rice	½ to ¾ cup	
Dry cereal	1 ounce	

*These amounts were established by the U.S. Department of Agriculture to meet specific nutritional requirements. For the milk group, serving sizes are based on the calcium content of 1 cup of milk. For the meat group, serving size is determined by protein content. Thus, rather than eat 2 cups of cottage cheese (milk group) or 4 tablespoons of peanut butter (meat group), it would make more sense to eat half those amounts and count each as half a serving in their respective groups. If cottage cheese (½ cup) is consumed as a meat substitute, you may count it as a full meat serving and a quarter of a milk serving.

Source: Jane Brody, *Jane Brody's Nutrition Book* (New York: Norton, 1981), p. 18.

A Suitable Diet

Every person's body uses food in a unique way, for different people metabolize food (turn it into energy) at varying rates, and their ability to digest foods, their levels of activity, and their eating habits also vary. A diet that is right for one person may therefore be unsuitable for another.

Eating habits are very important, because over time people and their bodies adapt to shortages and excesses of certain nutrients in their diets. These shortages and excesses are sometimes the result of cultural patterns, and sometimes of personal habits. In the United States, for example, diets commonly lack enough of certain vitamins because most Americans do not like to eat the fruits and vegetables that are rich in these vitamins. Moreover, one American does not like to eat this, another does not like to eat that. If these individual and social dietary deficiencies are not very great, most people's bodies can adjust to them. This "nutritional conditioning" makes it difficult to define a single optimum diet for a hypothetical person representing an average of all people. Before the science of nutrition can define the best possible diet for a person, it must learn more about the effects of nutritional conditioning, especially in early childhood, and how that early conditioning affects people throughout their lives.

Recommended Dietary Allowance (RDA)

Despite the basic problem of establishing dietary requirements that are perfect for everyone, the U.S. government has tried to determine how much of many nutrients is needed by four population groups: infants (birth to 12 months); children under 4 years of age; children over the age of 4 and adults; and pregnant and nursing women. For each of these groups the government suggests a so-called Recommended Dietary Allowance (RDA) of the nutrients. These allowances (except the one for calories) tend to be set a little high, so that anyone who follows them will get enough. But people who are sick or undernourished may need more or less than the RDA of some nutrients.

Vegetarianism

Throughout history, poverty has made many of the world's people vegetarians. But more and more people are now taking up vegetarianism as a matter of choice. It is possible for vegetarians to get enough of the essential nutrients, but it is harder for them than for meat eaters, so vegetarians have to be much more careful.

Some vegetarian diets are simply dangerous, for instance, the Zen macrobiotic diet, which in its most extreme form puts its followers on a regimen of cooked brown rice. Those who adopt a vegetarian diet should be sure they are still getting enough proteins by eating eggs and

Recommended Daily Dietary Allowances,[a] Revised 1980

Food and Nutrition Board, National Academy of Sciences – National Research Council

Designed for the maintenance of good nutrition of practically all healthy people in the U.S.A.

	Age (years)	Weight (kg)	Weight (lbs)	Height (cm)	Height (in)	Protein (g)	Fat-Soluble Vitamins			Water-Soluble Vitamins							Minerals					
							Vitamin A (µg RE)[b]	Vitamin D (µg)[c]	Vitamin E (mg α TE)[d]	Vitamin C (mg)	Thiamin (mg)	Riboflavin (mg)	Niacin (mg NE)[e]	Vitamin B6 (mg)	Folacin (µg)[f]	Vitamin B12 (µg)	Calcium (mg)	Phosphorus (mg)	Magnesium (mg)	Iron (mg)	Zinc (mg)	Iodine (µg)
Infants	0.0-0.5	6	13	60	24	kg × 2.2	420	10	3	35	0.3	0.4	6	0.3	30	0.5[g]	360	240	50	10	3	40
	0.5-1.0	9	20	71	28	kg × 2.0	400	10	4	35	0.5	0.6	8	0.6	45	1.5	540	360	70	15	5	50
Children	1-3	13	29	90	35	23	400	10	5	45	0.7	0.8	9	0.9	100	2.0	800	800	150	15	10	70
	4-6	20	44	112	44	30	500	10	6	45	0.9	1.0	11	1.3	200	2.5	800	800	200	10	10	90
	7-10	28	62	132	52	34	700	10	7	45	1.2	1.4	16	1.6	300	3.0	800	800	250	10	10	120
Males	11-14	45	99	157	62	45	1000	10	8	50	1.4	1.6	18	1.8	400	3.0	1200	1200	350	18	15	150
	15-18	66	145	176	69	56	1000	10	10	60	1.4	1.7	18	2.0	400	3.0	1200	1200	400	18	15	150
	19-22	70	154	177	70	56	1000	7.5	10	60	1.5	1.7	19	2.2	400	3.0	800	800	350	10	15	150
	23-50	70	154	178	70	56	1000	5	10	60	1.4	1.6	18	2.2	400	3.0	800	800	350	10	15	150
	51+	70	154	178	70	56	1000	5	10	60	1.2	1.4	16	2.2	400	3.0	800	800	350	10	15	150
Females	11-14	46	101	157	62	46	800	10	8	50	1.1	1.3	15	1.8	400	3.0	1200	1200	300	18	15	150
	15-18	55	120	163	64	46	800	10	8	60	1.1	1.3	14	2.0	400	3.0	1200	1200	300	18	15	150
	19-22	55	120	163	64	44	800	7.5	8	60	1.1	1.3	14	2.0	400	3.0	800	800	300	18	15	150
	23-50	55	120	163	64	44	800	5	8	60	1.0	1.2	13	2.0	400	3.0	800	800	300	18	15	150
	51+	55	120	163	64	44	800	5	8	60	1.0	1.2	13	2.0	400	3.0	800	800	300	10	15	150
Pregnant						+30	+200	+5	+2	+20	+0.4	+0.3	+2	+0.6	+400	+1.0	+400	+400	+150	h	+5	+25
Lactating						+20	+400	+5	+3	+40	+0.5	+0.5	+5	+0.5	+100	+1.0	+400	+400	+150	h	+10	+50

a The allowances are intended to provide for individual variations among most normal persons as they live in the United States under usual environmental stresses. Diets should be based on a variety of common foods in order to provide other nutrients for which human requirements have been less well defined. See p. 23 for heights weights and recommended intake.

b Retinol equivalents. 1 Retinol equivalent = 1 µg retinol or 6 µg β carotene. See text for calculation.

c As cholecalciferol. 10 µg cholecalciferol = 400 I.U. vitamin D.

d α-tocopherol equivalents. 1 mg d-α-tocopherol = 1 α T.E. See text for variation in allowances and calculation of vitamin E activity of the diet as α-tocopherol equivalents.

e 1 N.E. (niacin equivalent) is equal to 1 mg of niacin or 60 mg of dietary tryptophan.

f The folacin allowances refer to dietary sources as determined by Lactobacillus casei assay after treatment with enzymes (conjugases) to make polyglutamyl forms of the vitamin available to the test organism.

g The RDA for vitamin B12 in infants is based on average concentration of the vitamin in human milk. The allowances after weaning are based on energy intake (as recommended by the American Academy of Pediatrics) and consideration of other factors such as intestinal absorption. see text.

h The increased requirement during pregnancy cannot be met by the iron content of habitual American diets nor by the existing iron stores of many women. therefore the use of 30-60 mg of supplemental iron is recommended. Iron needs during lactation are not substantially different from those of non-pregnant women. but continued supplementation of the mother for 2-3 months after parturition is advisable in order to replenish stores depleted by pregnancy.

various kinds of dairy products. They should also reduce the number of "empty" calories they eat. (Empty calories come from foods—for example, soda and alcohol—that provide calories but few or no nutrients.)

Nutritional Fallacies

Food can be pleasurable for the person who eats it and profitable for the people who supply it. Pleasure and money are the two chief breeding grounds of myths and fallacies. And food is a subject that abounds in them.

Misinformation

The catalog of nutritional nonsense is so long that no book could ever do justice to it. Here are a few of the most common errors:

- Vitamins and minerals provide energy. Wrong: Energy is produced when fats, carbohydrates, and proteins are metabolized. We need vitamins and minerals for good health, but, no, they do not provide energy.
- Carbohydrates are more fattening than proteins and fats are. Wrong: Ounce for ounce, carbohydrates have the same number of calories as protein.
- You need nutritional supplements every day to stay healthy. Wrong: A well-chosen diet, one that includes the right number of servings from each major food group, supplies all the nutrients you need. Taking some vitamins and minerals to excess can be harmful.
- "Vitamin-enriched" products are more healthy. Wrong again: First, the extra vitamins may be useless or even harmful. And some vitamin-enriched products, like prepared cereals, also contain a great deal of sugar. Eating them is therefore not terribly good for your health, no matter how many vitamins they contain.

Food Quackery

Sometimes misinformation about food is worked up into a system. The U.S. government estimates that more than 10 million Americans spend more than $500 million a year on nutritional nostrums. Taken together, vitamin products, organic foods, special dietary foods, and food supplements may be the most expensive kind of quackery (see Chapter 18) in the United States. The reason is simply that there is a great deal of money to be made by promises of health, beauty and long life—whether they are true or false.

Fad diets, one of the major forms of nutritional quackery, are described in Chapter 9. Vegetarianism is not in principle a system of quackery, although in its extreme forms it can be. *Organic foods,* foods grown without chemical pesticides or fertilizers, should be viewed with suspicion: They have no more nutrients than ordinary foods do and often cost twice as much. Besides, foods grown with chemicals do not differ in appearance from organic foods, for the most part, so you can never really know that what you are buying is organic.

Malnutrition

Nutritional fallacies are one reason for poor nutrition. Poverty is another, yet so too is wealth. How can this be?

We saw in Chapter 7, Exercise, that the body needs energy to function. The body gets its energy from food, and that energy is measured in calories (see Chapter 9 for a fuller explanation). In the course of merely staying alive an adult uses up almost one calorie an hour for each kilogram (2.2 pounds) of body weight—59 calories an hour, for example, for a person of 130 pounds. Physically demanding activities (like swimming and basketball) use up more calories than sitting still does.

Since the very beginning of human life, many (perhaps most) people have gotten fewer calories than they needed. In the past, only rich people got more than they needed. Today in the United States, eating too much and getting too many calories is no longer a privilege of the rich. Both those who get too many calories and those who get too few have a problem—a problem called *malnutrition*, which simply means

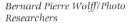
Bernard Pierre Wolff/Photo Researchers

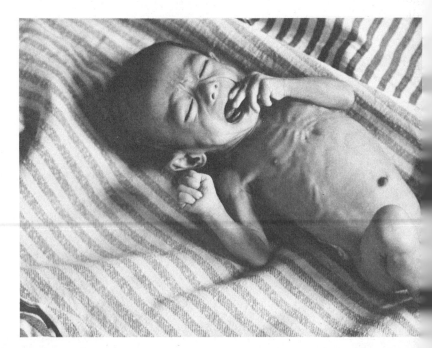

any deviation from a person's caloric needs. *Undernutrition* is the more narrow term: It means the deficiency of nutrients that accompanies a deficiency of calories. In plain English, it is starvation.

Undernutrition

The effects of undernutrition are catastrophic, especially when it begins in infancy or childhood. Starving children weigh less and do not achieve their full adult height—if they survive to adulthood, which they often do not. Their lives are shorter, on average, than the lives of people who were fed adequately as children. Their mental development is set back, sometimes irreversibly, for childhood malnutrition prevents the full complement of brain cells from developing.

Overconsumption

You have already read how this country's eating habits have changed, mainly for the worse. Overconsumption of fats and refined sugars—and of all the other nutrients—is an important cause of disease in this country.

How important could improved nutrition be? Consider these facts: One out of every three men in this country dies of heart disease or stroke (see Chapter 10) before the age of 60. One in every six women can expect the same fate. Perhaps 25 million people suffer from high blood pressure and almost 5 million from diabetes (see Chapter 10). A government report estimates that a real improvement in the national diet could reduce heart and vascular disease by 25 percent. Though some of the evidence linking disease with diet is still controversial, there is very little doubt that improved nutrition can make you healthier and perhaps wealthier (through reduced medical costs), if not wiser. Here are some of the things you can do:

- Keep your consumption of carbohydrates to about 55 to 60 percent of your total intake of calories. Make sure that a substantial proportion (40–45 percent) comes from complex carbohydrates: whole grains, fruits, and vegetables.
- Reduce overall fat consumption.
- Keep your consumption of saturated fats to about 10 percent of your total intake of calories; polyunsaturated fats should account for another 10 percent. Substitute nonfat milk for whole milk. Eat little of foods rich in cholesterol, such as butterfat and eggs.
- Keep sugar consumption at about 15 percent of your total intake of calories.
- Keep salt consumption at 3 or so grams a day. (A gram of salt is about one-third of a teaspoon.)
- Eat more fish and poultry than other kinds of meat.

Shopping

As we have noted in many places in this book, ours is a time of great choices. Before the invention of the train (in the early 19th century), most foods could not travel more than a few miles without spoiling, so even the richest people were mainly restricted to the foods grown in their own areas. Today, trains, ships, and planes bring all of us the foods of every country in the world. Since we have so much to choose from, life has become more difficult, but also more rich. Some choices have little to recommend them: It is a commonplace today that food often is less tasty than it used to be. Anyone who has ever eaten a garden tomato and a "corporate tomato" knows that this is not mere nostalgia. That is why you should think as you shop. Here are some simple and useful guidelines:

- Check the unit price of a brand—its price for each unit of weight or volume—and compare it with the unit price of other brands. Unit price is the truest measure of cost. Larger sizes often have lower unit prices.

- Remember that generic and unadvertised products and private labels (those sold under the retailer's name) can often save you money and may be comparable in quality to nationally advertised brands.

- Be aware of the cost of convenience foods. Generally, they cost more than their fresh counterparts, contain additives for longer shelf life, and have fewer nutrients because of their commercial processing.

- Learn to calculate the cost per serving of cooked meat, as opposed to the price per pound of the same meat before cooking. Bone, fat, and waste make a big difference in what you really get for your dollar.

- When you buy fruits and vegetables, buy in season. Do without items when they are in short supply. The later into the season you buy fresh fruit and vegetables, the cheaper they are.

- Look at the date stamped on a product to ensure some freshness. This is the last date on which it may be sold.

- Be sure to check the ingredients of all the packaged foods you buy; the law requires that they be listed from the ingredient of greatest amount to that of least amount. Many foods also come with nutritional information.

Do not be influenced by advertising: Advertisements tell you little about the true nutritional value of foods. The most heavily advertised foods are often the least nutritious (and the most expensive for each serving).

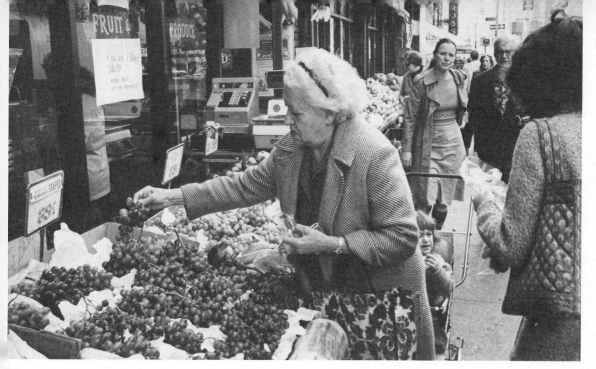

Christa Armstrong/Photo
Researchers

SUMMARY

The human body needs some 50 nutrients, including different
kinds of fats, proteins, vitamins, minerals, and carbohydrates; and
water. You can get these nutrients from the four basic food
groups: meats, fruits and vegetables, grains, and milk. Your daily
diet should include appropriate servings from each group. No diet
suits everyone, because metabolism and past food habits, which
are unique to each person, shape each person's nutritional needs
as an adult.

Some of the nutrients—fats, carbohydrates, and proteins—are
used by the body to provide energy. The energy content of food is
measured in calories. People who do not get enough calories suffer—terribly—from undernutrition, and people who get too many
calories become overweight. Both undernutrition and overconsumption, and the medical problems associated with them, are
found in the United States.

Pleasure and profit give rise to food fads and food quackery.
One way to make sure you buy food wisely is to read the information printed on food packages, information that describes the ingredients and nutritional content; another way is to buy only fresh
foods and prepare them yourself.

Suggested Readings

Caliendo, Mary Alice. *Nutrition and Preventive Health Care.* New York: Macmillan, 1981. Discusses the relationships among food, health, and disease. Delves into the U.S. health-care system, the American diet, and issues in nutrition education.

Meded, Medical Education Programs, Ltd. *The Medicine Called Nutrition.* Englewood Cliffs, N.J.: Best Foods, 1980. A comprehensive source about contemporary nutrition, how it helps to prevent diseases, and how it helps to treat them.

Runyon, Thora J. *Nutrition for Today.* New York: Harper & Row, 1976. Provides basic information on nutrition and presents an interesting view of the social and natural sciences on nutrition.

Wenck, Dorothy, Baren, Martin, and Dewan, Sat Paul. *Nutrition.* Reston, Va.: Reston, 1980. Includes a 37-page chart of the nutritive value of foods. Devotes a chapter to practical suggestions on how to obtain the dietary goals of nutrition.

Whitney, Eleanor, and Hamilton, Eva May. *Understanding Nutrition.* St. Paul: West, 1977. A very readable yet technical presentation of the science of nutrition. An excellent resource for those interested in detailed information.

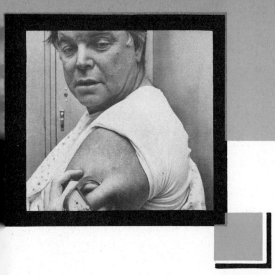

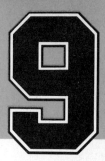

Weight Control

chapter objectives

When you have finished reading this chapter you should be able to:

1. Appraise your weight and apply sound diet and exercise practices to maintain a desirable weight
2. Recall the causes of obesity
3. Evaluate popular diets
4. Recognize that a physician's supervision is needed in any effort to lose a great deal of weight
5. Recognize that there are many ways of losing weight, some better than others

Perhaps 40 percent of the people of the United States are not on good terms with the bathroom scale. Of course, no specific weight is ideal for everyone; your "ideal weight" has to take into account your height, sex, age, level of activity, and build. Most people who weigh more than they should are only moderately overweight—between 10 and 25 percent over the ideal. But a minority of overweight people have a more serious problem—*obesity.* Obesity is not a matter of weight but of body fat. Between 10 and 14 percent of an average male college student's total weight consists of body fat—between 16 and 20 percent for the average female college student. Men who have 25 percent more body fat than the average, and women who have 30 percent more of it, are obese. Not all cases of overweight are caused by excess fat, for a heavily muscled person weighs more than a lightly muscled person of the same height.

Obesity is a disease; it has symptoms. People who are obese may tire easily, and they may often be short of breath and have pains in their legs, back, and feet. More than people of average weight, they suffer from hypertension and heart attacks (see Chapter 10), gall bladder and liver diseases, diabetes (see Chapter 10), appendicitis, and other serious diseases. They may suffer mentally, too, because our culture has imposed rigid limitations on what is portrayed as attractive or acceptable. Therefore they may feel unattractive and may withdraw from social contacts.

Dieting: A Way of Life

We saw in Chapter 7 that to be successful, an exercise program has to become part of your life, not a rare and marvelous event. That is also true of dieting. People who look for "secret" diets are looking for frauds. The real and fundamental facts about weight control are well known and are not controversial. These facts are as follows: The food

BLONDIE
© *King Features Syndicate, Inc.*

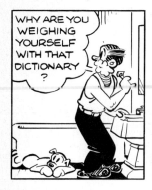
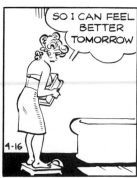
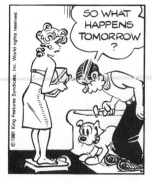
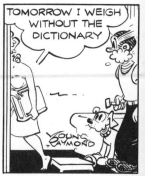

Metropolitan Life Insurance Company Table of Desirable Weights (in Pounds) for Men and Women of Ages 25 and Over (Indoor Clothing)

Height (with shoes on— 1-in. heels)	Small Frame	Medium Frame	Large Frame
Men			
5 ft. 2 in.	112–120	118–129	126–141
5 ft. 3 in.	115–123	121–133	129–144
5 ft. 4 in.	118–126	124–136	132–148
5 ft. 5 in.	121–129	127–139	135–152
5 ft. 6 in.	124–133	130–143	138–156
5 ft. 7 in.	128–137	134–147	142–161
5 ft. 8 in.	132–141	138–152	147–166
5 ft. 9 in.	136–145	142–156	151–170
5 ft. 10 in.	140–150	146–160	155–174
5 ft. 11 in.	144–154	150–165	159–179
6 ft. 0 in.	148–158	154–170	164–184
6 ft. 1 in.	152–162	158–175	168–189
6 ft. 2 in.	156–167	162–180	173–194
6 ft. 3 in.	160–171	167–185	178–199
6 ft. 4 in.	164–175	172–190	182–204
Women			
4 ft. 10 in.	92–98	96–107	104–119
4 ft. 11 in.	94–101	98–110	106–122
5 ft. 0 in.	96–104	101–113	109–125
5 ft. 1 in.	99–107	104–116	112–128
5 ft. 2 in.	102–110	107–119	115–131
5 ft. 3 in.	105–113	110–122	118–134
5 ft. 4 in.	108–116	113–126	121–138
5 ft. 5 in.	111–119	116–130	125–142
5 ft. 6 in.	114–123	120–135	129–146
5 ft. 7 in.	118–127	124–139	133–150
5 ft. 8 in.	122–131	128–143	137–154
5 ft. 9 in.	126–135	132–147	141–158
5 ft. 10 in.	130–140	136–151	145–163
5 ft. 11 in.	134–144	140–155	149–168
6 ft. 0 in.	138–148	144–159	153–173

Note: For women between 18 and 25, subtract 1 lb. for each year under 25.
Source: The Metropolitan Life Insurance Company.

we eat provides the energy that the body and its organs need to function. The body has the ability to store energy for times when additional amounts of it are needed, and for times when food is scarce. But this ability is the root of the weight problem, since body fat is the form in which energy is stored. It is stored in this way when you take in more potential energy (food) than you use through physical exertion. *The way to lose weight is to make sure that your intake of energy (food) does not exceed your output of it (physical exertion). You can—and should— do this in two ways: By eating less food but more of the right kinds of food, and by getting more physical exercise.*

This is the truth, the whole truth, and nothing but the truth. When you hear or read anything else, ignore it.

Metabolism.   We have seen that the way you use energy through physical exertion helps to determine whether or not you gain weight. But the rate at which the body uses energy is only in part—though in large part—determined by conscious, and therefore controllable, activities like exercise. It is also determined by each person's *metabolism—* the chemical reactions within each cell that transform nutrients (see Chapter 8) into energy. The rate of metabolism varies from person to person and also from time to time. It is easiest to determine the rate of a person's metabolism when that person is awake but at rest. This *basal metabolic rate* (BMR) is the minimum expenditure of energy needed to maintain the activities of the cells and such functions as respiration (breathing) and circulation (of the blood). Generally, the higher the BMR, the more rapidly will the body use its fuel, or food. The unjust and unfair facts are that people with high BMRs can eat more and exercise less, without getting fat, than people with low BMRs.

Causes of Overweight

Perhaps as many as 15 percent of all children and teenagers are seriously overweight, and among adults the percentage is even greater. Why do some people manage to balance their inputs and outputs of energy, while others do not?

Genetic Causes

Genetic Traits.   Among the physical traits we inherit is *body type,* or *body build.* Some people tend to be plump, while others have a slimmer, taller body build. People who tend toward plumpness, the *endomorphs,* need to watch their weight much more than do people who are slender, the *ectomorphs.* People who are muscular, the *mesomorphs,* are also less likely to have weight problems than endomorphs. Few people are just one type; most everyone has some traits of each.

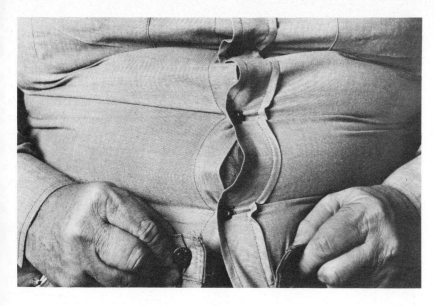

Bob Adelman

Is Obesity Inherited?   Studies have shown that about 75 percent of the children of two obese parents are obese themselves. If only one parent is obese about 50 percent of the children are also obese. If neither parent is obese only about 9 percent of the children are obese. These statistics do not really show whether obesity (or overweight in general) is inherited genetically, because families pass on their eating, exercise, and work habits—all of which are cultural, or environmental—as well as their genes (see Chapter 13).

Physiological Causes

Some researchers believe that people become overweight and obese because the appetite-control mechanism of their brains, the apostat, fails to work correctly. When a normal person eats, the apostat responds by shutting down the appetite. When it fails to do this, the result is often excessive eating and thus overweight.

Environmental Causes

As we just saw, families transmit ways of behaving to their members. So, too, does each culture. Overweight and obesity, even if they result in part from genetic or physiological causes, also can be traced to the lessons we learn from our culture.

The Convenience Culture.   In office buildings we ride elevators rather than walk up one or two flights of stairs; parents drive their kids to the neighbor's instead of telling them to ride bikes or walk; home gardeners use power mowers rather than old-fashioned blade mowers.

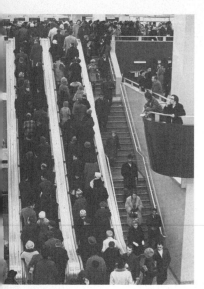

The easy life.
George E. Jones III / Photo Researchers

Alas, Americans have become less and less active, and they have become more and more reliant on machines—especially the automobile—to do the work their ancestors had to do with their own muscles.

As if this profusion of conveniences were not problem enough, Americans now eat foods high in fat and in refined starches and sugars—all of which are high in calories (see Chapter 8). They are eating fewer of the foods called complex carbohydrates—whole grains, fruits, and vegetables—foods that have fewer calories and greater nutritional value. This combination of less physical exertion and more empty calories has left many Americans "overweight and out-of-shape."

Infant Overfeeding.   Plump babies have commonly been regarded as healthy babies. That is why some parents overfeed their babies—mainly bottle-fed babies—and encourage them to overeat. Babies who eat more food than they need—especially during the first six weeks of life—are likely to become overweight or obese in their teens. Some studies indicate that as many as 80 percent of overweight children become obese adults.

Psychological Causes

In Unit One and Unit Two you read about many kinds of behavior—drug taking, for instance, that can be used as ways of coping with stress. Overeating is yet another coping strategy. In other words, it can be used to fight loneliness, frustration, anger, depression, and other unhappy feelings. But as overeaters gain more and more weight their self-images may wane, for our culture glorifies slimness; then all the problems that caused them to overeat in the first place may become even worse.

Some overweight and obese people handle their emotional problems through "game playing" (see Chapter 3). The object of the game is self-deception. For example, game-players may pretend that dieting would be futile because their metabolisms are too low to permit them to lose weight. Some game-players try to blame their excess weight on others or on life problems they use as an excuse to avoid dieting.

Game playing is sometimes used by psychologists to help overweight and obese patients lose weight by consciously acting out their games and thus gaining insights into their behavior.

Diets and Dieting

We saw in Chapter 8 that pleasure in eating and the desire to make money from it have joined to create a flourishing subculture of nutritional nonsense. Now, *all* human pleasures and wishes have created special classes of businesses to cater to them, and the wish to lose weight is no exception. And in this field, too, the nonsense is very great.

SELF-ASSESSMENT DEVICE 9-1: ARE YOU OVERWEIGHT?

The chart below provides a fairly simple way to determine whether you are overweight. Find your weight in the left-hand column and your height in the right-hand column, and draw a straight line between the two numbers. If it falls within the "acceptable" range, in the middle of the chart, your weight is all right. If the line falls in the overweight or obese range, consult a physician.

This chart can only give you an idea of whether you are overweight. It is not a scientific measure of healthful weight. Even if you come out in the "acceptable" range on the chart, talk to your physician if you think you may have a weight problem.

Here's another simple test to determine whether you are overweight: Pinch the skinfold on the back of your upper arm, beside your navel, or on your back, just below the shoulder blade. If you get more than one inch you are probably overweight.

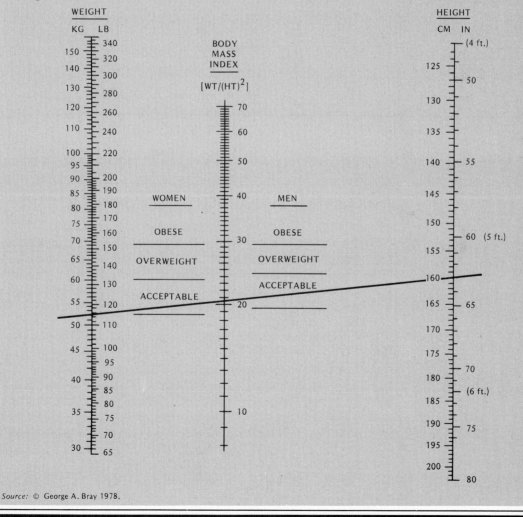

Source: © George A. Bray 1978.

The Dieter's Secret Prayer

Many dieters have a secret prayer: "Please let me lose weight without having to eat less—or exercise more." That prayer was seemingly answered some time ago in a diet pill, one that many people must have bought in the belief that they would be liberated from any need for self-control. The package, at any rate, said nothing about dieting. But when you bought the package and opened it up you found a circular discreetly tucked into it. In the circular the manufacturer recommended that the would-be weight loser hold down calories to a fairly strict thousand or so a day. The appetite-control aids were *supposed* to make it easy for dieters to do so, but the product was not effective. Dieters were left, once again, to go one-on-one with the calorie.

The dieting public, though, remains steadfast in its yearning to lose weight instantly and permanently, without effort. So far, the only people lucky enough to attain anything like an instant loss of weight are the astronauts; and they, of course, regain their weight as soon as they reenter Earth's atmosphere. Nonetheless, the dieter's prayer keeps diet pills on the market.

Beware of all nonprescription diet preparations. And be cautious about prescription products handed out by physicians. Some prescription products may be helpful in getting dieters started, but in the long run, only healthy eating habits and regular physical activity keep the pounds off.

But if you really do want to lose weight, the road, although straight and narrow, is yet clear and certain.

Fad Diets: How to Go Nowhere Fast

High-protein diet, low-carbohydrate diet, high-fat diet, low-fat diet, Scarsdale diet, Atkins diet . . . there seems to be no shortage of choices. Some of these diets promote one kind of nutrient (fats, carbohydrates, or proteins), and others prohibit the eating of foods from one food group or other. But most nutrition experts believe that a well-balanced diet—one that contains low- to moderate-calorie foods from *all four* food groups (see Chapter 8)—is essential for good health.

Many fad diets cannot be followed safely for more than a few weeks. Nor is a fad diet likely to be geared to your particular dieting needs—needs based on your present weight, the amount of exercise you do or may be able to do, and your medical history. And fad diets do not teach you new eating habits that help you maintain a healthful weight for many years to come. Fad diets do not often make claims about their effects in the long run; instead they promise to help you lose weight right at the start—and quickly. And often, people on fad diets *do* lose several pounds in the first week or two—but what they are losing is water, not fat. In the first stages of a diet, notes Jean Mayer (1920-   ), a famous nutritionist, as your actual consumption of calories falls below your body's energy needs, you will first start to use up the small stores of glycogen [stored carbohydrates] in your liver and muscle to get the glucose it [your body] needs for energy. When that's gone, you begin to burn up your fat, but you also break down some of the protein in your lean body tissue. Later on, usually in a week or two, the loss of protein stops and your body will finally be utilizing more and more of that excess fat for its energy. This is the point you've been working toward in your reducing diet.

Meanwhile [before the fat loss begins], you will probably have shed pounds according to the bathroom scale. But where did those pounds come from? Well, the glycogen in your liver and muscles and the protein in your lean tissue exist in combination with water. When the glycogen and the protein go, so does the water. In this way, you lose water weight in those beginning weeks without actually dropping fat.[1]

What this means is that diets that do not get you to continue dieting beyond 4 weeks or so—and fad diets often do not—will not have much effect on your figure.

And what about the claim of some fad diets that "calories don't count"? As Mayer points out, it is really a question of who is doing the counting. If a diet specifies the precise amounts of each food you can eat at each sitting, the calories have already been calculated by the diet maker, at least if the diet is at all rational.

Let us take a look at the major types of fad diets.

High-protein.   On a high-protein diet you would eat mostly meat, fish, chicken, eggs, cheese, and so on (see Chapter 8). The idea is that eating large quantities of proteins—and also fats, since many high-protein foods are also high in fats—causes the body to rid itself of a good deal of water. It is a good bet, therefore, that the weight you lose on a high-protein diet is mainly water. And since the high-protein diet discourages you from eating large quantities of fruits, vegetables, and whole grains, you would be missing important vitamins and minerals, and not getting enough fiber. Too much protein, besides, can cause severe problems in people with kidney conditions, for it forces the kidneys to work overtime excreting the nitrogen found in the protein.

On a "liquid-protein" diet, you get most of your nourishment from a bottle of processed protein—which is low in some vitamins, minerals, and fiber—not from real food. A number of deaths have been associated with such products.

Low-carbohydrate.   Low-carbohydrate diets are in some ways similar to high-protein diets: They are both short on vitamins and minerals, since you have to avoid grain products, fruits, and vegetables.

[1]Jean Mayer, "The Fad Diet Bust," *Family Health* 10, No. 7, pp. 42–43, n.d.

High-carbohydrate. On a high-carbohydrate diet, it is proteins and fats that are given short shrift. Of course, the complex carbohydrates—fruits, vegetables, and whole grains—are very nutritious and *should* be a prominent part of almost any diet (see Chapter 8). But sticking almost exclusively to carbohydrates can cause trouble for people with hypoglycemia or diabetes (see Chapter 10). And, of course, many high-carbohydrate foods—especially sweets—are high in calories.

High-fat. It may seem odd, but eating a lot of foods that are rich in fats—butter, cream, and vegetable oils, for instance—can make you lose weight quickly, even though fats are high in calories (see Chapter 8).

The reason is that eating too much fat causes diarrhea. Much of the fat is therefore eliminated from the body—undigested—along with vitamins, minerals, and other important nutrients. Of course, on a high-fat diet you probably would not be getting enough of those nutrients in the first place. High-fat diets are quite dangerous.

Low-fat.   A low-fat diet, like all the other diets that prohibit one thing or stress another, is simply not well-balanced. Fats are needed for energy; they protect the skin and other parts of the body, and they are vital to the body's metabolism.

Macrobiotic.   The macrobiotic diet excludes all foods of animal origin and, when practiced most strictly, comprises sesame seeds and seaweed. Several deaths have been attributed to this diet.

Diet Pills.   All the fad diets we have discussed are *unhealthy* diets, but at least they *are* diets: They introduce awareness and order into eating, albeit the wrong kind of awareness and order. Diet pills do not even do that; they claim to release the dieter from the need to make any conscious choices at all—by suppressing the appetite. Do the pills work? Are they safe? Independent studies suggest that diet pills offer little, if any, help in controlling weight.

Dieting Gone Mad

Most people start to diet because they want to feel better about themselves. But for a certain kind of young woman, mostly between the ages of 10 and 20, the decision to go on a diet initiates a kind of hate affair with herself, in the form of a psychological condition called *anorexia nervosa*. It is not that these young women do not get hungry; they do, but simply forbid themselves to take in more than a handful of calories a day. For them, the goal of dieting is not merely to lose a certain number of pounds to reach the weight suitable for their height and body build. Losing weight becomes instead an end in itself, an obsession, a mania. Eventually the anorectic's limbs become as thin as the celery that is often her only regular food.

Some anorectics seem to be driven by self-hatred, by an attempt to punish themselves through self-denial. Others have had unpleasant experiences with boys or men or may be afraid of their own developing sexuality—a sexuality they try to escape from by becoming thinner and thinner. Still others may be trying to punish someone, especially parents. (Some young women resent it when their parents suggest that they weigh too much. The daughter becomes anorectic and thus obeys her parents and, at the same time, defies them.)

Many victims of anorexia can be treated through psychotherapy (see Chapter 3). But for some, the course of self-starvation progresses all the way to death.

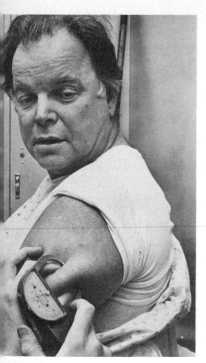

If you fail the pinch test . . .
Bob Adelman

When dieters stop taking the pills, they often regain any weight they might have lost. And like all strong drugs, diet pills can have serious side effects, including allergic reactions, addiction to the pills themselves, and high blood pressure with all its symptoms.

A Real *Diet*

Does *anything* work? And now for the good news: Yes! Despite all the mumbo-jumbo and sheer fraud that surrounds dieting, the keys to weight reduction are sure and simple. You can influence your body weight in two ways: by controlling your intake of energy, that is, food, and by controlling your output of energy, that is, physical exertion. The way to lose weight is to ensure that your energy output exceeds your energy input. You can control your energy output by exercising systematically (see Chapter 7). You can control your energy input by remembering that *calories do count,* for calories are simply the measure of the energy contained in food. The more energy you take in, the more energy you will need to burn up—or you will gain weight.

If your weight causes you concern; if you feel you have problems because you are fat; if you tire easily because you are carrying extra pounds; if you find that your weight is more than 20 percent greater than the weights set for your height (see chart); if you fail the pinch test —it is time to lose a few pounds.

How Much, How Soon?   If you are moderately overweight, losing 1 or 2 pounds a week is sensible and realistic. To lose 1 pound a week you must burn up 3,500 calories without replacing them. Each pound of body fat is the equivalent of 3,500 calories. To lose one pound you must reduce caloric intake or increase your level of activity enough to burn this amount. This means taking in 500 fewer calories a day (3,500 calo-

Table 9–1.   Daily Caloric Requirements*

Age in Years	Males	Females
1–3	1,300	1,300
4–6	1,700	1,700
7–10	2,400	2,400
11–14	2,700	2,200
15–18	2,800	2,100
19–22	2,900	2,100
23–50	2,700	2,000
51–75	2,400	1,800
76+	2,050	1,600

*These are average requirements for typical work levels. A person's basic, or basal, requirement per day, merely to survive, is about 1,650 calories. Moderate activity can increase the daily requirement by 500–600 calories; laborers and athletes may need as much as 3,500–6,000 more than the average requirement per day. (Dale Hanson, *Health Related Fitness.* Belmont, Calif.: Wadsworth, 1970.)
Source: Food and Nutrition Board, National Academy of Sciences-National Research Council, *Recommended Dietary Allowances*, 9th ed. (Washington, D.C.: National Academy of Sciences, 1979.)

Table 9–2. Amount of Exercise Needed to Burn Up Certain Foods

Food	Calories	Running	Tennis (Singles)	Swimming	Riding Bicycle	Walking	Reclining
Apple, large	101	5	8	9	12	19	78
Bacon, 2 strips	96	5	8	9	12	18	74
Banana, small	88	4	7	8	11	17	68
Beans, green, 1 cup	27	1	1	2	3	5	21
Beer, 1 glass	114	6	9	10	14	22	88
Bread and butter	78	4	6	7	10	15	60
Cake, 2 layer, 1/12	356	18	31	32	43	68	274
Carbonated beverage, 1 glass	106	5	8	9	13	20	82
Carrot, raw	42	2	3	4	5	8	32
Cereal, dry, ½ cup, with milk, sugar	200	10	17	18	24	38	154
Cheese, cottage, 1 tbsp.	27	1	1	2	3	5	21
Cheese, Cheddar, 1 oz.	111	6	9	10	14	21	85
Chicken, fried, ½ breast	232	12	20	21	28	45	178
Chicken, TV dinner	542	28	47	48	66	104	417
Cookie, plain	15	1	1	1	2	3	12
Cookie, chocolate chip	51	3	4	5	6	10	39
Doughnut	151	8	12	13	18	29	116
Egg, fried	110	6	9	10	13	21	85
Egg, boiled	77	4	6	7	9	15	59
French dressing, 1 tbsp.	59	3	4	5	7	11	45
Halibut steak, ¼ lb.	205	11	17	18	25	39	158
Ham, 2 slices	167	9	14	15	20	32	128
Ice Cream, 1/6 qt.	193	10	16	17	24	37	148
Ice Cream Soda	255	13	22	23	31	49	196
Ice Milk, 1/6 qt.	144	7	12	13	18	28	111
Gelatin, with cream	117	6	9	10	14	23	90
Malted milk shake	502	26	44	45	61	97	386
Mayonnaise, 1 tbsp.	92	5	7	8	11	18	71
Milk, 1 glass	166	9	14	15	20	32	128
Milk, skim, 1 glass	81	4	6	7	10	16	62
Milk shake	421	22	37	38	51	81	324
Orange, medium	68	4	5	6	8	13	52
Orange juice, 1 glass	120	6	10	11	15	23	92
Pancake with syrup	124	6	10	11	15	24	95
Peach, medium	46	2	3	4	6	9	35
Peas, green, ½ cup	56	3	4	5	7	11	43
Pie, apple, 1/6	377	19	33	34	46	73	290

Source: Neil Solomon, M.D., Ph. D., with Sally Sheppard, *The Truth about Weight Control: How to Lose Weight Permanently* (Briarcliff Manor, N.Y.: Stein & Day, 1971), p. 147.

ries ÷ 7 days) than you have been doing—either by eating 500 fewer calories *or* by increasing your physical activity enough to burn up 500 calories. You can also combine a reduced calorie intake with increased physical activity. In fact, this is the best way to lose weight.

Meals and Snacks.   Avoid heavy meals, especially in the evening. It is generally better to eat three or four low- to moderate-calorie meals than to skimp on breakfast and lunch, then gorge at dinner. It is all right to eat snacks as long as you remember to include them in the total number of calories you eat each day. (By the way, an apple is just as filling as a bag of potato chips and has many fewer calories. It also has some vitamins, minerals, and water—all of which will help keep you nourished while you are "eating less." There are many other exchanges you can make.)

To figure out how much to eat at each meal, first find how many calories you are eating now, and then subtract 500 calories (or fewer, if you plan to exercise). Then subtract any calories you eat as snacks and divide the remainder by 3. The result is the number of calories you should eat at each meal.

Water.   Never attempt to lose pounds by dehydrating yourself. At the beginning of a diet the body often loses water, as it does when you are physically active. If you are thirsty, drink plenty of water (or, if your diet permits, juice or skim milk).

"Spot Reduction."   Concentrating weight loss at any one part of the body is a myth. Gadgets aimed at minimizing (or maximizing) for instance, are worthless. Exercises of all kinds help build and use muscle tissue so that you get a better muscle to fat ratio. The best type of exercise, aerobics (see Chapter 7), works out muscles throughout the body.

Respect Your Individuality.   Dieting should not be viewed as a competitive event. Even on the same diet, people lose weight at differing rates—depending on their age, sex, body build, present weight, height,

Snacking.

Bob Combs/Photo Researchers

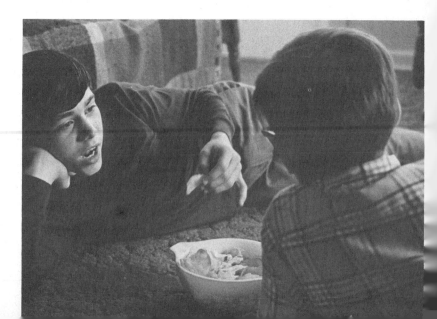

basal metabolic rate, and other factors. Heavy people and tall people, for instance, usually lose weight more quickly than others do. If you are unsure and cannot set a realistic goal, get a physician's advice and follow it, regardless of how much weight others may be losing.

Be Patient.   Do not become frustrated, because you don't slim down overnight. Do not aim for a dramatic weight loss, just a steady one. If you lose 1 pound each week, that's 52 in a year—a lot of pounds. Do not worry if you do not lose weight at a precise, steady pace; the body converts its stored fats into energy unevenly.

Reward Yourself.   When you lose weight do something you like to do for its own sake. Also, reward yourself emotionally by feeling good about yourself. Do not depend on other people to recognize that you have lost weight; no one will care as much about this as you do.

Other Ways to Lose Weight

Sometimes the plan we have described just is not enough, or it does not work at all. In that case you might have to consider some other ways of losing weight.

Strength in Numbers: Diet Groups.   When you are trying to change less than desirable eating habits, it sometimes helps to have support from others who are trying to do the same thing. Some of these groups are run by professionals, such as physicians, nutritionists, and the like; some are run by nonprofessionals. At meetings, members exchange ideas, discuss the problems they have had in trying to control their weight, and, in general, offer support and encouragement to one another.

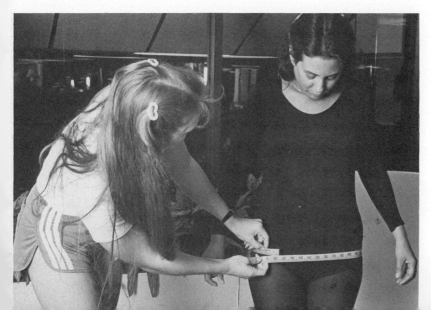

Progress.

S. Oristaglio/Photo Researchers

Behavior Modification.   For most people, eating is not just a biological need, but a major activity in the day's routine. Studies have shown that people with severe weight problems are more likely than others to be *preoccupied* by food—that is, to think about it constantly—and to eat, not so much because they are hungry, as in response to certain food-related "cues" (or stimuli) around them. Some overweight people feel that a meal is not truly a meal unless they have two or three helpings of everything. And the eating habits of many overweight people are completely controlled by the clock; they take meals and snacks at certain times, even when they are not hungry or when the only foods available are high in calories.

Some therapists use behaviorist techniques (see Chapters 1 and 3) to help overweight people become aware of the cues that provoke their eating. Their new-found awareness helps them to resist these cues and to become the masters, not the slaves, of food they eat. This, of course, is at the heart of any good diet.

Fasting.   Fasting as a means of losing weight means taking in nothing but water, vitamins, and minerals. It is used only when cases of extreme obesity have not responded to any other method, and it is unusual even then. In any case, fasting is only a short-term treatment, and when the fast ends a carefully controlled diet must be worked out (and followed) to maintain the new weight level or reduce it further.

Surgery.   When obesity does not respond to less extreme measures it is sometimes treated by surgery. These surgical techniques shorten the digestive tract and thus limit the surface that absorbs nutrients (and therefore calories). Surgery of this sort is risky and can be even more dangerous than obesity itself.

A diet group meeting.

Josephus Daniels/Photo Researchers

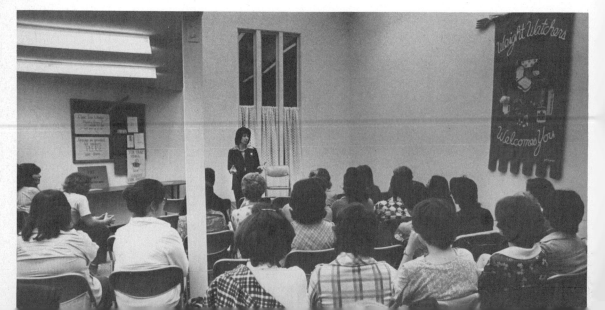

Table 9-3 Comparison of Various Weight Reduction Methods

Method	Description	Promised Goals	Advantages	Disadvantages
Balanced Deficit	Reduction of energy intake Avoidance of concentrated sweets and foods of high fat content	Steady rate of weight loss	Nutritionally adequate No known medical risks Fosters development of appropriate eating behaviors (if not below 1,000 kcal/day)	Relatively slow weight loss
Weight Watchers	Weekly group meetings Reduction of energy intake by standardized meal plan	Steady rate of weight loss	Encouragement in group situation Nutritionally adequate Provides structured plan, beneficial for some	Relatively slow weight loss Does not provide for individual preferences in foods and life style
Behavior Modification	In conjunction with energy-restricted diet	Weight loss Changes in eating behaviors	Opportunity to learn new eating behaviors Allows for personal preferences in foods and lifestyles	Does not work for all individuals
"Liquid Protein"	High-protein/low-carbohydrate/low-fat diet Use of predigested protein	Rapid weight loss	Short-term rapid weight loss	Medically risky Nutritionally imbalanced Does not foster development of appropriate eating behavior Weight loss not maintained
Starvation	Intake restricted to water and vitamin/mineral supplements for extended period of time	Rapid weight loss	Rapid weight loss for massively obese	Requires hospitalization Medically risky Loss of lean body mass Maintenance of weight loss usually not sustained
Drugs	Amphetamines	Reduction in appetite leading to weight loss	"Easy and painless"	Weight loss not sustained Potentially serious side effects Does not foster appropriate eating behaviors
Surgery	Decrease of intestinal absorption area	Weight loss	Effective for massively obese Steady weight loss for 1-2 years	Surgical risk Serious medical side effects in many people

Source: Adapted from Patricia A. Kreutler, *Nutrition in Perspective* (Englewood Cliffs, N.J.: Prentice-Hall, 1980), pp. 207-208. By permission.

SUMMARY

Food is the body's fuel, the energy on which it runs. You gain weight when you take in more energy (measured in calories) than you burn up as fuel. To lose weight you have to cut down on calories by eating less, getting more exercise, or both.

About 40 percent of the people of the United States are overweight to some extent. Genetic, physiological, and mental problems are partly causes of overweight, and so too is a technology that does not demand physical effort from most people.

Your ideal weight depends on a number of factors, including age, sex, height, body build, extent of physical activity, basal metabolic rate, and medical history. The best way to determine your ideal weight is to see a physician, a nutritionist, or a dietician.

The correct way to lose weight is to change your eating habits and exercise patterns. But that takes time and effort. That is why so many people try fad diets that forbid some foods or stress others. Those diets frequently are low in vitamins, minerals, and fiber; and most people do not stick with them. They work best at the beginning, because many of them cause the body to lose water. The pounds you get rid of in this way often are soon regained.

Certain people find that they simply cannot cut down on calories by themselves—or at all. Some of them find diet groups useful; others are helped by behavior modification techniques. Fasting and surgery are for extreme cases only.

But for most people there is really no substitute for diet and exercise. Good luck!

Suggested Readings

Guthrie, Helen Andrews. *Introductory Nutrition,* 4th ed. St. Louis: Mosby, 1979. Chapters 20 and 21 provide basic information about dieting.

Kreutler, Patricia. *Nutrition in Perspective.* Englewood Cliffs, N.J.: Prentice-Hall, 1980. Another good source for basic diet information.

Williams, Sue Rodwell. *Nutrition and Diet Therapy,* 3rd ed. St. Louis: Mosby, 1977. A source presenting realistic information on how to go about dieting.

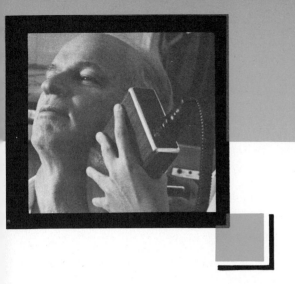

Noncommunicable Disease

chapter objectives

When you have finished reading this chapter you should be able to:

1. Define disease
2. Describe the causes, rates of incidence, and symptoms of various noncommunicable diseases
3. Recognize the role of risk factors in chronic diseases

Disease is many things and can be defined in many ways. The definition is sometimes based on the cause (perhaps a virus or an injury); on the part of the body affected; on the body's responses (fever, for example, or the death of cells); or, finally, on what most people actually notice: the discomforts that result, such as pain, fatigue, a stuffy nose, diarrhea, itching, and the like. In short, *disease is the whole pattern of responses made by an organism to the abnormal functioning of cells, whatever the cause.* Sickness and health depend on the complex interaction of many forces and biological responses. Focusing on these interrelated responses is called the *holistic* concept of health.

Classifications of Disease

Diseases affect not only the body as a whole but all of its constituent parts, as well: organ systems, organs, tissues, and cells. The most basic level of disease is the cellular level, and here the real explanation of disease must be found. The process of cell destruction that often accompanies disease is known to scientists as cell pathology. Pathological changes are called *local illnesses* when they affect only a single group of cells that make up one of the body's organs (the heart or the lungs, for example) or one of the body's systems (the nervous system and the digestive system, among others). Lung cancer and appendicitis are two well-known local diseases. Diseases that involve many systems or even every system in the body are called *systemic illnesses.* The common cold is a systemic illness because it disrupts the normal functions of many body systems.

Diseases can also be classified according to their causes, or *agents.* Some agents of disease are living microorganisms, like bacteria, which may be transmitted through *communicable* diseases (see Chapter 11) from host to host (human or animal). Much has been done to bring these diseases under control. These successes, along with an increase in the average age of our people, largely explain why most Americans now die of *noncommunicable diseases,* diseases that cannot be transmitted.

Incidence and Prevalence

The number of new cases of a disease that develop during a specified period of time is the *incidence* of that disease. During the winter season, for instance, many cases of flu develop, so within that period the incidence of flu is high. Incidence is a measure of acute, short-term diseases.

Long-term diseases are not seasonal in nature, so the number of people who develop them during a period of time is not really important. The *prevalence* of long-term diseases—in other words, the number of people in a given population who have a long-term disease at a particular time—is what we want to know. Prevalence is used as a measure of chronic diseases, like arthritis, cancer, and heart disease (see below), and of long-term communicable diseases, like tuberculosis.

Risk Factors

It is often quite easy to say what causes a communicable disease; for example, anyone who eats food containing the toxins produced by the bacterium known as *Clostridium botulinum* will get a disease called botulism—and two-thirds of those people may be dead within the week. The causes of noncommunicable diseases are more elusive. Many researchers think that smoking causes lung cancer, but they are not sure how; the only thing that is clear is that people who smoke have much higher rates of lung cancer than people who do not smoke—and this is not quite the same thing as proven cause. A *risk factor* is a physical condition, like high blood pressure, or a practice, like smoking, that is statistically associated with a disease. To put it another way, risk factors increase the likelihood that people will contract certain illnesses. For example, studies of Americans show that cancer and heart disease are most common among people who have great stress at work or at home, who eat diets high in animal fats, smoke cigarettes, lead inactive lives, or live in areas with high levels of environmental pollutants (see Chapter 19).

The message is clear: If you want to live longer, look to your diet, life style, and environment. Of course, living longer does not mean that you will avoid noncommunicable disease entirely. Everyone dies of something in the long run; living longer simply means postponing the day when you succumb to a chronic illness. To paraphrase Joseph Addison, an 18th-century essayist, life is a bridge that spans the dark river of death. At one end of the bridge are the many trapdoors of diseases permanently sealed by medical science, diseases that once were killers. At the far end of the bridge, however, lie the trapdoors of those diseases that have so far eluded all efforts to cure them. If you live long enough to get past the first set of trapdoors, as most do, pass through life's in-

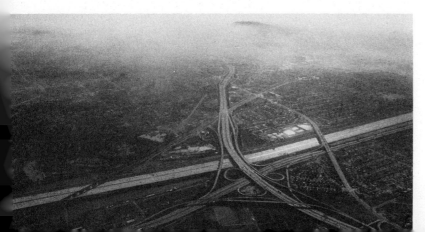

Environmental pollution is a risk factor for cancer and heart disease.

Georg Gerster/Photo Researchers

cidental dangers, and survive to old age, the trapdoors at the far end must open for you at last.

In Addison's day very few trapdoors had been sealed. Today many have been. But even now there are still many trapdoors at the far end of the bridge—and most of them are noncommunicable diseases, the subject of this chapter. We will now consider the several categories of noncommunicable diseases.

Inherited Diseases

Genetic Diseases

Some unfortunate travelers begin their life's journey with inborn diseases that have been transmitted to them through their genes. Although these *genetic* (inherited) diseases are transmitted from parent to child, they are noncommunicable because they cannot be contracted by contact. There are three basic inheritance patterns. In the dominant gene pattern, only one gene (from either the father or the mother) brings about the disease, Huntington's chorea, for example. Each child of such parents has a 50 percent chance of getting the disease. In the recessive pattern, both parents must be carriers of genes causing an illness, such as sickle cell anemia. Each child of such parents has a 25 percent chance of getting the disease. The third pattern is sex-linked inheritance, which occurs when the female parent carries the genes, but the disease ap-

Sickle Cell Anemia

Some ethnic groups suffer more from certain diseases than others do. In the United States, for example, 1 black person in 600 (a very high figure) has a condition known as sickle cell anemia, in which a large proportion of the body's red (oxygen-carrying) blood cells take the shape of sickles or crescents, rather than the normal disc shape. Another 1 black in 12 carries the gene for the sickle cell trait and, therefore, can pass it on genetically.

The effects of sickle cell anemia include pallor, weakness, shortness of breath, and jaundice. In severe cases, the victims must have blood transfusions to survive. Why is this problem more prevalent among blacks than whites? Scientists have found that the sickle cell trait offers protection against malaria. Since blacks originally lived in areas where malaria was rampant, those with that trait were more likely to survive to reproduce. Their numbers therefore increased and the sickle cell trait spread.

pears only among her male children. Hemophilia is such a disease. Each male child has a 50 percent chance of getting the disease.

People born with extra or missing chromosomes may have multiple defects. *Polygenic* disorders, those that are caused by the interaction of many genes, are less predictable: Inheritance may predispose people to them, but they are not inevitable; only if inheritance is combined with the appropriate environmental factors will the disease occur. *Diabetes* and *hypertension* (see below) are polygenic disorders.

Congenital Defects

Some defects that are present from birth are not transmitted genetically but are caused by "accidents" that wound the fetus while it is in the mother's womb (see Chapter 13). Such *congenital defects* include malformations of the heart, limbs, and mouth. Also congenital in origin are abnormalities of the nervous system such as spina bifida (protruding spinal cord), and deafness in the children of mothers who were infected with *rubella* while they were pregnant. Some of these defects tend to recur in some families, so scientists believe that a polygenic predisposition to them may interact with other causes.

Congenital defects are common. For instance, about 1 baby in 500 is born with congenital dislocation of the hip. One baby in 700 is born with clubfoot, a deformity in which the foot is twisted out of shape or position. Deformities of the lip and palate (roof of the mouth) occur in 1 out of 600 births (this rate is twice as high among whites as among blacks). Serious malformations of the nervous system occur in 1 to 3 babies for each 1,000 born, depending on the abnormality. Congenital malformations of the heart (abnormal "holes" between the chambers) are also common, affecting as many as 1 in 100.

Late-appearing Genetic and Congenital Diseases

Parents fear genetic defects in their offspring. When a new baby is born they and the obstetrician or midwife (see Chapter 17) look to make sure it has all the fingers, toes, limbs, and organ systems that it is supposed to have. Yet, even if it does, hidden genetic predispositions and congenital problems can manifest themselves later on, in childhood, adolescence, and adulthood. Stomach and intestinal ulcers, for example, are often due to a congenital weakness in the lining of the stomach and intestines. Coronary artery disease is attributed by some researchers to a genetic predisposition to accumulate fatty deposits in the blood vessels. Epilepsy, a disease marked by seizures, may be due either to genetically caused imbalances between the right and left portions of the brain or to defective brain chemistry. Genetic abnormalities can cause some cells to grow in a rapid and uncontrolled manner—cancer (but not all kinds are genetic in origin). Even mental illnesses (see Chapter 3) are attributed by some researchers to genetic biochemical problems of the nervous system.

Diabetes.   Late-appearing genetic diseases almost always have multifactoral causes; in other words, their appearance or nonappearance can be explained by a combination of genetic and environmental factors. Consider *diabetes mellitus,* which is caused mainly by an inherited inability to produce enough of the hormone insulin. The body's cells (especially the liver and muscle cells) need insulin to store and use glucose, and also to store and use fats, since fats can only be used as energy if a certain amount of glucose is used at the same time. When insulin is not available, glucose builds up in the blood and is then filtered out from it by the kidneys, so that glucose appears in the urine. The fats that are not used break down into products called ketoacids, which can intoxicate or destroy the delicate tissues of the brain and cause "shock" (diabetic coma) or even death. The unused fats also form deposits on the walls of the arteries and block them up. After a time, cells that depend on those arteries for oxygen and nutrients wither and die. The diabetic may now be struck by a heart attack, a stroke, gangrene of the limbs, or blindness.

Although this inherited inability to produce enough insulin is present at birth in almost 2 out of 100 babies born, the incidence of diabetes increases with age: Diabetes is diagnosed in 2 out of 1,000 people under the age of 24, but in 33 out of 1,000 people aged 45 to 54, and in 69 out of 1,000 aged 65 to 74. What does this age-related increase suggest? Some researchers think that early occurring (juvenile-onset) diabetes is only minimally controlled by genetic factors. Because cases of juvenile diabetes tend to appear after epidemics of mumps and other viral diseases (see Chapter 11), it appears that viruses may trigger diabetes in predisposed children or that viral infection may destroy the pancreas cells that produce insulin. If juvenile diabetes is indeed virus-triggered, it might be possible to control it with vaccines (see Chapter 11).

Adult-onset diabetes seems to be marked by a greater than normal production of insulin, although that amount is still not enough for the needs of diabetics. Juvenile diabetics can be helped by injections of insulin. But although adult diabetics may benefit from insulin, they still develop clogging of the arteries. In addition to taking insulin, affected adults appear to benefit from losing weight, not smoking, and avoiding certain foods, such as refined sugars and animal fats (see Chapter 8).

Disorders of Blood Flow: The Cardiovascular Diseases

The example of diabetes illustrates the importance of good blood flow. Blood carries oxygen and nutrients to all of the body's cells and carries away their waste products. The blood circulates throughout the

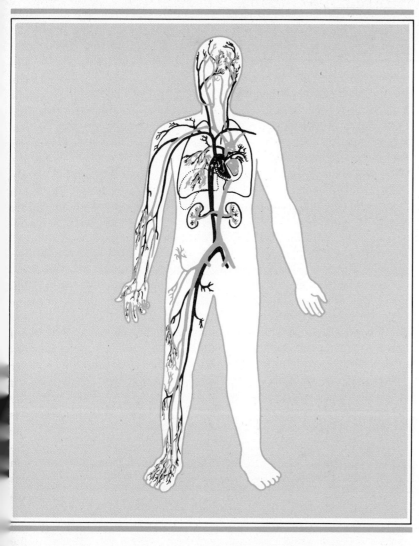

Figure 10–1. The Circulatory System.

body because contractions of the heart muscle push blood through the vessels, and at an amazingly fast rate; a blood cell passing through the big toe, for example, could make a complete circuit to the heart, through the lungs, and back to the toe in a minute or less. Any abnormality in the blood cells, the blood vessels, or the heart itself can disastrously affect the workings of the entire body. Diseases of the heart and the blood vessels—*cardiovascular diseases*—are now the chief cause of death in the United States. In 1980, about 985,000 people died from them.

"Cardiovascular" is a compound word, and the problems of the heart ("cardio") and the problems of the blood vessels ("vascular") are different, but related. The heart can fail to work properly for several reasons. Some hearts are too weak to pump out all the blood inside them, and other hearts do not pump properly, because the nerve impulses that cause the heart to beat become interrupted. In some cases, the heart's own arteries (the coronary arteries), which supply it with blood, may become blocked (an occlusion). The chief problem of the blood vessels is blockage, or the closing up of a vessel so that the blood cannot flow freely. For example, fatty deposits build up in the arteries, so that they become narrow and even close up completely. Therefore the arteries cannot send enough oxygen and nutrients to the cells, and the cells cannot work properly. Meanwhile, the heart has to pump against increased resistance from narrowed arteries, so blood pressure goes up. People who are genetically predisposed to cardiovascular disease stand a good chance of dying from it—if other diseases or accidents do not get them first. Yet the onset of cardiovascular disease can be delayed, if not prevented altogether, by healthier living—in other words, by exercise (see Chapter 7), proper diet (see Chapter 8), and not smoking.

Since 1970, the rate of death from cardiovascular diseases has declined dramatically. Some of this decline is due to better medical care—speedy intervention during heart attacks, more effective drugs to treat high blood pressure, sophisticated surgical techniques to increase blood flow to clogged arteries. The rest is attributable to our greater concern for nutrition, exercise, weight control, and stress control, and to lower rates of cigarette smoking.

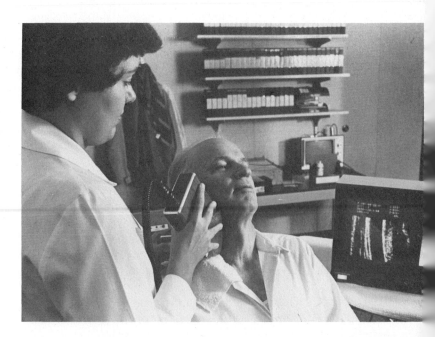

Looking at arteries through an ultrasonic scan.

Will McIntyre/Photo Researchers

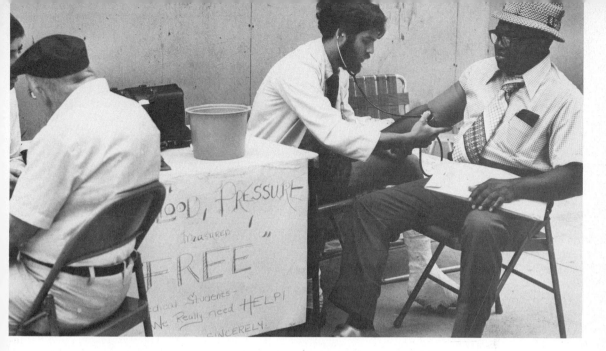

Checking blood pressure. Black men seem to be especially prone to cardiovascular diseases.
Rhoda Galyn/Photo Researchers

Not all risk factors can be controlled. Older people, especially black men whose fathers and other close male relatives have died from cardiovascular diseases, are prone to develop them, too. Since these people cannot change their age, race, sex, or family history, such risks cannot be controlled. But other risks can be: high blood pressure, high cholesterol levels, cigarette smoking, overweight, and sedentary life styles.

Studies have shown that some people who are predisposed to cardiovascular problems start to develop them even in childhood. The earlier these problems are discovered and treated, the better the chance of preventing heart attacks and stroke. Community screening programs have become important for this reason. Such programs have identified over 20,000,000 Americans with high blood pressure.

Your Heart in Sickness and in Health

What is it about the heart and blood vessels that makes them so prone to disease, even at early ages? A look at the anatomy (structure) and physiology (function) of the cardiovascular system will help explain the problem.

The heart of a healthy person is just a little larger than a fist and weighs less than 1 pound. But it works 24 hours a day, 7 days a week, 52 weeks a year to pump blood to all the body tissues. With so much work to do, it is no wonder that this compact pump sometimes shows signs of wear. Certain parts of the heart are quite vulnerable to damage. One such part is the pumping mechanism itself. The heart is divided into a "right heart" and a "left heart." The right heart receives "used" blood (laden with carbon dioxide and other wastes) from body organs and pumps it to the lungs, where carbon dioxide is exchanged for oxygen. The other wastes go on to the kidneys, which filter them out. This reoxygenated blood then travels to the left heart, which pumps it out (through a large blood vessel known as the aorta) to the

Figure 10–2. The Heart and the Way it Works.

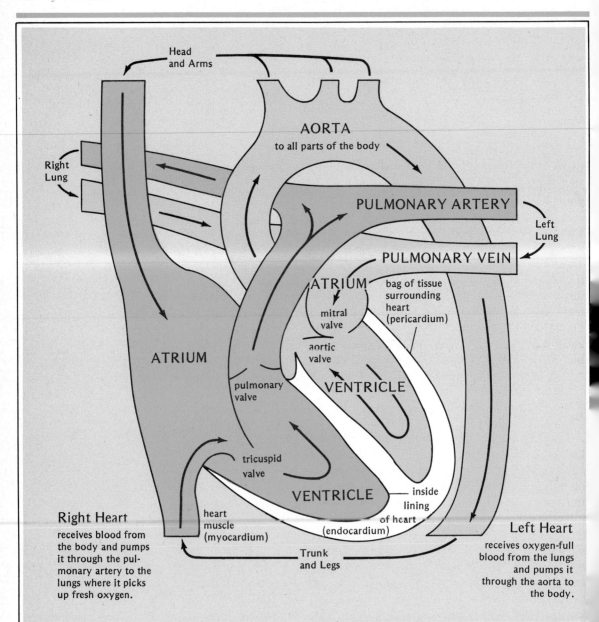

HEAD and Arms

AORTA
to all parts of the body

Right Lung

PULMONARY ARTERY

Left Lung

PULMONARY VEIN

ATRIUM
bag of tissue surrounding heart (pericardium)

mitral valve

aortic valve

ATRIUM

pulmonary valve

VENTRICLE

tricuspid valve

VENTRICLE

inside lining of heart (endocardium)

heart muscle (myocardium)

Right Heart
receives blood from the body and pumps it through the pulmonary artery to the lungs where it picks up fresh oxygen.

Trunk and Legs

Left Heart
receives oxygen-full blood from the lungs and pumps it through the aorta to the body.

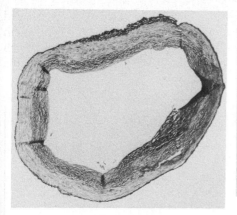
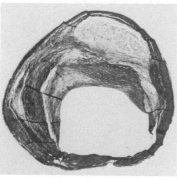
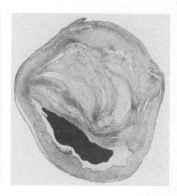

(Left) Normal Artery; (Center) Fatty Deposits in Vessel Wall; (Right) Plugged Artery with Fatty Deposits and Clot. *Heart Facts 1981/American Heart Association*

many small arteries that supply the body. Any disruption in the regular rhythm or force (pressure) of this pumping system weakens every organ and organ system.

Valve Disorders. Other vulnerable parts of the heart are the *valves,* which regulate the flow of blood through the heart and into the arteries. The valves permit blood to flow out of the heart, and they prevent it from flowing back in between contractions. When they are damaged by infectious diseases, fail to close completely as a result of congenital defects, or simply wear out, the blood *does* flow back into the heart. This in turn reduces the outflow of blood and therefore the amount of nutrients reaching distant cells. Physicians can hear the blood as it flows back and call the sound a "heart murmur."

Atherosclerosis and Essential Hypertension

The large blood vessels (arteries and veins) and the small ones (capillaries) have their problems, too. As we have seen, fats sometimes accumulate in the arteries (atherosclerosis). When vessels clog, the flow of blood slows. The heart, however, keeps pumping at the same rate, so the pressure on these vessels increases. High blood pressure is also called *hypertension.* Continued clogging causes the cells to receive less than their normal supply of oxygen and nutrients, so the cells "send a message" for the heart to pump harder. This message stimulates the adrenal glands, which produce hormones that control the heart rate, among other things. The heart does pump harder, but the arteries continue to clog and the cells get even less blood. Again they send the message for the heart to pump harder, and the vicious cycle of "essential" (that is, incurable) hypertension continues.

Figure 10–3. Estimated Prevalence of the Major Cardiovascular Diseases in the United States.

Source: Heart Facts 1981. American Heart Association, p. 11.

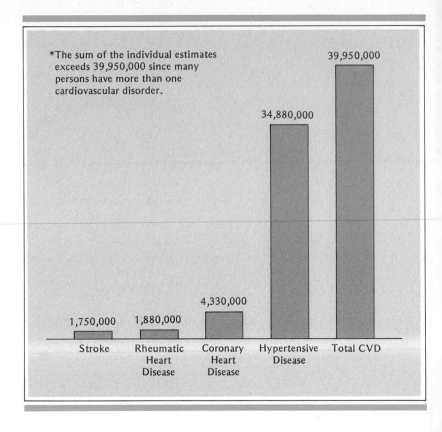

*The sum of the individual estimates exceeds 39,950,000 since many persons have more than one cardiovascular disorder.

| | | | | 39,950,000 |

Stroke — 1,750,000
Rheumatic Heart Disease — 1,880,000
Coronary Heart Disease — 4,330,000
Hypertensive Disease — 34,880,000
Total CVD — 39,950,000

Rehabilitation of stroke victims.

Josephus Daniels / Photo Researchers

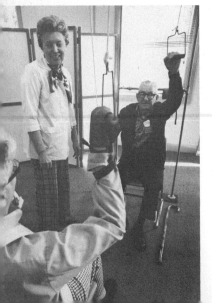

Stroke

Atherosclerosis not only interferes with the flow of blood to the cells but also causes the blood vessels, after years of degeneration, to become brittle and, therefore, subject to breakage. When the brain's blood vessels get blocked or break, or when abnormal growths, called *neoplasms* (see below), press upon them, the cells of the brain begin to die. When brain cells die, the functions that they control—the ability to walk, for example, or to speak—are disturbed or stopped. Precisely which function is affected depends on the part of the brain that is affected.

The disruption of the blood supply to the brain and the resulting death of some brain cells is called a *stroke* (or cerebrovascular accident). Strokes occur suddenly and some victims lose consciousness. If breathing and heart function are not artificially stimulated, they can die within minutes. Even if help does come in time, many brain cells may die from lack of oxygen, and the victim may lose many physical and mental powers—for a time or permanently. Not all strokes are severe, but minor strokes can occur in a series over the years, and they may culminate in a major stroke.

Heart Attack

Atherosclerosis can clog all arteries, including the coronary arteries, which supply oxygen and nutrients to the heart itself. The heart is a specialized muscle. Like other muscles, its cells require large amounts of nutrients and oxygen. If they are not supplied or if the supply is reduced, the muscle works less hard and the heart's pumping power decreases. The weakened heart often fails to beat regularly.

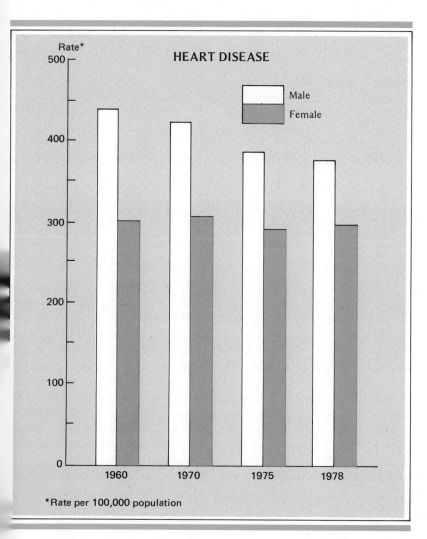

Figure 10–4. Death Rates from Heart Disease: 1960 to 1978.

Source: U.S. Bureau of the Census, *Statistical Abstract of the United States, 1980* (101st ed.), figure 2.4, p. 81.

New Organs for Old

Noncommunicable diseases of the heart, bones, and other organs are often incurable, even by surgery to remove the damaged areas. But what if doctors could remove an entire organ and replace it with a brand new one? Far from science fiction, this possibility has become a reality for many patients. During the last 10 years, millions of Americans have pledged that their organs may be removed for transplant after they die, and doctors are ready to use them. Today, about 25 tissues and organs are commonly transplanted—including bones, skin, corneas, kidneys, blood vessels, livers, and even hearts. If you think that the Bionic Man and Bionic Woman are figments of the imagination, you should know that surgeons are now at work to perfect transplants of arms, legs, and other parts of the body.

Another consequence of the narrowing of the blood vessels that lead to the heart may be sudden clogging, which shuts off the heart's blood supply. The cells of the heart muscle may then die in great numbers, and the victim becomes frightened, weak, short of breath and feels a crushing pain in the chest—in short, a *heart attack*, or *coronary thrombosis*. The heart muscle is often permanently destroyed, a *myocardial infarction*, and the damage hits so quickly that many patients die before reaching a hospital. In some cities, special ambulances or firefighter units speed trained technicians to the side of heart attack victims (see first aid and safety appendix). These technicians administer oxygen to heart attack victims, so that their hearts and vital organ cells stay alive; the technicians can also try to "jolt" the heart back into regular beating, with electric shocks. If the victims are lucky, they reach the hospital alive and are given more sophisticated treatments; among them are heart–lung machines, fluid-replacement therapy, powerful drugs, controlled diets, and exercises.

Patients who survive heart attacks can lead normal lives. But the heart is so important that losing heart muscle tissue can cause problems that show up mainly at times of physical or emotional stress. At these times the heart has to work harder to meet the body's demands for additional oxygen and nutrients. A normal heart does have a sufficient reserve of strength to meet such demands. But after a heart attack the blocked blood vessels that caused the attack may stay blocked, and so the heart muscle may receive too little oxygen. It quickly tires, and this causes the strong pressure and squeezing pain in the chest called *angina pectoris*.

The Dreaded Disease: Cancer

Even though cardiovascular disease kills more Americans than anything else, cancer is the most feared of diseases. Anyone who has ever lost a friend or a relative to cancer will understand this fear, yet much of it may not be justified, for many cancer victims survive. Since concern about cancer is so great, Americans have invested billions of dollars annually in cancer research. These vast research programs create the impression that cancer is a plague of modern times. But on the contrary, cancer may actually be one of the most ancient and universal of diseases. It was recorded as early as 500 B.C., and it afflicts every living species, including plants. But it is most common among human beings. In the United States alone, 1 person out of 4 develops cancer and 1 out of 6 dies from it. Nearly 420,000 a year die from cancer, and nearly 60 million Americans now alive will become its victims. And cancer's impact is increasing: In 1900 it ranked 6th as a cause of death in this country, but today it is 2nd—behind cardiovascular disease.

What Is Cancer?

Oddly enough, cancer in itself does not really kill people: it brings about death indirectly. Unlike the agents of contagious diseases—agents such as bacteria and viruses (see Chapter 11)—cancers are not foreign to the bodies they attack. They are actually cells of that same body, cells that in some unknown way devote themselves solely to reproducing and not to performing useful work. Those cells choke out normal cells by using nutrients that would normally be used by them or put pressure on organs and make them work poorly or not at all. Cancers thus grow and multiply, while useful cells die. It is this malnutrition of normal cells that causes the victim to weaken, waste away, and die.

125 Danger Signs of Cancer

Breast

- Hard lump in breast—may be fixed or movable
- Lump under arm
- Dimple in skin of breast
- Thickening or reddening of skin on breast
- Discharge from nipple
- Ulceration of nipple
- Inverted nipple, if nipple previously was erect
- Change in size of breast—swelling or shrinking
- Sore on breast or nipple that doesn't heal
- Persistent breast pain or sense of discomfort

Lung

- A smoker's cough which has become persistent or violent
- A nonsmoker's cough which hangs on for more than two weeks
- A chest pain that is persistent and unrelated to a cough
- A wheezing sound in breathing
- Bloodstained sputum
- Change in color or volume of sputum

Female Reproductive Organs

- Vulva: Itching, burning, pain
- Vagina: Painless bleeding following intercourse or exam; bladder pain; frequent urination
- Neck of uterus: Unusual bleeding or discharge; pelvic pain
- Body of uterus: Unusual bleeding especially if past menopause; lower abdominal and back pain

Skin

- Any lesion which forms a scab, rescabs, and fails to heal
- A scaly thickening which develops in a small area, usually on face, neck, or hands
- A molelike growth that increases in size, becomes ulcerated, and may bleed easily
- A pearly or waxy growth
- Any sore, blister, patch, pimple, or other blemish that does not show signs of healing within two or three weeks

Head and Neck

- Nose: Reddish, easily bleeding mass in nasal passage or cheek
- Salivary glands: Lump below ear and jaw; occasional pain or tenderness; hard consistency; facial palsy

Head and Neck (cont.)

- Mouth: White patches, sore that does not heal; lump or thickening; bleeding; difficulty in chewing or swallowing food; restricted movement of tongue or jaw; discomfort in wearing dentures
- Upper throat: Velvety-red patches; open sores in mouth; difficulty in breathing; earaches.
- Lower throat: Difficulty in swallowing; lumps in neck; difficulty in breathing; earaches; cough; bad breath
- Thyroid: Lump in neck; persistent hoarseness; difficulty in swallowing
- Larynx: Hoarseness; lump in throat; difficult or painful swallowing; pain in ear; shortness of breath; harsh and noisy breathing
- Esophagus: Difficulty in swallowing; pressure; burning pain in middle chest

Gastrointestinal

- Signs of blood in stool or urine (this is always a warning—must see doctor immediately)
- Change in bowel habits; increased use of laxatives; change in stool size
- Sense of incomplete evacuation
- Gas pains or cramps
- Constant indigestion or heartburn
- Abdominal pain or distended feeling
- Burning sensation when urinating
- Need for frequent urination
- Vomiting
- Feeling of lump or mass in abdomen

Brain and Spinal Cord

- An unusual kind of headache, more painful than usual. A constant ache or soreness, located in the back, front or side of the head or behind the eyes. Often present upon waking
- Vomiting, usually in the morning
- Impaired speech
- Hearing loss or ringing and buzzing in ears
- Loss of smell
- Muscle weakness of the face

- Abnormality in functioning of the eye
- Balance problems, or lack of coordination in walking
- Changes in personality
- Convulsion or epileptic seizure
- Inability to sleep for long periods
- Drowsiness

Male Reproductive Organs

- Prostate: Urination problems; blood in urine; pain in lower back, pelvis, upper thighs
- Testicle: Enlargement or change in consistency of testicles; dull ache in abdomen, dragging or heaviness; enlargement of breast, tender nipples
- Penis: Pimple, sore, nodule, wart, etc. on penis, usually tip. Bleeding associated with erection. Erection without desire

Adult Leukemia and Lymphoma

(*Hodgkin's Disease and Non-Hodgkin Lymphoma*)

- An enlarged lymph node in the neck, armpit, or groin
- Pain in abdomen, back, or legs
- Persistent fatigue
- Fever
- Loss of weight
- Night sweats
- Itching
- Nausea and vomiting
- Pain in certain areas of body after alcohol ingestion

Childhood Cancer

- Acute Lymphocytic Leukemia: Fatigue; weakness; pallor; low-grade temperature; bleeding gums; frequent nosebleeds; bone or joint pain; enlargement of lymph nodes, liver or spleen; pinpoint-size red or deep-purple spots on the skin and/or infection that doesn't respond well to antibiotics and persists

How Cancers Grow

Unlike normal cells, cancer cells never stop dividing. This uncontrolled growth is called *hyperplasia.* Moreover, cancer cells cannot perform useful functions. Cancerous white blood cells, for example, cannot fend off bacteria and viruses, the proper job of white blood cells. This lack of normal functioning is called *anaplasia.* What anaplastic cells *can* do is break off from their original areas of accumulation (called a *neoplasm*) and float freely through the lymph ducts and bloodstream. Wherever they land, these cancer cells attach themselves and soon begin to produce new growths. The breaking off of cells and their growth at remote sites is called *metastasis.* Cancer cells metastasize because they do not stick together well.

All cancers are hyperplastic, anaplastic, and metastatic. But not all neoplasms are cancerous. Some neoplasms—the noncancerous ones—are surrounded by capsules or membranes, and they are full of normal cells—neither anaplastic nor metastatic. These so-called *benign tumors* frequently cause no disruption to surrounding tissues unless the tumors press on vital organs. Unlike their *malignant*—cancerous—counterparts, benign tumors usually grow slowly, and if they are removed by surgery they usually do not grow anew.

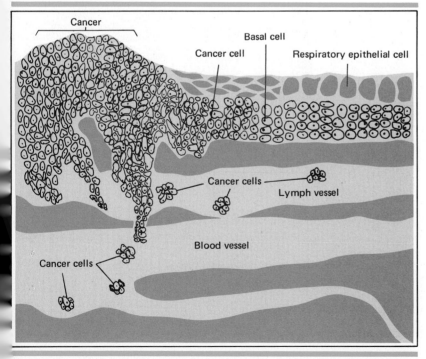

Figure 10–5. Cancer cells grow and then break away from the source; they enter the bloodstream and land at new sites—where they start new growths.

Figure 10–6. Death Rates from Cancer: 1960 to 1978.

Source: U.S. Bureau of the Census, *Statistical Abstract of the United States, 1980* (101st ed.), figure 2.4, p. 81.

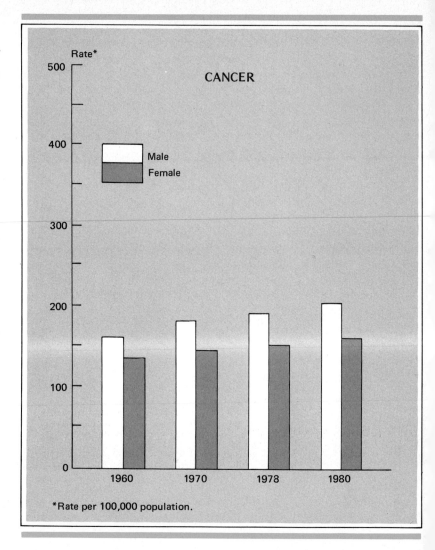

Is Death Inevitable?

In 1981, over 800,000 people were told they had cancer. According to statistical projections, some 270,000 of these victims—about one-third—will still be alive in 1986. Researchers estimate that 134,000 of the cancer victims who died in 1980 could have been saved by early treatment. Half of those who get cancer could and should survive. Indeed, about 2,000,000 Americans now alive actually *have* been cured of it.

Still other cancer victims could have avoided the disease altogether by paying attention to risk factors. Most lung cancers, for example, are caused by cigarette smoking. Most skin cancers result from too much exposure to direct sunlight. Quitting the habit (see Chapter 6) and avoiding excessive sun (or using sun-screening lotions) would prevent many of these cancers. Other cancers could be prevented by eliminating or reducing contact with cancer-causing *(carcinogenic)* substances in the environment (see Chapter 19). Some cases of bladder cancer, for instance, have been traced to dyes used in many industries; lung cancer is common among asbestos workers; and some stomach cancers are caused by heavy use of smoked, pickled, or salted foods.

The Warning Signs

In order to survive cancer, you have to recognize its signs early and get immediate treatment. Luckily, cancer often produces early symptoms; unluckily, they often resemble those of common, and less serious ailments. Many cancer victims do not seek treatment until their tumors have progressed beyond simple remedy.

Here are some of the early symptoms of cancer:

- Changes in bowel or bladder habits (prolonged constipation, "gas" pains, or diarrhea; a frequent need to urinate; or a weak flow of urine.
- Sores that do not heal, either on the skin or in the mouth.
- Unusual vaginal bleeding or vaginal discharge, even if no pain is involved.
- A thickening or lump in the breast or some place else, again, usually painless and often very small.
- Persistent indigestion or difficulty in swallowing—hard to recognize as cancer-related because these problems are so common today.
- An obvious change in a wart or mole—another very minor problem that can prefigure a cancer called melanoma.
- A nagging cough or hoarseness—again, an everyday ailment important only if it persists for 3 weeks or more.

Most people would feel quite foolish to go to a doctor every time they had stomach pains or coughing spells. They would be right to feel foolish. Recognizing the difference between a short-term problem and an unusually persistent one is easy, and it is the persistent problems that may be signs of cancer.

A Varied Assortment

Cancers come in many shapes and sizes. All told, there are over 100 distinct kinds, each with its own symptoms and treatment. From all these kinds, scientists have distinguished four big categories:

- *Leukemias:* Diseases in which the bone marrow produces abnormally large numbers of white blood cells (leukocytes). Leukemias affect people of all ages and are the most common kind of cancer in children.
- *Lymphomas:* Diseases in which the spleen and the lymph nodes, organs that help the body to resist infectious disease, produce an abnormally large number of lymphocytes, a special kind of white blood cell.
- *Sarcomas:* Solid tumors growing from connective tissues—cartilage, bone, and muscle. This type of malignancy is not common; it affects fewer than 2 percent of cancer patients.
- *Carcinomas:* Solid tumors growing from the epithelial tissues—the skin, glands, and nerves in the breasts, and on the linings of the respiratory, gastrointestinal, urinary, and genital systems. Cancerous epithelial tissues account for over 85 percent of all cancers.

Leukemia.   In 1960, it was not common for a victim of leukemia to survive as long as 5 years (a period that predicts a long-term cure). Yet by 1980, as many as 50 percent to 75 percent of the victims of some kinds of leukemia survived that long. Nonetheless, about 16,000 people died from leukemia in 1980. Part of the reason for these deaths is that scientists have not been able to identify leukemia's causes. The risk factors seem to include hereditary predisposition; too much exposure to radiation and to certain chemicals, like benzene; and certain viral diseases—but their specific roles are not yet known.

As with many cancers, the symptoms of leukemia—fatigue, paleness, weight loss, repeated infections, easy bruising, and nose bleeds—mimic those of some minor conditions. But some forms of leukemia progress slowly, without any warning signs until the advanced stages, when extreme fatigue, massive hemorrhages (bleeding), and persistent infection suggest the possibility of cancer. Blood tests and examination of marrow cells (usually extracted from the chest) show whether or not leukemia is to blame.

Treatment with anticancer drugs *(chemotherapy)* can wipe out large numbers of abnormal white blood cells, and blood transfusions and antibiotics can help tide the body over until normal cells recover. But although chemotherapy *can* substantially remit (or reduce) the symptoms of cancer, it often produces such unwanted side effects as nausea, weight gain, mood changes, and loss of hair. Most of these unpleasant effects go away when the period of concentrated chemotherapy is over, and patients may then stay free of disease for months, and even years. Others may have relapses caused by isolated cancerous white blood cells that survive and later reproduce. More chemotherapy may control

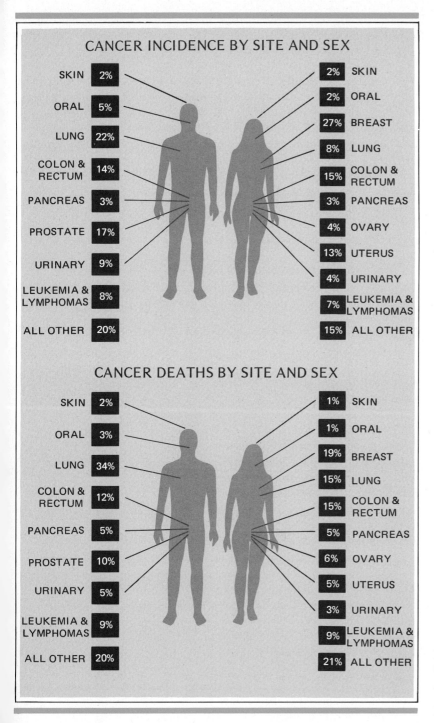

Figure 10–7. The 1981 Cancer Estimates.

Source: Cancer Facts & Figures 1981. American Cancer Society, p. 7.

these relapses, but not always, and some victims of leukemia then die from hemorrhages or infections.

Lung Cancer.   Despite the mystery of leukemia's causes, progress has been made in controlling it. Less progress has been made in controlling lung cancer, usually a carcinoma. About 90 percent of its victims die before the end of 5 years. More than 100,000 people died of lung cancer in 1980, and most of these cases of lung cancer could have been avoided, for they struck down men who smoked cigarettes. The clear fact that smoking is a very significant risk factor for lung cancer should make it easily controllable, but many smokers will not or just cannot break the habit (see Chapter 6 for advice on quitting).

Some progress has been made in treating lung cancer, and the proportion of 5-year cures should rise. But the best thing to do about lung cancer is to avoid it—by not smoking.

Breast Cancer.   Breast cancer, a carcinoma, is the most common cancer to affect only women. Indeed, among women aged 40 to 44 years, it is the leading cause of death. About 1 woman in 4 will develop breast cancer sometime in her life. But there is good news too: 85 percent of those whose cancers are found in the early, localized stages of the disease survive for 5 years (up from 78 percent in the 1940s). For those who learn the bad news in the late stages or for those who refuse early treatment, the chance of survival is only 56 percent, a rate unchanged since the 1940s.

The American Cancer Society recommends a breast x-ray examination (or a mammogram) every year for women over the age of 50. (It also suggests that women between 35 and 40 should get at least one mammogram, to have a baseline measure of their normal breast contours.) But some researchers think that mammograms are themselves carcinogenic. In any case, only after a tumor is discovered should a woman under 35 get a mammogram. Other helpful examination techniques include thermography (infrared detection of breast "hot-spots" that may indicate cancer) and monthly manual breast examination.

If a cancer is found, most doctors recommend an operation to remove the lump and the adjacent breast and lymph node tissue. This procedure—known as mastectomy—can involve total removal of the breast, its underlying muscles, and the associated lymph nodes (radical mastectomy), or less drastic removal of only the lump (lumpectomy) or the breast. Recent studies indicate that combining surgery with radiation therapy or chemotherapy, or both, offers the best chance of long-term survival.

Although breast cancer can be treated effectively, it cannot yet be prevented; in fact, it is becoming steadily more common. Some researchers think that women who have children before the age of 30 are to some extent protected against breast cancer, and that a first pregnancy after that age increases the risk of it. According to them, the fact that many young women now delay childbearing explains the increase in breast cancer. Other researchers believe that viruses may play a role in the disease's spread, and still others focus on such possible risk factors as heredity, obesity, an excess of estrogen in the bloodstream, or high-fat diets.

Cancer of the Uterus and Cervix.   Only a woman has a uterus and a cervix (see Chapter 13), so only women get uterine and cervical cancer. Sexual relations at an early age and a large number of sex partners increase the risk of cervical cancer. The risk is lower for women whose sex partners have been circumsized, presumably because circumcision decreases the amount of smegma (a thick secretion) that may accumulate under the foreskin of the penis. Smegma may also contribute to cancer of the penis. Late menopause (after age 55), the use of birth control pills, diabetes, high blood pressure, and obesity appear to increase the risk both of cervical and uterine cancer. Some of the risk factors for cervical and uterine cancer can be controlled, but it is also possible that some women are genetically predisposed to these kinds of cancer.

The death rates for cervical and uterine cancer have fallen by more than 70 percent over the last 40 years, mainly because of better and earlier diagnosis. The diagnosis is made by examining cells from the cervix or the uterus under a microscope—the so-called Pap test—which permits physicians to detect potentially cancerous cells at an early stage. Sexually mature women should take a Pap test at least once every 3 years. About 85 percent of all cases of cervical cancer, and 40 percent of all cases of uterine cancer, can be discovered early; and when this is done the 5-year survival rates are as high as 78 percent and 86 percent, respectively. Cervical and uterine cancer are usually treated through *cryotherapy* (the application of extreme cold) or radiation therapy, or both.

The Cancer that Nobody Talks About.   In the United States, the most common kind of cancer is a disease that nobody wants to talk about: cancer of the colon (lower intestine) and the rectum. It is understandable, for although we depend on these organs, we are embarrassed by them. But it is also silly—and even tragic—for this kind of cancer can be detected early (by unusual bleeding in the stool or changes in bowel habits), and it is quite treatable—about 70 percent of all victims survive when treated promptly. The current survival rate, however, is only 50 percent, mainly because thousands of victims neglect the early symptoms. An instrument for examining the rectum and colon (a proctosigmoidoscope) makes it possible to diagnose, without exploratory surgery, 60 percent of all these cancers. An even simpler examination can be performed by a physician during an office visit. Research suggests that a diet high in beef or low in roughage (see Chapter 8) may be risk factors, so changes in diet might prevent many cases.

The treatment for these kinds of cancer almost always requires the removal of a part of the colon. Some people then need a special incision, from the colon to the outside of the body (a colostomy), to permit bowel wastes to be discharged.

Is There a Cure in Sight?

As we have seen, cancer is not just one disease: It has many forms and many causes. It is therefore not likely to be cured by any single treatment, even in the future. At present, more people are being cured each year, and 5-year survival rates are up for many kinds of cancer. But recovery from cancer still requires early detection and prompt treatment. And cancer will continue to be a problem in our society because our population is getting older, because other diseases have been wholly or partly cured, and because new carcinogens will affect us.

Allergies

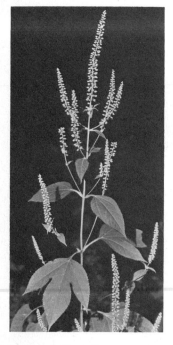

Ragweed—its pollen causes many people much suffering every fall.

A. W. Ambler/Photo Researchers

One of the greatest indignities of having allergies—sometimes greater than the disease itself—is the fact that people who do not have them do not take them seriously. In September, when these people see others suffering from the allergy called Hay Fever, they think, "It's only an allergy." *Only* an allergy! People who *have* allergies know that they are serious business, even if they usually are not fatal. Believe it or not, 5 to 10 percent of the *world's population* suffers from serious and sometimes crippling allergies.

What are these wretched allergies, anyway? They are diseases of the body's immune system, its mechanism for fighting off foreign substances, or *antigens.* When an antigen enters the body and injures its cells, it can respond in two ways. One way is called the *inflammation response:* The flow of blood to the site of the injury increases, and the injured cells release a substance called histamine (along with other cell chemicals). These permit blood plasma and white blood cells to escape, through the capillaries, to the site. There they produce swelling, redness, and higher body temperature—the inflammation response. A second reaction is triggered, in addition, only by certain kinds of antigens, such as viruses: the formation of *antibodies,* chemicals that counteract particular antigens. When the body has finished dealing with the threat of an antigen, the inflammation response subsides, and the antibodies are absorbed by the cells. Should the same antigen again invade the body, it is rapidly neutralized with these remaining antibodies.

In some cases many antibodies are released, and the inflammation response is particularly severe and persistent—more so than the threat of the antigen really warrants. This is called an allergy. In some allergic reactions, massive amounts of plasma escape from the blood vessels, and the victim's life is threatened by a sudden fall in the blood pressure. But most allergies are just intensely annoying. They may drive you crazy, but they don't kill you.

Discoveries made during the last 50 years have revolutionized the treatment of allergies. But many allergy sufferers who could be helped never go for treatment, and many treatments that could be used to help them never reach the general public. Vast numbers of patients need treatment, and there are few allergists to treat them. Physicians who do not specialize in the treatment of allergies are usually not familiar with the newer therapies.

The C.O.L.D. that Kills

Chronic obstructive lung disease—C.O.L.D., in short—is not one disease, but several: asthma, emphysema, and chronic bronchitis. All cause shortness of breath and difficulty in breathing.

Asthma is a kind of allergy that causes recurring, but not constant, obstruction of air passages. But it does not permanently destroy the lung tissues. Bronchitis is an irritation of the bronchial (lung) airways, through which the lungs get air. This irritation causes a continuously excessive production of mucus, which provokes an irritating cough. Bronchitis often results from long-lasting attacks of asthma, attacks in which violent episodes of coughing break the delicate air sacs of the lungs. This permanent destruction makes patients more susceptible to other illnesses and shortens their lives. Emphysema is the destruction of the smaller and finer air sacs (alveoli) of the lungs, where oxygen exchanges occur. Air is trapped in the broken alveoli, and this inhibits breathing, so not enough oxygen is supplied to the bloodstream. The victims are short of breath, their muscles waste away for lack of exercise, and large amounts of mucus are produced within the lungs. As these descriptions show, the three C.O.L.D.s are sometimes hard to tell apart.

The most common cause of bronchitis and emphysema is cigarette smoke, which over time destroys the lungs' cleaning mechanism. Mucus that is secreted within them builds up and closes off the bronchioles, the lungs' airways. The victim becomes starved for air, and any kind of work becomes difficult. Other causes of C.O.L.D. are respiratory infections and air pollution.

C.O.L.D. in its various forms can be treated if it is discovered early. Bronchodilator drugs and steroid (hormone) preparations can relieve asthma by opening clogged airways. Antibiotics and vaccines can cure and prevent the infections that often accompany C.O.L.D. Inhaled moisture can relieve dryness. Emphysema patients can be given oxygen.

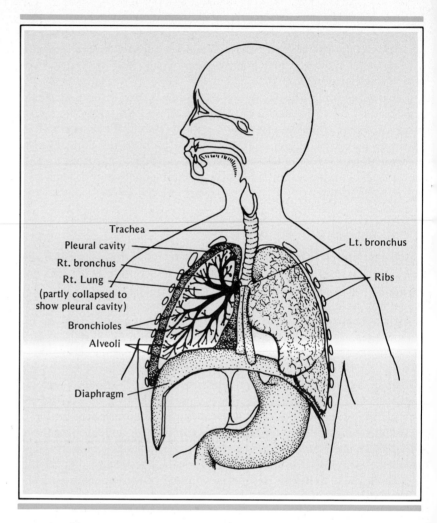

Figure 10-8. The Respiratory System.

Trachea

Pleural cavity

Rt. bronchus

Rt. Lung
(partly collapsed to
show pleural cavity)

Bronchioles

Alveoli

Diaphragm

Lt. bronchus

Ribs

Exercise therapy can teach C.O.L.D. victims to breathe more effectively. But in the late stages, their chances for recovery are slim.

Arthritis: Crippler of the Young and Old

The lungs are delicate, so it is easy to see that they are prone to injury when abused. But even the hard tissues of the bones, and the joints between bones, are subject to wear, tear, and destruction from many sources, including the disease called *arthritis*. There are two forms of this disease, and both develop over time.

Rheumatoid arthritis, the more dangerous form, commonly begins with feelings of stiffness in the hands or feet. The stiffness is worst in the morning but lessens during the day. As the disease progresses, the affected joints swell and cause aches and pains that limit movement. Over the years, rheumatoid arthritis actually "eats away" the bones. It is probably caused by an allergic reaction whose exact mechanism is still disputed. Osteoarthritis, the second form of the disease, and the most common kind of arthritis, does have proven causes—including hereditary defects, poorly formed joints, injuries, and poor bone alignment within a joint. In the early stages of the disease, the joints ache after physical exertion, but the pain stops when exertion stops. Gradually, the pain becomes more frequent and persistent, and the joints stiffen, becoming fixed in deformed positions. X-rays of such joints show that the spaces between bone endings are closing up and becoming hard and dense.

Neither kind of arthritis is curable. In the early stages, mere rest sometimes makes arthritis victims feel better. In the later stages, pain-killing and anti-inflammatory drugs may be helpful. If the pain and lack of movement become more and more severe, surgery may be needed to relieve them by removing damaged or inflamed bone tissue. Virtually every arthritis patient can be helped to be more comfortable and more mobile.

A young victim of arthritis is receiving therapy.
Stanford University/UPI

Diseases of the Digestive Tract

Although most people do not think of tooth decay as a disease, it is one; in fact, it is the most common noncommunicable disease of the digestive tract. The first permanent molars of more than 95 percent of all American children begin to decay a few years after they emerge from the gums. Over 20 million people in this country will lose all their teeth when they get older, because of tooth decay. Much of this decay and destruction can easily be prevented by flouride (found in toothpaste, in drinking water, and in mineral supplements), by regular brushing and flossing of the teeth, and by carefully regulating sugar consumption, mainly the eating of syrupy, sticky foods. In fact, almost everyone could reach old age with a full set of teeth, not "choppers."

Teeth are harder, and therefore less difficult to protect, than the softer organs of the digestive system: the esophagus, the stomach, and the intestines. It is amazing that they survive at all, considering the fluids and solids, hot things and cold, alcohols and acids that we throw into those delicate tissues.

At times, we all eat something that is just too much to handle, and the stomach and intestines cry, "Ouch." This is *gastritis* (or, in everyday language, heartburn and upset stomach). The protective tissues of the stomach and intestines can recover from gastritis fairly quickly. But if it occurs often and for a long time, these tissues can wear away, so that the walls of the stomach and intestines are exposed to direct contact with digestive acids, which cause as much pain in your stomach as they would on your skin. The result is a crater-like indentation called an ulcer, a problem that affects more than 20 million people in this country.

Antacids (see Chapter 18), bland food, and peace and quiet can stop the pain in many cases. To prevent ulcer craters from bleeding and turning into very dangerous wounds, some people require stronger drugs than antacids, and some even need surgery.

Diseases of the Nervous System

When your stomach is hurt, at least you know where the pain is coming from. When your brain, spinal cord, or nerves are hurt, the symptoms are so varied that it is hard to know what is causing them. For this reason, diseases of the nervous system are hard to diagnose and treat.

Consider Joyce, a woman in her early twenties. While playing racquetball one day, she had trouble seeing the ball. The next day her blurred vision had not cleared and she stumbled into things, so she went to see a doctor. Tests disclosed some minor oddities in her brain-wave patterns and in the fluid around her spinal cord. The diagnosis: multiple sclerosis (MS), a disease in which the outer coating of the brain and the nerve cells breaks down, so that the movement of messages from the nerves to the organs they control is disrupted.

In a week's time, with no treatment, Joyce's symptoms went away and she returned home. Five months later, she had another brief attack of blurred vision, along with a feeling of weakness in her left leg. As her doctor explained, the symptoms of multiple sclerosis tend to come and go. Some patients have one or two attacks and never experience a third. Other patients are hit with constant attacks that sometimes cause death within months or years.

Although many unscientific cures (such as fad diets) have been used to treat multiple sclerosis, as yet no scientifically proven cure exists. Since most patients have only mild and fleeting symptoms at first, the lack of an effective treatment does not prevent them from leading more or less normal lives.

Other nervous system disorders can be treated effectively but are just as serious as MS. Patients who develop Parkinson's Disease, which causes shaking and other difficulties in movement, can take drugs that relieve their crippling symptoms. Unfortunately, these drugs do nothing to stop the process of brain degeneration, and they eventually lose effectiveness. Scientists have recently made real advances in unravelling the mysteries of brain chemistry. Newly discovered substances called chemical transmitters seem to hold the key to many incurable diseases of the nervous system.

SUMMARY

The term disease embraces the entire pattern of responses made by a living thing to the abnormal functioning of cells. Local diseases affect only one of the body's organs or systems; systemic illnesses involve many. Communicable diseases can be passed by direct or indirect contact. Noncommunicable diseases cannot be transmitted by contact.

One way to avoid noncommunicable diseases is to eliminate from your life the risk factors that are associated with each disease, by changing your diet, life style, and physical environment. Some risk factors, like heredity, cannot be changed or controlled.

Inherited (genetic) diseases are transmitted from parents to children at the time of conception. They are noncommunicable because they cannot be contracted through direct or indirect contact. Many inherited diseases are caused by more than one gene or chromosome. Individuals may then be predisposed to a disease, but it does not always and inevitably develop in them.

Congenital defects, the result of accidents during fetal development, are often visible at birth. Some of them have partly genetic causes. Some congenital and genetic diseases, like diabetes, are not apparent at birth, but emerge in childhood, adolescence, or adulthood.

Cardiovascular diseases—diseases of the blood chemistry, blood vessels, and heart—kill more people in the United States than anything else. Among these diseases are hardening and blockage of the arteries, high blood pressure, and heart valve disorders. These three can lead to chest pain (angina), heart attack, and stroke.

Cancer, the second-ranked killer, causes death by robbing normal tissues of nutrients and by replacing useful cells with useless ones. Cancer cells that travel through the body and create new tumors sap the victim's strength and make the victim more prone to infection and death. Fortunately, new methods of detection and treatment are continuing to lower cancer's mortality rate.

Other noncommunicable problems—allergies, lung disorders, arthritis, tooth decay, gastritis, ulcers, and nervous system disorders—are also responding to earlier detection and better treatments. Yet we can expect the rates of incidence for these diseases to rise because people are living longer, and noncommunicable diseases are mainly diseases of older people. But we can also expect to see new drugs and new diagnostic methods that will lessen the impact of these diseases, even if the diseases themselves are inevitable.

Suggested Readings

Berkow, Robert, and Talbott, John H. *The Merck Manual.* Rahway, N.J.: Merck, 1977. This manual is expressly designed to meet the needs of a general practitioner in selecting medication. It is an excellent resource for anyone interested in explanations of diagnosis and therapy.

Burke, Shirley R. *Human Biology in Health and in Disease.* New York: Wiley, 1975. This book discusses the basic structure and function of the human body and some of the common disease processes affecting the various organ systems.

Groer, Maureen E., and Shekleton, Maureen E. *Basic Pathophysiology: A Conceptual Approach.* St. Louis: Mosby, 1979. This book is directed to those interested in health-related fields. The authors use a conceptual approach to present the information concerning the areas of medicine, nursing, and health.

Myers, Julian S. *An Orientation to Chronic Disease and Disability.* London: MacMillan, 1965. This book is useful for a background in medical information.

U.S. Department of Health, Education, and Welfare. *Healthy People: The Surgeon General's Report on Health Promotion and Disease Prevention.* Washington, D.C.: Government Printing Office, 1979. This informative resource concerns the prevalence, prevention, and characteristics of health and health care in the United States.

U.S. Department of Health and Human Services. *MMWR: Morbidity & Mortality Weekly Report Annual Report.* Atlanta, Ga.: Public Health Services/Centers for Disease Control. This publication gives the annual disease and fatality rate year by year. U.S. Department of Health and Human Services. *Sexually Transmitted Diseases.* Atlanta, Ga.: Public Health Services/Centers for Disease Control, Number (CDC) 81-8195. This is a source for basic statistical information about sexually transmitted diseases and the extent of the problem in the United States.

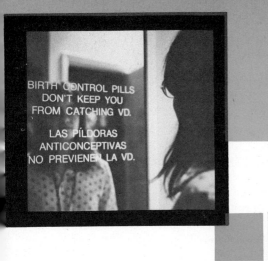

BIRTH CONTROL PILLS
DON'T KEEP YOU
FROM CATCHING VD.

LAS PÍLDORAS
ANTICONCEPTIVAS
NO PREVIENEN LA VD.

Communicable Diseases

chapter objectives

When you have finished reading this chapter you should be able to:

1. Identify the various agents of disease and the diseases they cause
2. Explain the process of infection
3. Describe methods of controlling communicable disease

It's Infectious, but Is It Communicable?

Most people know a lot about infectious and communicable diseases—mainly as victims of them! Some of these diseases cause so much discomfort and even suffering that it is hard to believe that they are caused by tiny living creatures—by microorganisms, in fact. But they are. When a microorganism capable of causing a disease gets into the body and begins to reproduce, its entry is called an *infection*. The "invading" microorganism is called a *parasite;* the human, plant, or animal body it enters is its *host.*

Human sociability, and breathing, eating, and drinking, help these organisms to reach many human hosts. And we are excellent hosts, in many senses of the word: The mucous membranes of the human nose, throat, digestive tract, and reproductive organs supply all the moisture, warmth, and nutrition that a lonely microorganism could want. You might even wonder why it is that human beings are not always sick.

The main reason is *immunity,* the medical term for all those defenses that the body uses to fight infection. Humans have a natural immunity against many organisms and can acquire immunity against many others. The body protects itself against infection in two ways: inflammation, a generalized response, and the immune reaction, a specific one (see Chapter 10). Those two responses produce such symptoms as sneezing, fever, rashes, nausea, and diarrhea—visible effects of the struggle between the invading organism and the body. Our bodies are subject to many infections, but only an infection severe enough to create reactions of this sort is called an infectious disease.

Another reason why humans stay fairly healthy is that not all infectious diseases are *communicable*—not all of them, in other words, can be transmitted from host to host. For example, germs on a rusty nail may cause a serious infection in someone who steps on the nail, but that infection will not travel to people who meet the infected person. All communicable diseases are infectious, but not all infections can be communicated.

Americans: How Sick Are We?

Epidemiologists (scientists who study the occurrence of disease in human populations) estimate that each year an average American comes down with at least one infectious disease that requires medical attention. Over half of all infections are respiratory (breathing-related) illnesses, most often caused by viruses (see below); and on average we get four of these illnesses each year. Most of them are not treated. In children, the average is higher: six or more.

People with infectious diseases usually stay home in bed, and that means lost school time and work time—in 1977, about 38,132,000 days and 27,200,000 days, respectively. Lost work time cost wage earners and employers about $1.3 billion in lost income.

The cost in human lives is even higher: In the United States, infections are the fourth leading killer of the elderly, after heart disease, cancer, and stroke. Infectious diseases kill people of every age, but the greatest number of victims are the very young and the very old.

Many communicable infections hit hard at adolescents and young adults, even if these infections do not kill them. In 1979, for example, people between the ages of 15 and 24 accounted for over 630,000 reported cases of gonorrhea (see below), over 4,500 of rubella (German measles), and over 2,000 of tuberculosis.

The Process of Infection

Every case of infection represents a chain of events, and each event is necessary for disease to break out. Now, it is often said that a chain is no stronger than its weakest link, and the chain of infection is no exception: If broken at any point, no disease will develop.

The chain of infectious disease has six links, in this sequence:

1. *A causative, or etiological agent.* This is the invading organism—a virus, an animal or plant parasite, or a bacterium (see below).
2. *A reservoir, or source, of the causative agent.* Like other living creatures, agents of disease have to live someplace, and these places are

---

Ring-Around-the-Rosy

You have all heard it, probably recited it, and perhaps even joined hands and gleefully pranced through a Ring-Around-the-Rosy.

Remember the words? "Ring around the rosy, pocket full of posey, ashes, ashes, all fall down." Just what does this mean? Well, it has been handed down from the 14th century, when the "black death" wiped out about a fourth of Europe's population and filled streets with corpses. Here's an interpretation:

"Ring around the rosy": These are the swollen red inflammations that surrounded the initial bite of the flea that transmits plague from rats.

"Pocket full of posey": Posey means the flowers people wore in their pockets or lapels to sniff when a funeral passed by or a corpse crossed their paths. The sweet smell warded off what people believed was the cause of plague, the foul odor from the bodies of plague victims.

"Ashes, ashes": The skin of a person dying of plague was often gray or black. This is the origin of the term "black death."

"All fall down": Fatalities from plague were amazingly high—perhaps three-quarters of the population in some parts of Europe.

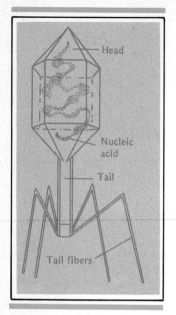

Figure 11–1. A virus.

Figure 11–2. The three basic shapes of bacteria: (A) Spirilli, (B) Cocci, (C) Bacilli.

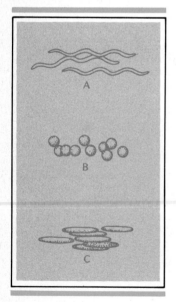

called the *reservoirs* of disease. Humans are the most common reservoir of communicable diseases that affect humans. Rodents, domestic animals, and insects also act as reservoirs of human diseases.

3. *A mode of escape from the reservoir.* If infectious organisms could not escape from their reservoirs, infections would never spread. In fact, most infections easily escape into the air through breathing, speaking, coughing, sneezing, and spitting; and they escape into the general environment through feces and urine or through discharges from open sores.

4. *A mode of transmission from the reservoir to a new host.* Once an infectious organism escapes from its host (or carrier), it cannot cause a new infection unless it manages to travel to a new host. The way it makes that trip is called its mode of transmission. Direct contact, by such means as inhaling the breath of an infected host or touching, is one mode; another is indirect transmission through "mechanical" carriers, such as insects that bite, blood (from transfusions or reused hypodermic syringes), and infected food and water.

5. *A mode of entry into the new host.* Just arriving at the body of a new host is not enough; the infectious organism must get inside. Most do so through the same routes they used to get out of their old hosts. Organisms that escape through the lungs, for example, usually enter new hosts through the lungs. The chief modes of entry are the "respiratory route" (through inhalation), the "anal/oral route" (through body wastes that get into food or water and are then eaten), and the "reproductive route" (in which organisms enter the body during sex).

6. *A susceptible host.* Even if a powerful invading organism escapes from its reservoir, is transmitted to a new host, and makes a successful entry, that host's natural immunity may prevent an infection from occurring. If it does not, the host is said to be susceptible to the infection.

The forces of infection continually struggle with the forces of resistance. When the forces of infection are stronger we get sick; when the forces of resistance are stronger we are well. Let us examine this battle in more detail.

The Invaders

Agents of infection, that is, infectious organisms, come in many shapes and sizes, from the submicroscopic viruses that cause the common cold to the tapeworms that grow large enough to fill human and animal intestines.

Viruses. The smallest agents, *viruses,* are submicroscopic organisms that invade living cells and multiply within them. Viruses themselves are *not* cells; they are extremely small particles that easily pass through cell membranes. Then they take control of the host cells, turning them into miniature factories that ignore their normal body functions and work only to produce viruses. Like living things, viruses can reproduce, but they can do so only under special circumstances; otherwise they are inert. Scientists have found over 300 viruses that infect humans. About 150 of them cause respiratory infections, such as influenza (flu) and colds. Other viruses cause smallpox, measles, rubella, polio, and rabies, to name but a few diseases.

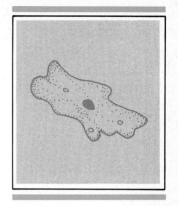

Figure 11–3. A protozoon.

Rickettsiae. Closely related to viruses are the *rickettsiae,* which also inhabit body cells. Unlike viruses, they can survive and function outside of cells, but they cannot multiply outside of them. All rickettsiae are transmitted by joint-footed insects (arthropods), such as ticks and fleas. The only common rickettsial diseases that occur in the United States are Rocky Mountain Spotted Fever, carried by ticks, and typhus, carried by lice.

Bacteria. Bacteria are one-celled plants that come in round shapes, called *cocci;* rod shapes, called bacilli; and spiral shapes, called spirilla. They cause many fatal diseases. Bacteria can live and reproduce outside of body cells; they are commonly found in colonies on the skin and mucous membranes.

Chlamydia. The chlamydia make up a category of organisms with features of both viruses and bacteria. Like viruses, they can reproduce only in living cells. Like bacteria, they have cell walls, but their metabolic activities (see Chapter 9) are much more limited than those of bacteria. Chlamydia are responsible for most cases of blindness (Trachoma) and for certain *sexually transmitted diseases* (see below).

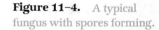

Figure 11–4. A typical fungus with spores forming.

Protozoa. One-celled animals called *protozoa* multiply within human and animal hosts much as bacteria do. Many protozoa live in the intestinal tract. Because they often escape through the feces, protozoan infections are common in places with poor sanitation. Two well-known protozoan infections are malaria, which is carried by insects, and amoebic dysentery, which is spread by contaminated water.

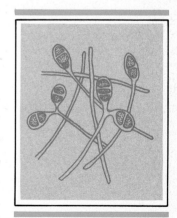

Fungi. Between bacteria and protozoa are the *fungi,* multicelled plants that exist both in the microscopic forms called "yeast" and in large colonies called "mushrooms." Fungi travel by spores in the air. The spores can grow both on living things, including humans, and on

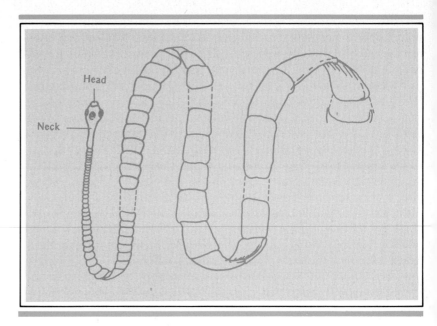

Head

Neck

Figure 11–5. A tapeworm.

inanimate objects, such as food or damp walls. You may be familiar with such fungal infections as ringworm, "jock itch," and athlete's foot.

Worms. Worms are another category of multicelled organisms that infect the human body. Intestinal roundworms—such as the tiny pinworm, which causes intense rectal itching—infect about 40 percent of all white children in North America and 80 percent of the children in some parts of Europe. Flatworms, including the intestinal tapeworm, deprive their hosts of nutrients by absorbing food from the intestinal tract. Schistosoma, filaria, and other worms live in the blood and the lymph. Their eggs spread to many organs, where they mature and cause painful irritations and inflammations.

Human and Animal Reservoirs

Infectious organisms would die out if they did not have warm, moist, food-filled reservoirs where they can grow and multiply. Human beings are the chief reservoir of human diseases, since most of their agents grow best in our bodies. These human reservoirs include both the sick and the healthy, for seemingly healthy people are often infected by agents they unknowingly transmit to others. Animals, too, are reservoirs of organisms that infect human beings: Rabies and anthrax infections, for example, are spread to humans through contact with wild and domesticated animals; and some insects become infected through contact with other animals or with humans and then spread those infections.

Finally, plants, soil, manure, compost, dust, and other nonliving substances can also act as reservoirs. In a hospital, for example, such infectious diseases as diphtheria and scarlet fever may spread from patient to patient through the dust and fluff from bedclothes and linens.

Direct and Indirect Transmission

Microorganisms can easily escape from their reservoirs and travel to new hosts, either by direct or indirect means. Sexual intercourse is an avenue of direct transmission for such communicable diseases as syphilis and gonorrhea. Cold and flu viruses are transmitted directly when droplets of infection-laden moisture are sneezed, coughed, or breathed directly from one person to another.

Objects that transmit disease indirectly—including toys, clothing, bedding, and surgical instruments contaminated by an infected person—are called fomites. Infections may also be spread indirectly, through water, food, milk, blood, and other so-called vehicles.

Etiology

Infectious agents, reservoirs, and modes of transmission combine in many ways to produce disease. With such a wide assortment of suspects, it's not surprising that epidemiologists must often undertake complex detective work to discover the *etiology* (source and responsible agent) of infectious diseases.

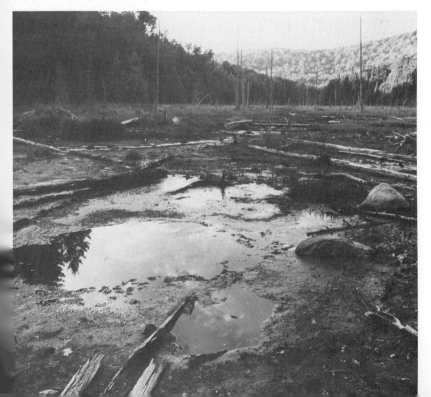

A reservoir of disease.

Laurence Pringle/Photo Researchers

Agent-Host-Environment Relationships

So far, we have followed the chain of infection from agent, to reservoir, to mode of transmission. Now we come to the susceptible host. Not all living things *are* susceptible, however. For on the battlefield of infection, human beings often come out on top. Sometimes human defenses manage to overcome the microbes. More frequently, some characteristic of the infectious agent or something in the environment stems the tide of disease before it can attack a new host.

Infectivity.   The ability of microbes to lodge and multiply in human hosts—their *infectivity*, in other words—varies a good deal. Some microbes, like the chickenpox virus, infect just about everyone who is exposed to them. Other organisms, like Hansen's bacillus (which causes leprosy) cannot infect a host without a long exposure.

Virulence.   Even organisms that are highly infectious do not necessarily make their hosts very sick. *Virulence* is the ability of an organism to sicken or kill its host. The common cold, although it is highly infectious, is rarely fatal or even severe. Untreated rabies, however, is almost always fatal.

Factors in the Environment

An infectious disease cannot occur unless an agent can leap across the environment it shares with its host. Some changes in the environment encourage diseases and some discourage them. Air pollution (see Chapter 19), for example, is a threat to health. And weather conditions can trap polluted air in densely populated areas and cause many people to become sick. Weather also affects disease-producing organisms directly, since higher temperatures usually speed their reproduction, while cold weather slows it down. The more organisms may be present in food, air, and water the greater is the chance of infection.

Conditions in our *social* environment affect the spread of disease, too. The kinds of food people eat, and the ways in which those foods are prepared, can promote or hinder intestinal infections from worms and food poisoning caused by protozoa and bacteria. When people move frequently from place to place they expose themselves to new microorganisms, to which they may not have immunity. Technical advances in medical care and medical treatment influence disease statistics; so do improvements in housing and sewage, the enforcement of laws to control water pollution and food storage, and attempts to educate people about diseases and how to prevent them. Finally, social values, habits, and beliefs affect the level of infectious disease. In the United States, for example, greater social acceptance of casual sexual relations has increased the incidence of sexually transmitted diseases.

Epidemics.   Environmental conditions create two kinds of transmission patterns, and therefore two kinds of epidemics—unusually high levels of a communicable disease. A "common source" epidemic follows the exposure of a group of people to the same agent at the same time, as in cases of food poisoning. A "propagated," or "progressive," epidemic results from the direct or indirect transmission of an agent from one host to another, perhaps over a long period of time. Gonorrhea, for example, is transmitted from host to host by sexual contact. The ability to distinguish between these two patterns is important for controlling epidemics and also for treating their victims. In a common source epidemic, victims begin to show signs of disease at more or less the same time, but in a propagated epidemic, the victims fall sick in the same order in which they were infected, one after the other.

The Protectors

The sum of all the body's defenses against infection is called resistance. Certain people are highly resistant to almost every illness, other people are particularly susceptible (sensitive) to illness and seem to be sick frequently, still others have resistance to certain infections but not to others. Finally, some people might have resistance to an average dose of an infectious organism but not to an overwhelming dose.

Defense Mechanisms.   The body's first line of defense against disease consists of the skin and the mucous membranes. The second line of defense is made up of the white blood cells, which surround and destroy invading organisms. White blood cells are called "nonspecific" defense factors because they are always present in the body and react to any threatening agent. In addition, the body also produces "specific" factors in response to chemicals in the invading organisms. These chemicals are called *antigens,* and they prod the host's body to produce chemical substances called *antibodies,* which combat, destroy, or neutralize the harmful effects of infectious agents. The production of these antibodies is called *immunity.*

Natural versus Acquired Immunity.   Many people have high levels of antibodies to certain infectious agents, although they have never had the diseases those agents cause. How could this happen? One possibility is that the antibodies were acquired in response to an extremely mild infection during childhood. Or these people might have a natural, inborn immunity, one present at birth and acquired from their mothers' antibodies, then kept throughout life. In any case, natural immunities are quite common. One result is that many animal diseases never develop in humans, because we have a natural species immunity to those diseases. And many human diseases cannot be transmitted to animals, because of their own species immunity.

"Inherent insusceptibility"—a physiological state that makes some people, with or without antibodies, quite resistant to infection—seems at first to be inborn but is not: It is created or supplemented by fitness, good nutrition, and adequate sleep.

Active and Passive Immunization.   We can now become immune to some diseases even if we lack natural immunity to them, for injecting very small numbers of disease agents (or their products) into healthy people stimulates the production of antibodies, without causing serious illness. Such injections are called *active immunization,* and the injected material is a vaccine. Most American children receive immunization (vaccines) against smallpox, polio, diphtheria, tetanus, and pertussis. Other vaccines protect us against mumps, measles, and rubella.

Physicians can also inject protective antibodies directly into the body of someone who lacks them—*passive immunization.* In this case, the immune system of the person who is injected does *not* produce antibodies.

Herd Immunity.   Another kind of immunity is conferred on some people simply because they live among populations with high levels of immunity to certain diseases. For example, areas that have just been struck by epidemics of polio, measles, or chickenpox become safer for everyone because many of the people who live in them develop immunities, so fewer people are left to transmit the infection. This is called a herd immunity. But as babies are born and as nonimmunized men and women move into such a community, the number of people who are not immune increases, so the herd immunity is diminished.

Immunization.
Omikron/Photo Researchers

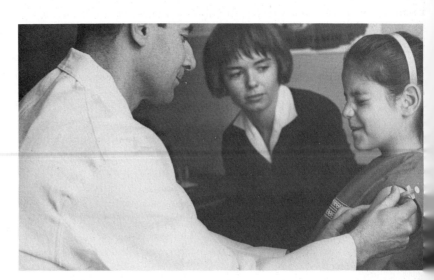

A Battle without End.   Each moment of your life, the forces of disease struggle against those of resistance. The state of your health at any moment depends on the strength of each side. When the balance between the invaders and the protectors is upset, you become sick. But the body fights back by producing new antibodies, which make you well in the short run and then continue to protect.

Some Common Communicable Diseases

Infectious diseases can be classified in many ways: among others, by the symptoms they cause (such as fever, coughing, and itching); by the ways they are transmitted (sex, for instance); and by their causal agents (viruses, bacteria, fungi, and so on). Most people are chiefly aware of their symptoms. But symptoms vary from case to case, so this would not be a clear sort of classification. The way a disease gets transmitted is much more clear and important as a classifier. But some diseases can be transmitted in two ways or more, so the categories in this classification cannot be quite separate. All infectious diseases, however, have one and only one causal agent, so classifying them by their causal agents eliminates the overlap between categories. That is why in this section all diseases (except the sexually transmitted ones) are classified by causal agent.

Viral Diseases

The Common Cold.   There are more colds in the United States than people, since most people get more than one cold each year. Why do we not develop immunity against colds? In fact, we do; in the course of a year we rarely catch the same cold virus twice. Unfortunately, there are many cold viruses, and they have an amazing ability to change their form through mutation (genetic variation), so there is always a new one to catch.

Omikron/Photo Researchers

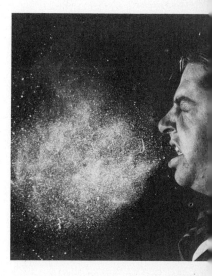

"Catching Cold." People talk about "catching colds," but colds actually catch people. Cold viruses circulate through the air. The virus gets into your body when you inhale the virus or touch a contaminated surface with your hand and then bring it into contact with the mucous membranes of the eyes, nose, or mouth. (That is why colds make themselves known through itchy eyes, stuffy noses, and scratchy throats.) If the very same virus were to make contact with the mucous membranes of the digestive tract or the genital organs, it would not grow; cells have specialized receptors that match only certain viruses.

Once the cold virus enters receptor cells, the virus alters those cells to make them produce more viruses. The viruses multiply quickly. The host cell dies and splits apart, spilling out thousands of new viruses, which infect neighboring cells. The cold symptoms mount. Besides the

Feed a Cold . . . with Chicken Soup

Popularly advertised cold pills and capsules cannot cure colds, but that old standby, hot chicken soup, just might. Scientists at the Mount Sinai Medical Center in Miami have found that chicken soup speeds the flow of mucus through the nasal passages and thus slows the reproduction of cold viruses. The moral is clear: Listen to your mother.

discomfort in your nose and throat, you may develop fever, a congestion headache, and general achiness. At bottom, these symptoms are good news; however unpleasant they may be, they are a sure sign that your body is fighting the infection. Fever raises the body's temperature, so that viruses multiply less quickly and white blood cells work more efficiently. It also increases the circulation of blood, and thus of antibodies, to injured cells. The cells destroyed by the invading virus release substances called histamines, which alter the blood vessels near the site of an injury to permit plasma (with its antibodies and white blood cells) to move to the injured area. The blood vessels deliver extra proteins, which help to replace dead cells and heal the damage. And the body makes a chemical called interferon, which impairs the virus's ability to reproduce within cells.

Taken together, these reactions are called the inflammation process. If you have paid attention to advertisements for cold remedies, you might think that the way to end a cold is to reduce the inflammation that accompanies it. The truth is that inflammation-reducing products diminish some symptoms but actually do little to fight colds. They might even slow down the healing. Products designed to reduce low-grade fevers also work against the body's defense mechanisms. Fevers higher than 102 degress Fahrenheit may be dangerous, though, and should be treated by a physician.

Rather than fight the body's healing process, why not help it along? You can do that in these ways:

- Drink plenty of water and other fluids, to soothe throat irritation and to prevent dehydration.

- Keep warm, to reduce tension and to keep your body heat high enough to keep down the reproduction of the virus.

- Avoid stress, because relaxation keeps blood flowing evenly and lowers the body's supply of cortisol, a hormone that inhibits the production of antibodies.

- Get plenty of rest and an adequate diet, so the body has enough energy to heal itself.

You can add cold and cough remedies to this natural regimen, but you cannot expect them to cure you; they can only give short-term relief for symptoms. As the old saying has it, "A common cold lasts 2 weeks if you treat it, and 14 days if you don't."

An Ounce of Prevention. The best way to deal with colds is not to get them in the first place. If possible, keep your distance from people with colds. If you are around sick people, be more careful about washing your hands and about personal hygiene in general. Eat well-balanced meals. Try not to get chilled or overtired, not because cold or fatigue causes colds—they do not—but because they can lower the body's resistance. And do not expect any help from your physician: At the moment there are no effective vaccines against cold viruses, and after many years of fruitless work, researchers at the National Institute of Allergy and Infectious Diseases have given up hope of developing one. And at this point there is little evidence that vitamin C can prevent colds or diminish their symptoms to any great degree.

There is a little hope for the future. Some scientists hope to develop drugs that will surround virus particles and prevent them from attaching themselves to receptor cells; others are working to produce larger quantities of interferon outside of the body or trying to produce a chemical that works faster and more effectively than natural interferon to stop the reproduction of viruses. Until they succeed, preventing and curing colds will be up to you.

Influenza.   Another illness spread by viruses, with symptoms (in mild cases) similar to those of the common cold, but with higher fevers, is the disease called influenza. At the moment, two kinds of "flu" viruses are active: the Type A strain and the Type B strain. These strains mutate easily and strike in cycles—in the United States, Type A influenza epidemics occur every 2 to 3 years; Type B influenza, every 4 to 6 years. Humans act as the reservoir for these flu viruses, transmitting them through direct contacts, like talking, or through indirect contacts, like freshly contaminated fomites.

Once inside a new host, flu viruses take 1 to 4 days (the incubation period) to multiply to disease-producing levels. Such symptoms as chills, high fever, muscular pains, and dry coughing may appear suddenly—and recovery may be equally sudden. Some patients get better in only 2 days; others may require 6 or 7 days, even longer.

What to Do for Flu

During an epidemic, flu may strike 2 or 3 out of 10 people in a community. When it is that widespread, the risk of getting it is high. But you need not sit back and wait. People who have been immunized against flu have a 70 to 90 percent lower chance of developing it. Most people have little reaction to the vaccine, but some children (and a smaller number of adults) actually come down with a mild case of influenza. If you're not willing to take that chance, and you happen to catch the flu, all is not lost: A new drug called amantadine can provide quick relief to flu victims in as little as 24 to 48 hours.

There are no effective treatments for flu; as with colds, you can get some relief by staying in bed and drinking fluids. Influenza is easier to prevent than colds are, and that is a good thing because flu still ranks among the top 10 underlying causes of death. Another piece of good news: flu is preventable. Only one or two of the many thousands of flu viruses affect a population at any time, so it is possible to prepare vaccines against whichever strain is currently active. To be effective, the vaccines have to be given *before* a flu epidemic begins.

Viral Hepatitis.   The human liver is the second largest organ of the body, next in size to the skin, and it has no fewer than 40 functions. Among other things, the liver produces chemicals that help to digest food, to clot blood, and to destroy harmful chemicals in the blood.

Hepatitis is an infection that inflames the liver and prevents it from doing its many jobs. Hepatitis is not caused by viruses only; alcoholism, for example, will bring it on, too. Viral hepatitis, though, is highly infectious and is transmitted by two kinds of viruses: hepatitis A virus (HAV), transmitted in feces and in contaminated food or water; and hepatitis B virus (HBV), transmitted from host to host through sexual contact, blood transfusions, and contaminated hypodermic needles. There might be yet another virus, called hepatitis C. Types A and B hepatitis can both cause severe, even fatal, liver disease, with such symptoms as serious protein and vitamin deficiencies; small or large losses of blood; and the yellow tint in the skin, eyes, and urine called jaundice. Hepatitis also produces extreme fatigue, nausea, abdominal pain, and fever. As with most viral infections, there is no cure—only supportive treatment.

Herpes Infections.   The members of the herpes family are among the most versatile of viruses; they cause diseases as unlike as chickenpox and cold sores. The virus responsible for cold sores (fever blisters) on the lips, a virus called Type 1 herpes simplex, is transmitted among human beings from mouth to mouth or from hand to mouth. Evidence seems to indicate that after the first infection goes away, some Type 1 herpes simplex viruses may remain in the body in a latent (resting) state. In times of illness, stress, and other forms of lowered body resistance, these latent viruses begin to multiply and cause new cold sores.

Another member of the herpes family, varicella-zoster, causes two diseases: chickenpox and shingles. This virus enters the body through the oral route or the respiratory tract and causes cells to swell with viruses, producing the skin lumps we call "pox." In less than a week, the antibodies do their work, and they remain in the body to prevent further chickenpox infections. But some virus particles may remain latent in the nervous system and, when they are revived by stress, they produce painful skin blisters ("shingles") along its pathways.

Another herpes virus, herpes Type 2 (or genital herpes), is transmitted during sex (see the section, below, on sexually transmitted diseases). At first, the infection produces sores on genital tissues. These sores heal without treatment, usually within 2 weeks. But the virus remains latent in nerve cells and later bursts forth repeatedly in new skin sores. These painful infections, in embarrassing places, often cause great distress. Infected women can transmit genital herpes virus to their babies during childbirth and thus cause permanent and, in some cases, fatal damage to the child's nervous system. Women infected by genital herpes are also much more likely than noninfected women to develop cervical cancer (see Chapter 10).

The sexual revolution gave both sexes an equal opportunity to get genital herpes. About 5 million of this country's men and women have it right now, and half a million new cases occur each year. These numbers and associated problems make genital herpes the most important sexually transmitted disease in the United States. What is more alarming, no cure has been found. Herpes can be prevented, but only by avoiding sexual contact with anyone who might have been infected. That is not always easy to tell; the infection is not always obvious. Condoms (see Chapter 14) may help somewhat, but researchers see little hope of controlling herpes in that way. For the time being, pregnant women should be tested before childbirth for signs of any infection that could damage their babies.

Mononucleosis.   "Mono" is a privilege of the rich. Children who live in crowded slum areas almost always get a mild case of mono—which resembles a prolonged cold—early in life, and they are never bothered by it again. Children who are better off seldom get mono in childhood. When they reach young adulthood they may live in a crowded college dormitory and catch the disease from someone else. Since they are not protected against it, they often become seriously ill.

Mono is called the "kissing disease" because the virus that causes it lives in the saliva of its host. It spreads through mouth-to-mouth contact and through contaminated cups and cutlery. Once you get mono, the only things you can do are to take aspirin (to reduce fever), eat nutritious meals (to maintain strength), and get plenty of bed rest. Take heart: If mono does not affect the liver, where it can cause severe illness, most of its victims most often recover easily.

Rickettsial Diseases

In contrast to the many kinds of viral infections, rickettsial infections are few. In fact, only one such infection is at all common in the United States: Rocky Mountain Spotted Fever, transmitted by wood ticks that are born with the infection or have gotten it from biting infected animals. The disease's name is actually a misnomer, since most cases occur in the Appalachian Mountains, along the East Coast. Its symptoms include high fever, weakness, rashes, and impairment of the nervous system.

Most cases of Rocky Mountain Spotted Fever could be prevented by vaccination, by wearing protective clothing when entering tick-infested areas, and by carefully removing all ticks embedded in the skin. Check any pets that are tick-prone, too. The disease can be treated with antibacterial drugs, such as tetracycline and chloramphenicol.

Bacterial Disease / Sexually Transmitted Disease

Bacteria cause many kinds of diseases throughout the world. In the United States the most important bacterial diseases are the sexually transmitted ones. There are more than 20 sexually transmitted diseases (STDs), and the majority of them are bacterial infections. (We have already discussed one STD that is not bacterial, genital herpes.) Gonorrhea and syphilis are the two best-known bacterial STDs, but a newly prevalent member of this family, nongonococcal urethritis, is quickly becoming familiar to sexually active people.

Gonorrhea.   The gonorrhea bacterium makes its home in the male and female reproductive tract—the urethra in men, the uterus in women. Gonorrhea usually causes a pus-like discharge from the penis and the vagina, but in men the discharge is more noticeable. Men, and some women, also feel pain when they urinate. Antibiotics can clear up most gonorrhea infections, but some gonorrhea strains are now resistant to antibiotics, and these cases are very difficult to cure. If left untreated, gonorrhea can scar the insides of the reproductive organs of both sexes and cause sterility (see Chapter 13). Infected women who become pregnant expose their babies to infection during childbirth. A baby's eyes are particularly vulnerable to damage, so physicians generally place a silver nitrate solution into the eyes of every newborn child to destroy any gonorrhea organisms that might be there.

Syphilis.   A less common disease than gonorrhea, but an equally dangerous one, syphilis causes only minor symptoms in its first stage—small, usually painless sores called chancres on the genitals, mouth, or rectum. They are often overlooked. Second-stage symptoms are also mild—fever, body aches, and a variety of rashes. They are often overlooked too, and meanwhile the disease spreads to sex partners. The symptoms of third-stage syphilis, symptoms that may become apparent 15 to 20 years after infection, are rare—but they cannot be ignored, for they include blindness, insanity, vascular problems, and death. Recognition during the second stage is most common, and treatment with antibiotics can control the disease.

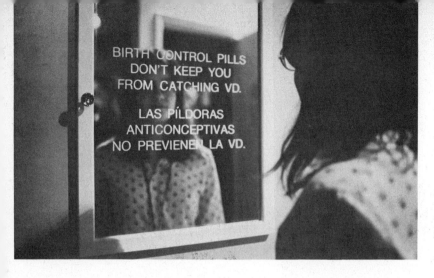

Venereal Disease Exhibit.
Dick Hanley/Photo Researchers

Nongonococcal Urethritis (NGU). Syphilis and gonorrhea are famous in song and story. Yet NGU, the most common sexually transmitted bacterial disease of young adults, is relatively obscure. Men with NGU commonly feel pain during urination, and this warns them that they are sick and need treatment. In women, however, the symptoms are not always apparent, and so women do not always learn that they have been infected. Sometimes they find out later in life, when they attempt to have children, for untreated NGU, like untreated gonorrhea, can cause pelvic inflammatory disease and sterility.

Genital Chlamydia Infection. Once upon a time chlamydia was classified with NGU, but it now has a notoriety all its own, as a separate disease. Most often, chlamydia infects the urethra, but it can attack other parts of the reproductive tract as well. In both sexes it can cause infertility, and it sometimes, during childbirth, infects the babies of infected mothers. Chlamydia often occurs alongside gonorrhea.

Sexually Transmitted Diseases and Sexual Freedom. Pain, inconvenience, bothersome symptoms of all sorts—what a price to pay for a sexual high. But that's the price some people pay, and worse.

It is unrealistic to suggest that young people abstain from sex. But you surely ought to be careful about it. At the very least, you should aim to lower the risk of STD infection. The more partners you have and the more sexual contacts they have had, the greater are your own chances of contracting an STD. If you have one steady relationship and others "on the side," be honest about casual sexual encounters. Tell your partner—and ask to be told by your partner—about any outside contacts or any suspicious symptoms. If you choose to have several sexual partners get periodic STD checkups from a physician or a health clinic. Such checkups are especially important for women, who may not be alerted to an STD infection by symptoms, which are usually less obvious in women.

If you take new partners, ask them about their past sexual contacts, and check them for discharges or genital sores *before* sex; you may be embarrassed, but better embarrassment than disease and pain. Do not have sex with anyone who seems to show signs of STD. Or make sure that the man uses a condom. Men who urinate right after intercourse often destroy and wash out gonorrhea organisms and avoid infection. A thorough washing after sex reduces the risk of syphilis.

If you are uncertain about your own sexual health or anyone else's, consult a physician or clinic. If you are too embarrassed to do so, call one of the local STD "hotlines," or the local health department.

Table 11–1.   Sexually Transmitted Diseases

The most common sexually transmitted diseases. Though some can develop without any sexual contact, all can be passed on this way

Disease	Usual Time from Contact to First Symptoms	Usual Symptoms	Diagnosis	Complications
Gonorrhea				
(Also called dose, clap, drip) Cause: bacterium	2-10 days sometimes 30 days	Local, genital discharge, pain; often no symptoms in men; usually no symptoms in women	Examination, smear for men; culture for women	Pelvic inflammatory disease, sterility, arthritis, blindness, eye infection in newborns.
Syphilis				
(Also called syph, pox, bad blood) Cause: spirochete	3-5 weeks; Average 21 days	First stage: painless pimple that disappears without treatment on genitals, fingers, lips, breast; Second stage: rash, fever, flu-like illness; Latent stage: none	Examination, blood test	Brain damage, insanity, paralysis, heart disease, death, damage to skin, bones, eyes, liver, teeth of fetus and newborns.
Herpes Simplex II				
(Also called herpes, virus) Cause: virus	About 1 week	Swollen, tender, painful blisters on genitals	Pap smear, examination, culture	Strong evidence linking infection to cervical cancer; severe central nervous system damage or death in infants infected during birth.
Non-specific Vaginitis				
Cause: (?) bacterium	1-2 weeks	Gray offensive vaginal discharge, usually *no* itching	Examination, smear, culture	Medical complications unknown.
Non-specific Urethritis				
Cause: chlamydia	1-3 weeks	Local discharge, frequent urination; often no symptoms	Examination: negative tests for gonorrhea	Medical complications unknown.

Table 11-1. Sexually Transmitted Diseases

Disease	Usual Time from Contact to First Symptoms	Usual Symptoms	Diagnosis	Complications
Trichomonas Vaginalis (Also called trich, TV, vaginitis) Cause: protozoa	1-4 weeks	Discharge, intense itching, burning and redness of genitals and thighs; painful intercourse.	Pap smear, examination, urinalysis	Gland infections in females, prostatitis in men.
Monilial Vaginitis (Also called moniliasis, vaginal thrush, yeast, candidiasis) Cause: fungus	Varies	Thick, cheesy, offensive discharge; itching, skin irritation	Examination, culture	Secondary infections by bacteria; mouth and throat infections of newborn.
Venereal Warts (Also called genital warts, condylomata acuminata) Cause: virus	Up to 2 months	Local irritation, itching	Examination	Highly contagious; can spread enough to block vaginal opening.
Pediculosis Pubis (Also called crabs, cooties, lice) Cause: louse	4-5 weeks	Intense itching, pin-head blood spots on underwear; small eggs or nits on pubic hair	Examination	No medical complications.
Scabies (Also called the itch) Cause: itch mite	4-6 weeks	Severe nighttime itching, raised gray lines in skin where mite burrows	Examination	May infest elbows, hands, breasts and buttocks as well as genitals.
Chancroid (Also called soft Chancre) Cause: bacterium	1 day to 2 weeks Average 4 days	Painful sores on the genitals; also, swollen, tender gland in the genital area, usually one side only	Examination, smear, culture	Scarring, permanent deformity.
Granuloma Inguinale (Donovaniosis) Cause: bacterium	1-10 weeks	Usually painless, beefy red, genital ulcers which spread slowly	Examination, smear	Scarring, tissue destruction.
Lymphogranuloma Venereum (LGV, Frei's disease) Cause: chlamydia	3 days to 3 weeks Average 10 days	Single, painless sore on genitals, joint pain and lymph node swelling	Examination, blood test	Large swelling of genitals and anal areas; rectal strictures.

Source: The Pennsylvania Department of Health.

Fungal Disease

Fungi live on moist surfaces, such as the floors of shower rooms, where they may infect human beings. Athlete's foot is a common fungal (or mycotic) disease, and so is ringworm, so named because of the raised, ring-like lesions it causes. Ringworm attacks the scalp, the groin, or the fingers and toes, and it causes itching; itching leads to scratching and thus to sores and even secondary infections. A less known, but equally annoying, mycotic disease is candidiasis—an infection of the vagina. This disease often follows treatment with antibiotics, which kill off bacteria that help control fungi.

Fungi are durable and stubbornly resist treatment, even with the most effective antibiotic drugs. Some antibiotics actually promote fungal diseases, like candidiasis.

Protozoan Diseases

In the past, most infectious protozoans caused diseases in obscurity. Yet one protozoan disease is famous: *malaria,* the most common infection in the Southern Hemisphere and probably in the world, though it is quite uncommon in the United States. A female mosquito that bites an infected host transmits the infection by biting new hosts.

Two protozoan diseases are becoming better recognized in the United States. Giardia is a species of protozoan found in streams and other bodies of water. People who drink the contaminated water become infected and may develop stomach pains or diarrhea, and sometimes liver inflammation. These symptoms usually clear up after drug treatment. The beaver is an intermediate host in the spread of giardiasis, so streams with beavers are often unsafe for drinking, however pure they might seem to be.

The other increasingly well-known protozoan disease is caused by a pest called *Trichomonas vaginalis,* which causes burning, itching, and discharges in the vagina. The male genital tract, too, can be infected by trichomonads—in fact, men are the most common source of transmission—but in them the symptoms are slight or unnoticeable. Trichomoniasis (infection by trichomonads) can be treated with a number of drugs.

Arthropod Infestation

Some joint-legged insects—arthropods—are parasitic on human hosts, much as viruses and bacteria are. Lice, for example, live and lay their eggs in the scalp and other hairy areas of the body and on furniture and combs, which can pass the infection to new hosts. Lice cause intense itching. Crab lice, which resemble tiny crabs, like to live in the genital area and can be passed from host to host during sexual intercourse.

Insects called mites burrow into such moist and warm crevices in the

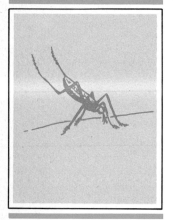

Figure 11–6.   The Anopheles mosquito, carrier of malaria.

skin as the area between the fingers and the folds of the wrists and the elbows, and they cause an infestation known as scabies. Like crab lice, scabies is transmitted directly from person to person, often during sexual contact; less frequently, it is passed on by contact with freshly contaminated underwear or bed linens.

Pain relievers applied directly to lice- and mite-infested areas can relieve itching. Sterilizing contaminated clothes helps to kill insect eggs, which can spread the infection. In addition, chemicals toxic to arthropods are put in certain shampoos, sprays, powders, and ointments.

Worm Infestations

The worms that infest human beings, including pinworms, tapeworms, and bloodworms, are big enough to be seen without a microscope, but small enough to infest human hosts in great numbers. Except for the common pinworm, worm infestations are relatively rare in temperate climates; they are a particular problem in tropical areas, especially where sanitation is poor.

Sometimes live worms or worm eggs are passed from host to host through food or water, or through objects contaminated with infested feces. This is the mode of transmission for pinworms and for many kinds of tapeworms. Undercooked meat or fish acts as a vehicle of transmission for other species of worms, such as the trichina worm (found in raw pork) and the fish tapeworm (in raw fish).

Good sanitation and thorough cooking can prevent most cases of worm infestation. If they do not, certain drugs are usually helpful. But they work by poisoning the worms with toxic substances that usually cause discomfort in the host as well.

Controlling Communicable Disease

Some of the ways of avoiding STDs—for example, avoiding infected people and other hosts—will also help you avoid other communicable diseases. Paying attention to your own body can help you become aware of (and cure) a disease at an early stage and prevent you from spreading it to others. But individual efforts at disease control are not enough. Physicians and public-health officials can help us by taking steps to control the reservoirs of disease and the transmission of disease agents. Other measures help reduce the susceptibility to infection of potential hosts.

Reservoir-oriented controls focus on human beings. Remember that people are the most important reservoirs for diseases that affect people. Public-health researchers attempt to locate and treat people with serious contagious diseases and try to contain reservoirs. One measure

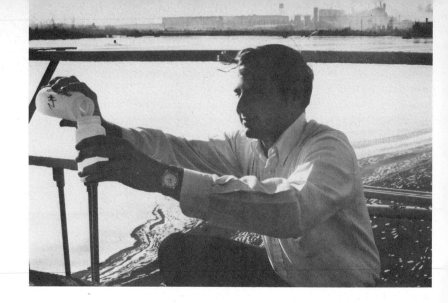

Public Health: checking the water.

Dick Davis / Photo Researchers

of containment, quarantine—limiting the free movement of infected people—is used rarely, and only for such serious infections as cholera, plague, and yellow fever. Quarantine can be quite effective, but controlling the movement of suspected carriers of disease is effective, too.

Quarantine during a 19th-century epidemic.

The Bettmann Archive

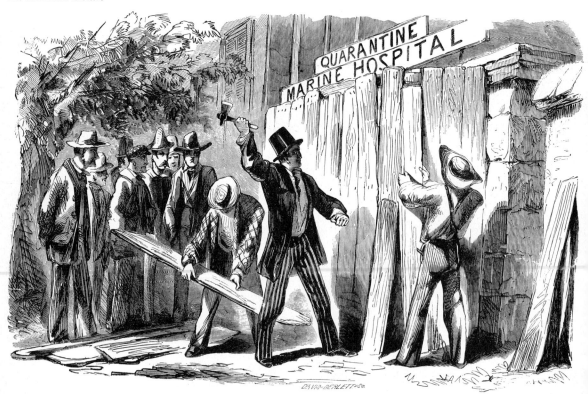

Transmission-oriented control measures include the improvement of sewage treatment, mandatory refrigeration of perishable foods, measures against air pollution, and chemical destruction of the nesting areas of ticks, mites, mosquitoes, and other carriers.

Host-oriented preventive methods are most popular in rich nations, such as the United States. Immunization against such diseases as diphtheria, tetanus, pertussis, poliomyelitis, mumps, measles, and rubella has brought them under control here—so successful, in fact, that many people have now asked if we still have to immunize young children against these infections. If you remember our discussion of herd immunity you will know the answer is definitely "yes": Because these diseases are now so rare, people do not build up immunity to them through exposure to infected hosts. If immunization programs lapsed, new cases would quickly spring up from remaining sources in the environment.

Yet, vaccination against smallpox is no longer thought to be desirable. Why? The unique characteristics of this disease offer a ready explanation. Smallpox is infectious only for humans, so no hidden reservoirs may be lurking in animals, insects, caves, or swamps. Thanks to many years of strict vaccination programs, there has not been one natural case of smallpox anywhere in the world since 1978. Smallpox has been defeated. With enough time and money, other infectious diseases could be defeated too.

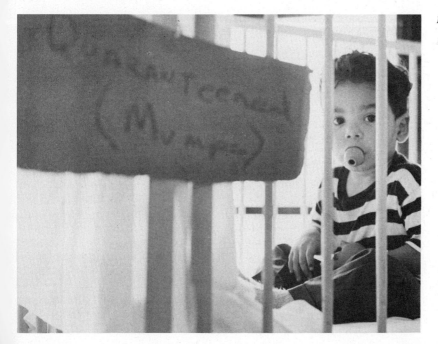

Bettye Lane/Photo Researchers.

SUMMARY

Infection is the entry of a disease agent into the body of a host. These agents include bacteria, viruses, rickettsiae, protozoa, worms, and fungi. Infectious diseases are common, but most are mild and quickly cured.

The agents of infectious diseases must have a reservoir, or source, to live, and to spread to new victims (or hosts) they need a means of escape from the reservoir, transmission to carriers (living or nonliving), a mode of transmission and entry to a new host, and, finally, a susceptible host. Infectious agents and hosts are locked in a constant conflict, with one trying to lodge and multiply and the other trying, through its defenses, to prevent the spread of disease. The outcome of the conflict is affected by factors in the physical and social environment.

The development of artificial ways of producing immunity has tilted the scale against disease. Although vaccines have not been developed for some persistent human infections, such as the common cold, immunizations do effectively prevent smallpox, diphtheria, tetanus, pertussis, mumps, measles, and rubella, among other diseases. New antibiotics and other drugs are also helping to control infections. Despite these medical advances, changes in cultural patterns—greater sexual freedom, for example—are working to increase the incidence of the sexually transmitted diseases, such as gonorrhea and NGU.

Suggested Readings

Berkow, Robert, and Talbott, John H. *The Merck Manual.* Rahway, N.J.: Merck, 1977. This manual is expressly designed to meet the needs of a general practitioner in selecting medication. It is an excellent resource for anyone interested in explanations of diagnosis and therapy.

Burke, Shirley R. *Human Biology in Health and in Disease.* New York: Wiley, 1975. This book discusses the basic structure and function of the human body and some of the common disease processes affecting the various organ systems.

Groer, Maureen E., and Shekleton, Maureen E. *Basic Pathophysiology: A Conceptual Approach.* St. Louis: Mosby, 1979. This book is directed to those interested in health-related fields. The authors use a conceptual approach to present the information concerning the areas of medicine, nursing, and health.

Myers, Julian S. *An Orientation to Chronic Disease and Disability.* London: Macmillan, 1965. This book is useful for a background in medical information.

U. S. Department of Health, Education, and Welfare. *Healthy People: The Surgeon General's Report on Health Promotion and Disease Prevention.* Washington, D.C.: Government Printing Office, 1979. This informative resource concerns the prevalence, prevention, and characteristics of health and health care in the United States.

U.S. Department of Health and Human Services. *MMWR: Morbidity & Mortality Weekly Report Annual Report.* Atlanta, Ga.: Public Health Services/Centers for Disease Control. This publication gives the annual disease and fatality rate year by year.

U.S. Department of Health and Human Services. *Sexually Transmitted Diseases.* Atlanta, Ga.: Public Health Services/Centers for Disease Control, Number (CDC) 81-8195. This is a source for basic statistical information about sexually transmitted diseases and the extent of the problem in the United States.

Sexuality

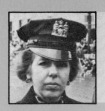

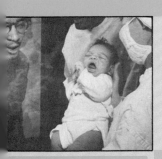

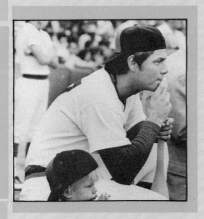

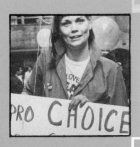

UNIT FOUR

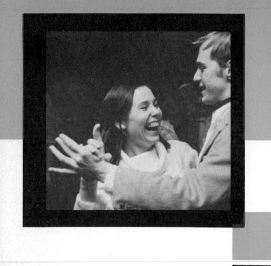

Sexuality

chapter objectives

When you have finished reading this chapter you should be able to:

1. Define sexuality and discuss its development
2. Argue logically for or against the statement "Anatomy is Destiny"
3. Compare and contrast aspects of intrapersonal sexuality and interpersonal sexuality

When a new baby is born, the first question asked is often: "Boy or girl?" From the moment of birth the sex of each human being is noted; we each become known as a sexual being. Throughout life your sexual identity determines—among many other things—the clothes you are expected to wear, the kinds of things you are expected to enjoy, the ways in which you earn (or do not earn) your living, and the people with whom you work and live. Sexuality is not just a biological fact; it is an essential part of the way humans deal with one another. This includes all the ways that women deal with themselves and others as women; the ways that men deal with themselves and others as men; and the ways that women and men deal with each other.

In many ways our culture makes it hard for us to enjoy our sexuality and share it with others. For one thing it encourages us to conceal our sexual needs and problems. But those needs and problems assert themselves anyway. Almost all of us think in private about sex and sexuality, and many people fear being "abnormal" or inadequate. Today, in addition, men worry about what it means to be a man, and women worry about what it means to be a woman. Let's look at that question first.

"Men's work!"

Ray Ellis/Photo Researchers

Sex Roles

All cultures—from the most primitive to the most advanced—have created jobs, rights, and privileges just for men and other jobs, rights, and privileges just for women. These jobs, rights, and privileges are known as *sex roles.* They are a part of each culture's most deeply held customs. They are what the culture expects from each man and each woman.

Sex roles differ from culture to culture, but certain traits seem to be shared by the modern Western ones. In them, women have the chief duty of keeping the home and caring for children and the other members of the family. Men have the duty of providing the family's food and shelter. This division of tasks tends to develop nurturing and dependent behavior in women and domineering, self-reliant behavior in men.

Does this mean that the women are passive and "motherly" and that the men are strong-willed and independent? Probably not, but there is some debate about this. Most women and men just conform to the sex roles (also known as sex-role *stereotypes*) that they learned from the day of their birth. Girls whose mothers and other female relatives spent their days raising children, cooking, and cleaning learned that these tasks are "suited" to women. Boys whose fathers and other male relatives had careers, and thereby provided their families' incomes learned that these jobs are "suited" to men.

Movies, TV, newspapers, and books reinforce children's ideas about how each sex should behave, and so do rewards and punishments. Boys

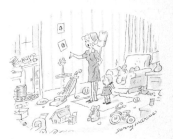

"Someday, if you're not careful, all this will be yours!"

Courtesy of Jerry Marcus and Good Housekeeping *Magazine.*

Table 12–1.   Masculine and Feminine Sex-role Traits

Masculine Traits	Feminine Traits
Athletic, strong	Weak, nonathletic
Worry less about appearance and aging	Worry about appearance and aging
Breadwinner	Domestic
Sexually experienced	Virginal
Unemotional, stoic	Emotional, sentimental
Logical, rational, objective, intellectual	Scatterbrained, inconsistent, intuitive
Leader, dominating	Follower, subservient
Independent, free	Dependent, overprotected
Aggressive	Passive
Success oriented, ambitious	Easily intimidated, shy

Source: Janet Saltzman Chafetz, *Masculine/Feminine or Human? An Overview of Sex Roles* (Itasca, Ill.: F. E. Peacock, 1974), p. 38.

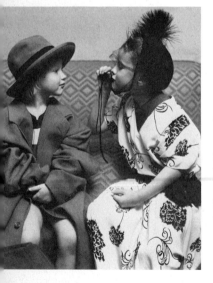

"Kiss me, you fool!"

Suzanne Szasz

are praised when they act like their fathers ("He's a real chip off the old block"), but not like their mothers ("He's just a mama's boy"). They are taught to act tough, not to cry or show their feelings, and they are encouraged to express their opinions and ideas. Girls are comforted and protected when their feelings spill over into tears. Girls who are quiet and sweet are called "ladylike." If they play roughly or loudly, or get dirty, they are told that "nice young ladies don't do that."

Despite these subtle and not-so-subtle pressures to behave as "real women and real men," many girls and women are active and assertive, just as many boys and men are quiet and not aggressive. These people are not always thought to be properly feminine or masculine, but research shows that it is quite normal for people to be both aggressive and submissive. What determines the balance of the two, in any person, is *socialization*—the way in which a person is brought up and taught to be a part of society. This explains why in some cultures boys grow up to be passive and emotionally expressive and why, in some, girls grow up to be bold and assertive.

Society Is Destiny

What we know about sex roles and socialization seems to refute the famous claim of Sigmund Freud that "anatomy is destiny." For most people, *cultural conditioning* is destiny. Most people assume that when children are born male or female they will just assume the proper role for their sex. But is it as simple as that? The research of John Money revolved around hermaphrodites—people whose bodies are partly male and partly female or not quite all male or all female. This condition results from hormone problems that occur during fetal life. Money observed that upon birth a sex was assigned to hermaphrodites, and some surgery and hormone therapy was given to reinforce their sense of sexual identity. Money saw that these people learned and adjusted to the sex roles assigned them; he concluded that these roles are learned, not a part of our personalities from conception. Money feels that we are born "psychosexually neutral" and that our culture shapes our sexuality.

Because our culture channels people into sex roles, the nurturing talents of men are mostly wasted, as are the administrative talents of women (to name just two).

We are not blind to this waste, but often we are slow to correct it. In our own culture women have fought for greater freedom of choice and action; many women now seek careers in the professions. As a result, men have become more free to choose careers that once were reserved for women only. Working women are no longer labeled "unfeminine" and "unfortunate" as they were only decades ago: Male nurses and secretaries are no longer automatically suspected of being gay.

Yet role stereotypes persist. Even after a hard day on the job, many women go home to cook, clean, and take care of the children. At work, few women are encouraged to seek positions of leadership or to get the training needed for highly technical jobs. The woman who does succeed in the world of business, the career woman, must often become more like a man—dressing in conservative suits, acting competitively, and avoiding friendships with women in clerical positions. The need to be somewhat "masculine" makes many of these women question their femininity; and those who enjoy their femaleness are troubled that the business world finds it less important than maleness.

Some career women come to envy and dislike men because men have an easier road to success than they have. Indeed, girls often envy boys and women often envy men. But men rarely envy women, and the reason is clear: Our culture rewards traditional male achievements, such as work skills or athletic ability, with money, power, and status; traditional female achievements, such as charm and housekeeping skills, are thought to be of value, not for themselves, but only for their help in attracting the attention of the right man.

Role Conflict in Women

Despite sex-role stereotyping, many women have gone to college and pursued careers. As a result they develop qualities that used to be thought of as purely male: individuality, independence, self-reliance, and competitiveness. Many career woman also enjoy social and sexual friendships with men. When they lead to marriage and children, as they often do, it is the women who are faced with severe conflicts. A career requires much time and much commitment—and so does a family. If there is not time and energy for both, some women feel that both aspects of their lives will suffer. They may not feel fully successful in

The Sex of Your Child

Can couples now plan the sex of their children and, more important, should they? In the past, couples tried to influence their children's sex by such techniques as eating certain foods before and during pregnancy and avoiding other foods; using one position or another during the sex act; timing the act close to ovulation; or douching with either mild acids or mild bases after intercourse, to change the acid level of the vagina.

More sophisticated methods have recently been devised, but neither for them, nor for the "do it yourself" method, is there any guarantee; a more advanced technique yet is required. The research continues. If it succeeds, one result might be a smaller population, since couples would be able to get a child of the desired sex the first time. Since most of the world's cultures prefer a male for the first-born, there would be a surplus of men. The consequences might be beyond belief.

Table 12–2.   Median Money Income of Year-round Full-time Workers with Income, by Sex and Age: 1970 to 1979

Age	Women			Men			Ratio: Women To Men		
	1970	*1975*	*1979*	*1970*	*1975*	*1979*	*1970*	*1975*	*1979*
Total with income	$5,440	$7,719	$10,548	$9,184	$13,144	$17,533	.59	.59	.60
14–19 years	3,783	4,568	6,715	3,950	5,657	7,518	.96	.81	.89
20–24 years	4,928	6,598	8,571	6,655	8,521	11,480	.74	.77	.75
25–34 years	5,923	8,401	11,155	9,126	12,777	16,824	.65	.66	.66
35–44 years	5,531	8,084	11,184	10,258	14,730	20,069	.54	.55	.56
45–54 years	5,588	7,980	10,934	9,931	14,808	20,464	.56	.54	.53
55–64 years	5,468	7,785	10,873	9,071	13,518	19,436	.60	.58	.56
65 years and over	4,884	7,273	10,664	6,754	11,485	16,107	.72	.63	.66

Source: U.S. Bureau of the Census, *Statistical Abstract of the United States, 1980* (101st ed.), table 768, p. 463.

UPI

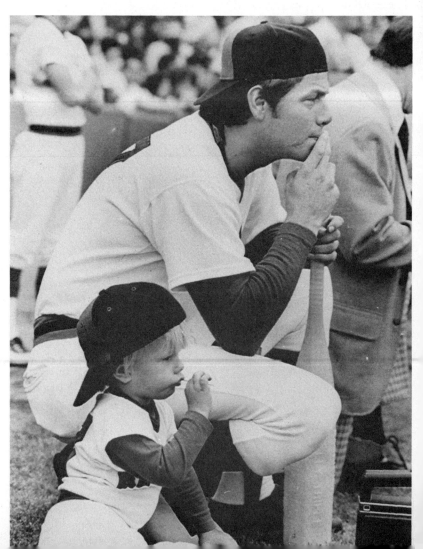

homemaking or child rearing because of the time they spend at work. They may not feel fully successful at work because they may not be free to choose projects or offers that keep them away from home. These women sometimes lose self-esteem and become angry, depressed, and unnerved by the conflict they face daily.

Sex-role Pressures on Men

Sex roles create problems for men as well as women. Since in our own culture women most often take care of children, boys are raised mainly by their mothers. Since we grow to love those who care for us, boys may come to love their mothers more naturally and more easily than they love their fathers. Boys soon learn, though, that they are expected to take their fathers as *role models,* or models of behavior. They learn, too, that the caretaking role of mothers is not really valued by

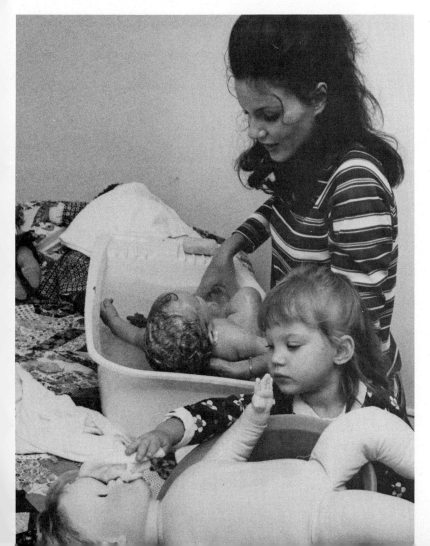

Erika/Photo Researchers

SELF-ASSESSMENT DEVICE 12-1: THE ATTITUDES TOWARD WOMEN SCALE (AWS)

THE ATTITUDES TOWARD WOMEN SCALE
SCORING INSTRUCTIONS

The Attitudes Toward Women Scale contains 55 items, each consisting of a declarative statement for which there are four response alternatives: Agree Strongly, Agree Mildly, Disagree Mildly, and Disagree Strongly. Each item is given a score from 0 to 3, with 0 representing choice of the response alternative reflecting the most traditional, conservative attitude and 3 the alternative reflecting the most liberal, profeminist attitude. Because the statement contained in some of the items is conservative in content and the statement in others is liberal, the specific alternative (Agree Strongly or Disagree Strongly) given a 0 score varies from item to item. Each subject's score is obtained by summing the values for the individual items. The range of possible scores goes from 0 to 165. The most conservative possibility is shown. The keyed responses should be covered before copies are made for participants, or items can be read aloud.

The statements listed below describe attitudes toward the role of women in society that different people have. There are no right or wrong answers, only opinions. You are asked to express your feelings about each statement by indicating whether you (A) agree strongly, (B) agree mildly, (C) disagree mildly, or (D) disagree strongly. Please indicate your opinion by marking the alternative that best describes your personal attitude. Please respond to every item.

(A) Agree strongly
(B) Agree mildly
(C) Disagree mildly
(D) Disagree strongly

Response keyed 0 (The most conservative alternative, scored 0, is shown)

A 1. Women have an obligation to be faithful to their husbands.

A 2. Swearing and obscenity are more repulsive in the speech of a woman than a man.

A 3. The satisfaction of her husband's sexual desires is a fundamental obligation of every wife.

D 4. Divorced men should help support their children but should not be required to pay alimony if their wives are capable of working.

A 5. Under ordinary circumstances, men should be expected to pay all the expenses while they're out on a date.

D 6. Women should take increasing responsibility for leadership in solving the intellectual and social problems of the day.

D 7. It is all right for wives to have an occasional, casual, extramarital affair.

D 8. Special attentions like standing up for a woman who comes into a room or giving her a seat on a crowded bus are outmoded and should be discontinued.

D 9. Vocational and professional schools should admit the best qualified students, independent of sex.

D 10. Both husband and wife should be allowed the same grounds for divorce.

A 11. Telling dirty jokes should be mostly a masculine prerogative.

D 12. Husbands and wives should be equal partners in planning the family budget.

A 13. Men should continue to show courtesies to women such as holding open the door or helping them on with their coats.

D 14. Women should claim alimony not as persons incapable of self-support but only when there are children to provide for or when the burden of starting life anew after the divorce is obviously heavier for the wife.

A 15. Intoxication among women is worse than intoxication among men.

A 16. The initiative in dating should come from the man.

SELF-ASSESSMENT DEVICE 12-1: (continued)

Response keyed 0	(The most conservative alternative, scored 0, is shown)
D	17. Under modern economic conditions with women being active outside the home, men should share in household tasks such as washing dishes and doing the laundry.
D	18. It is insulting to Women to have the "obey" clause remain in the marriage service.
D	19. There should be a strict merit system in job appointment and promotion without regard to sex.
D	20. A woman should be as free as a man to propose marriage.
D	21. Parental authority and responsibility for discipline of the children should be equally divided between husband and wife.
A	22. Women should worry less about their rights and more about becoming good wives and mothers.
D	23. Women earning as much as their dates should bear equally the expense when they go out together.
D	24. Women should assume their rightful place in business and all the professions along with men.
A	25. A woman should not expect to go to exactly the same places or to have quite the same freedom of action as a man.
A	26. Sons in a family should be given more encouragement to go to college than daughters.
A	27. It is ridiculous for a woman to run a locomotive and for a man to darn socks.
A	28. It is childish for a woman to assert herself by retaining her maiden name after marriage.
D	29. Society should regard the services rendered by the women workers as valuable as those of men.
A	30. It is only fair that male workers should receive more pay than women, even for identical work.

Response keyed 0	(The most conservative alternative, scored 0, is shown)
A	31. In general, the father should have greater authority than the mother in the bringing up of children.
A	32. Women should be encouraged not to become sexually intimate with anyone before marriage, even their fiancés.
D	33. Women should demand money for household and personal expenses as a right rather than as a gift.
D	34. The husband should not be favored by law over the wife in the disposal of family property or income.
D	35. Wifely submission is an outworn virtue.
A	36. There are some professions and types of businesses that are more suitable for men than women.
A	37. Women should be concerned with their duties of childrearing and housetending, rather than with desires for professional and business careers.
A	38. The intellectual leadership of a community should be largely in the hands of men.
A	39. A wife should make every effort to minimize irritation and inconvenience to the male head of the family.
D	40. There should be no greater barrier to an unmarried woman having sex with a casual acquaintance than having dinner with him.
D	41. Economic and social freedom is worth far more to women than acceptance of the ideal of femininity which has been set by men.
A	42. Women should take the passive role in courtship.
A	43. On the average, women should be regarded as less capable of contribution to economic production than are men.
D	44. The intellectual equality of woman with man is perfectly obvious.

SELF-ASSESSMENT DEVICE 12-1: (continued)

Response keyed 0	(The most conservative alternative, scored 0, is shown)
D	45. Women should have full control of their persons and give or withhold sex intimacy as they choose.
A	46. The husband has in general no obligation to inform his wife of his financial plans.
A	47. There are many jobs in which men should be given preference over women in being hired or promoted.
A	48. Women with children should not work outside the home if they don't have to financially.
D	49. Women should be given equal opportunity with men for apprenticeship in the various trades.
D	50. The relative amounts of time and energy to be devoted to household duties on the one hand and to a career on the

Response keyed 0	(The most conservative alternative, scored 0, is shown)
	other should be determined by personal desires and interests rather than by sex.
A	51. As head of the household, the husband should have more responsibility for the family's financial plans than his wife.
D	52. If both husband and wife agree that sexual fidelity isn't important, there's no reason why both shouldn't have extramarital affairs if they want to.
A	53. The husband should be regarded as the legal representative of the family group in all matters of law.
D	54. The modern girl is entitled to the same freedom from regulation and control that is given to the modern boy.
A	55. Most women need and want the kind of protection and support that men have traditionally given them.

Source: By Janet T. Spence and Robert Helmreich. Used with permission. A machine-scorable answer sheet is available from the Department of Psychology, The University of Texas, Austin, Texas 78712.

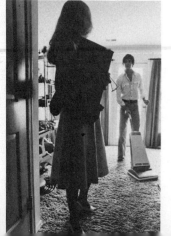

Bruce Roberts/Rapho/Photo Researchers

our culture. They may conclude that women are, then, less important than men are.

Because our culture undervalues female qualities, boys learn to hide those aspects of their personalities. They often conceal their emotions, play rugged games, and avoid friendships with girls, thus saying to the world: "There's nothing feminine about me." Although girls are sometimes criticized for being tomboys, wearing jeans and other "male" clothing, climbing trees, and competing in sports, such things are not forbidden to them or ridiculed. Boys would be ridiculed and bullied, though, if they played with dolls and wore "sissy" clothing. In this sense, boys are less free to explore traditional "female" qualities than girls are to explore traditional male ones.

When boys reach their teens, their confused feelings of love, hate, and fear toward women and femininity can cause them a few problems. Starting in their teens, boys must demonstrate their maleness in the bedroom, as well as on the playing field. As boys they may have feared that it was "sissy" to make friends with girls. But now having girl-friends becomes a test of male pride. Our culture makes this task easy since girls are taught to admire maleness; girls at this stage often prefer sports heroes to quiet or studious boys.

Yet the sports heroes and other aggressive types have their own problems. Although it is often easy for them to attract girls, it is not so easy to keep them; the "macho" personality cannot tolerate equality. Intimacy is hard to develop and maintain when a boy feels that he must dominate every contest and always be smarter and stronger than a girl. Then, too, although girls sometimes like their boyfriends to be aggressive and assertive with *others*, they most often want their boyfriends to be gentle and caring with *them*. This is a distinction that boys may not be aware of, and sometimes they try to promote their "male" toughness, which turns their friendships into "sexercise." Girls may then come to dislike this type of boy.

The Androgynous Personality

Would most boys and men be happier if they were freed from the need to play the tough guy all the time? And would girls and women be happier if they could express their aggressive feelings as well as their tender feelings? Do we need sex roles? Until recently these were not real questions; maleness and femaleness were taken for granted. But with World War II, more and more women began to work outside the home, and so more and more men had to take care of their children, on occasion, and do some of the housework. Traditional sex roles began to unravel long before the Women's Movement of the 1960s. Ours is still a sexist culture; but there are trends that may free today's children from stereotyped sex roles. Such trends should allow them to become complete human beings, who use all their skills and talents, not men and women who are limited in the traditional sense.

The old sex roles were taught through the old ideals of maleness and femaleness. Once the whole idea of sex roles was challenged, a new ideal was born. That new ideal is called the *androgynous personality*, from the Greek words *aner (andros)*, meaning man, and *gyne*, meaning woman. Such an ideal would encourage men and women to follow their natural (not social) personalities and to behave in ways that allow them to blend the male traits with the female traits that make them feel most comfortable. For men, this means taking on more family-centered tasks, if they want to, letting gentle and nurturing feelings show, giving and accepting support from both men and women. For women, it means more of a focus on personal fulfillment, pursuing employment goals, and using skills and talents outside the home. Androgynous friendships let people relax and "be themselves," to grow sexually, and to feel comfortable while exploring and sharing their sexuality with others.

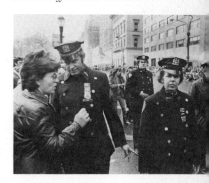

Michael Uffer/Photo Researchers

SELF-ASSESSMENT DEVICE 12-2: ARE YOU MASCULINE, FEMINE, OR BOTH?

Write down next to each item a number from 1 to 7 indicating how strongly you display that particular trait. On the first item, for example, put down a 1 if you believe that you are never or almost never self-reliant, a 7 if you believe that you are always or almost always self-reliant, or some other number in between to indicate how far you lean in the direction of self-reliance or lack of it. When you finish rating yourself on all 60 items, see the scoring instructions.

1. self-reliant
2. yielding
3. helpful
4. defends own beliefs
5. cheerful
6. moody
7. independent
8. shy
9. conscientious
10. athletic
11. affectionate
12. theatrical
13. assertive
14. flatterable
15. happy
16. strong personality
17. loyal
18. unpredictable
19. forceful
20. feminine
21. reliable
22. analytical
23. sympathetic
24. jealous
25. has leadership abilities
26. sensitive to the needs of others
27. truthful
28. will take risks
29. understanding
30. secretive
31. makes decisions easily
32. compassionate
33. sincere
34. self-sufficient
35. eager to soothe hurt feelings
36. conceited
37. dominant
38. soft spoken
39. likable
40. masculine
41. warm
42. solemn
43. willing to take a stand
44. tender
45. friendly
46. aggressive
47. gullible
48. inefficient
49. acts as a leader
50. childlike
51. adaptable
52. individualistic
53. does not use harsh language
54. unsystematic
55. competitive
56. loves children
57. tactful
58. ambitious
59. gentle
60. conventional

SCORING DEVICE

To score the test in Figure 10-8, first add up the numbers you have placed next to the items 1, 4, 7, 10, 13, 16, 19, 22, 25, 28, 31, 34, 37, 40, 43, 46, 49, 52, 55, and 58. Divide the total by 20. The result is your masculinity score. Next add up the numbers next to items 2, 5, 8, 11, 14, 17, 20, 23, 26, 29, 32, 35, 38, 41, 44, 47, 50, 53, 56, and 59. Divide the total by 20. The result is your feminity score. Now subtract the masculinity score from the femininity score—and divide the result, which may be plus or minus, by 23. You now have your final score, which can be interpreted as follows: Over +2, traditionally femine in tastes and behavior. Between +1 and +2, "near feminine." Between +1 and –1, mixed or androgynous (for the meaning of which see the text). Between –1 and –2, "near masculine." A minus figure greater than –2, traditionally masculine in tastes and behavior.

Source: Jerome Kagan and Ernest Haverman, *Psychology,* 4th ed. (New York: Harcourt Brace Jovanovich, 1980), pp. 387, 389.

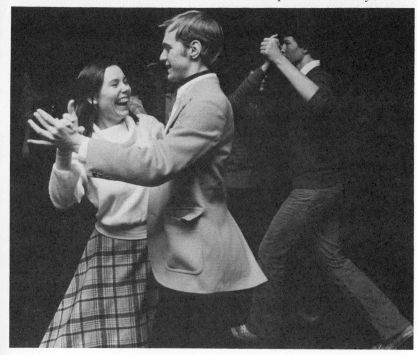

Frank Siteman/Stock, Boston

Physical Sexuality

Sexuality, as we have seen, includes all those ways in which women act as women and men act as men. So far, though, we have looked only at the social aspect of sexuality. We shall now look at its physical aspect. There is no real distinction between the physical and social aspects of sexuality, since different cultures regard different kinds of physical sexuality as "normal." So it is clear that physical sexuality is, in a great many respects, an extension of social sexuality. Nonetheless, there is a difference between the sexuality that lies behind the jobs we take and the clothing we wear, for example, and the sexuality of the sex act itself.

Physical sexuality is expressed in two ways. The sex drive within each person—the wellspring of the sexual impulse—is called *intrapersonal sexuality*. An example of intrapersonal sexuality is *masturbation*. Relationships with others, as long as they are to some extent mutual emotional and physical relationships, are called *interpersonal sexuality*.

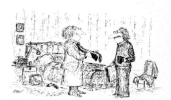

"Sweetie, will you help me with my tie?"

Drawing by Koren; © *1979 The New Yorker Magazine, Inc.*

Sexual Development

As humans mature, their sexuality unfolds and expands. A child's first task in sexual learning is to become familiar and comfortable with

Embarrassment and concern about human sexuality can tie the tongue of the most eloquent speaker. But almost every culture provides instant relief in two forms: euphemisms and "dirty" words.

Euphemisms are words and phrases that we substitute for the unmentionable. The word "unmentionable" is, in fact, itself a euphemism for "underwear," as in the sentence, "She packed just one dress and a few unmentionables." The substitution of "passing away" for "dying" and "large" for "obese" seems almost explicit when compared with sexual euphemisms like "rest room" (for "toilet," itself a French euphemism meaning "little piece of cloth") or "lady-in-waiting" (for "pregnant woman"). American newspapers tell us that a rape victim has been "molested"; the British press prefers to say that she was "interfered with." In the United States, homosexual behavior is "gay" or "queer"; in Great Britain, they say "poof" or "fluff."

At the other end of the spectrum are what we might call "euphemisms in reverse," substitutions of sexually explicit words for mild ones. Most substituted "dirty words" are designed to attract attention. When "He's an idiot" seems too mild, "He's a perfect #?!@" does the job nicely.

Why do we insult people by equating them with sexual terms, and at the other end of the continuum, why is it impossible to describe sexual matters without "skirting the issue"? Psychiatrists believe that dirty words and euphemisms emerge out of unhealthy attitudes toward sex and body functions. The increasingly common use of these expressions in an era of greater and greater sexual freedom suggests that we may not be very free at all.

Incidentally, the use of euphemisms is futile, as well as unhealthy, for each euphemism eventually becomes as explicit as the word it was meant to replace and must itself be replaced by a *new* euphemism. This is why we have so many words to describe the sexual and excretory functions.

its own body. At puberty the body changes so much that this sense of comfort has to be relearned. Girls learn to deal with menstruation, boys with ejaculation, and both sexes adjust to new sexual feelings—both of the mind and of the body.

Most children are very curious about their bodies and those of the opposite sex. This may lead to youthful exploring that may be punished by parents who mistakenly view a child's curiosity through adult eyes. After puberty we all have to overcome the guilt, shame, and fear of sex. We have to learn that some things that our culture frowns on, like masturbation and premarital intercourse, are quite common. As we set up our new friendships we have to shift the chief focus of our emotional lives from our families of birth to the freely chosen partner. We have to learn which sex acts we like and dislike, and we have to learn how to talk about sex with our partners. We must become responsible for our sexual behavior—by learning about birth control (see Chapter 14) and sexually transmitted diseases (see Chapter 11)—and we must act on what we learn.

The final task of sex education is understanding the emotions that go with physical sexuality, for few things (if any) involve the emotions as much as sex does. Through this understanding we learn how to enjoy its pleasures in a friendship that also provides love, trust, and closeness.

Learning to understand and express sexuality means, first of all, learning about intrapersonal sexuality, the inner source, as opposed to interpersonal sexuality, the shared experience. Let's begin by taking a look at intrapersonal sexuality.

Intrapersonal Sexuality

Intrapersonal sexuality starts to develop in infancy. An infant is curious, and one of the first things it explores is its own body. It soon discovers that touching and stroking certain parts of its body—the sex organs, or *genitals*—gives pleasure. With this discovery sexual life begins.

Masturbation. As a result of these earliest searches, the infant seeks pleasure from touching and stroking its genitals from time to time. In other words, the infant masturbates. The infant's parents may become aware of this and try to prevent it, sometimes with punishments. These punishments can create guilt feelings in the child and help to undermine its self-esteem.

In our culture, parents once tried to stop children from masturbating because it was thought to be sinful and a danger to health. Children were told that it could lead to insanity, stunted growth, hair on the palms of one's hands, warts, pimples, death, and damnation. To "save their children from themselves," parents tried to prevent them from masturbating, with everything from aluminum mitts to chastity belts.

Times have changed. Medical experts today agree that masturbation—whether frequent or not—causes no physical or mental harm. In fact, masturbation actually helps our sexual development. It teaches us the pleasures that sex organs can give and helps us to be comfortable about touching our own bodies. In the teen years and in adulthood, masturbating to climax, or orgasm, can reassure those who are insecure that they can function sexually. Masturbation also provides some release from sexual tension when we have no sex partner.

Health professionals are now so accepting of masturbation that according to Thomas Szasz, a well-known psychologist, "in the 19th century masturbating was an illness and not masturbating was a treatment; today not masturbating is a disease and masturbating is a treatment." Society as a whole has not kept pace with this changing tide of professional opinion. Many parents who were raised when masturbation was considered immoral still feel that way about it.

Despite these misgivings most of us do masturbate—studies show that this means almost all men and most women. It is common at every age, both among the married and the unmarried. In fact, most women find it easier to achieve orgasm, or sexual climax (see Chapter 13), this way than any other way.

Sexual Fantasies.   During masturbation many people imagine that they are having sexual intercourse with someone who excites them, a movie star, for example. A sexually stimulating scene of this kind, which takes the form of a daydream, is called a *fantasy.* The well-known 1948 and 1953 Kinsey surveys of sexual behavior showed that 50 percent of women and 72 percent of men said that they fantasized most of the times that they masturbated. During masturbation, melodies, objects, and smells that remind us of past sexual pleasures also tend to bring forth fantasies. Indeed, the mere thought of these memories can bring some people to orgasm. The most common fantasy-thoughts reported by women involved sex acts that most of them would never try in real life, like having intercourse with strangers or with more than one person at a time. These are common fantasies for men too. Although heterosexuals usually have heterosexual fantasies, and homosexuals have homosexual fantasies, at times people reverse their sexual preferences in their imaginations.

Fantasies can occur not only when you are awake but also while you sleep, in the form of dreams. Sexual dreams sometimes lead to orgasms during sleep, relatively often for men, but more rarely for women. In a man, an orgasm during sleep is called a *nocturnal emission.*

Some who research fantasies believe that they reveal our true sexual desires. Perhaps many of them do. But some do not: For instance, many women have fantasies about rape, but the thought of being raped is fearful both to women and to men. Some psychiatrists have interpreted

A remarkably high proportion of the American women who have sexual fantasies have them about Paul Newman.

UPI

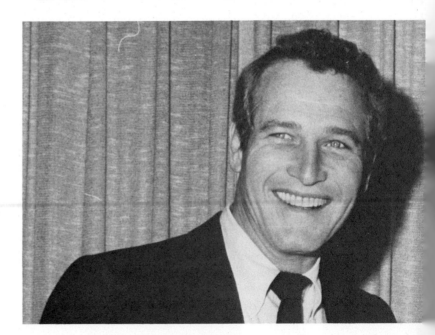

rape fantasies as women's attempt to "act out" this fearful situation, to deal with their worst worries and transform them into something less threatening. Others point out that women rarely see themselves as suffering in rape fantasies; they conclude that these fantasies permit women to imagine a vivid sex act that they can enjoy without any fear of engaging in it.

Freud and traditional psychiatrists believed that fantasy is neurotic. Today more psychiatrists are coming to think that fantasies are legitimate mental devices. Fantasies help us find out which sexual activities increase our pleasure. Through fantasy, each partner in sex can make some effort toward their own arousal, rather than relying wholly on the efforts of the other person. Fantasies also can heighten sexual pleasure: In a long-lasting marriage, for instance, fantasies can help replace sexual monotony with new-found excitement. Studies show that many married women use fantasies while making love with their husbands. These fantasies involve phantom lovers, forced sex, pretending to perform forbidden acts, and all the other subjects commonly reported as masturbation fantasies. These women may be content with their sex lives, but they are using their minds to make sex more pleasureful.

It is OK to fantasize. It is also OK not to fantasize. Many people never have fantasies yet still enjoy their sex lives.

Interpersonal Sexuality

We have seen that although fantasies are a part of *intra*personal sexuality, they can enrich *inter*personal sexuality. But sex with others is not always truly interpersonal. Many people are so self-centered in their attitudes about sex that they can *only* engage in *intra*personal sexuality, even when they have sex with a partner. Such people view their partners solely as a means to their own pleasure, not as people whose needs and desires also deserve attention.

Honesty.   Sexual relations without love are not always harmful. What is really needed in such cases is honesty—with yourself and with your partner. If you lead your partner to think that you are involved in a romantic way, when in fact you want sex and only sex, you are fooling yourself as well as your partner. But if both of you just want to use each other's bodies, no harm may be done. But what do you think it can mean when a person only wants a lot of sex of this kind?

Stages.   There are three overlapping stages to interpersonal sexuality. But each time we make love we do not always have to (or even want to) progress through all three: (1) first arousal, (2) then shared stimulation through kissing and touching to heighten each partner's sexual response, and (3) intercourse or masturbation to orgasm for both partners.

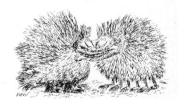

'You have a wonderful body.'

Drawing by Koren; © 1979 The New Yorker Magazine, Inc.

Homosexuality

If you have read the definition of interpersonal sexuality with some care, you may have noticed that it can be applied either to the love between men and women, *heterosexuality,* or to the love between people of the same sex, *homosexuality.* Homosexual women are called *lesbians.*

Most cultures condemn homosexuality to some extent. But in different cultures, at different times, it has been accepted. Although our own culture is not really one of those, Kinsey's surveys of 1948 and 1953 showed that in the United States many heterosexuals have homosexual fantasies and take part in homosexual acts. Most people cannot be grouped as two distinct populations—heterosexual or homosexual; most people have both tendencies.

These facts about homosexuality are gaining ground in the health profession; in the early 1970s, for example, the American Psychiatric Association removed homosexuality from its official list of mental disorders, and by so doing recognized homosexuality as a sexual preference, not an illness.

Variation

If homosexuality is no longer labeled an illness how might people look on other forms of sex that are not conventional, like sadism and fetishism? Are those who engage in them "variants," "deviants," or what?

When we pose the question in this way—"how might people look on" unconventional sexuality—we can see what the answer is. For "variation" and "deviance" are inherent in any act. Sex acts are called *deviant* only when they are regarded as such by a culture. Sometimes a culture changes its view; then an act ceases to be called deviant. Oral–genital sex (see Chapter 13) used to be regarded as deviant in our culture, for example, but it no longer is.

Ellis Herwig/Stock, Boston

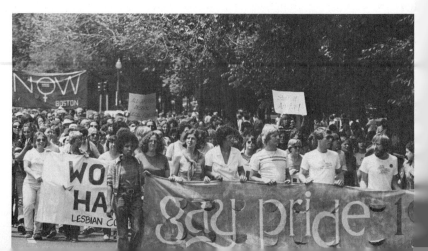

- *Masochism* is the desire to experience physical pain, a desire sometimes used to heighten sexual excitement during or before sexual intercourse. In its extreme forms the masochist typically wants to be whipped, cut, pricked, bound, or spanked in certain ritualistic fashions.
- *Sadism,* often considered the mirror image of masochism, is the desire to inflict physical pain on a sex partner, usually in a ritualistic manner. This pain may range from simple roughness during sex, to brutal torture. It is the agony and suffering of the victim that the sadist finds exciting.
- *Exhibitionism* is the display by men of their genitals to passing women—not as an invitation to sexual intercourse, but to demonstrate, to themselves and others, that they really are masculine. (Women may behave exhibitionistically, but as a sexual variation this is limited by definition to men.)
- *Voyeurism* means watching people while they are undressed or having sex. Voyeurs derive sexual pleasure from voyeurism only when they believe that the subjects do not know of the peeping and would not approve if they did.
- *Pedophilia,* the desire for sexual contact with children, usually suggests images of shadowy strangers lurking in schoolyards, waiting to abduct and rape unsuspecting children. But about 85 percent of such incidents involve a male parent, relative, family friend, neighbor or acquaintance—with a young girl.
- *Incest* means sexual relations between parents and their offspring or between brothers and sisters. All cultures define incest in some way and prohibit it.
- *Bestiality* is sexual activity with animals. Animals may be used when human partners are not available—as by teenagers on farms—but true bestiality, in which animals are preferred to human partners, is quite a rarity.
- *Fetishism* is a state of sexual excitement that can be aroused only by an inanimate object (dress, shoe, underwear, book, for example) or a part of the body (foot, hair, beard) not usually identified as erotic. True fetishism is very rare in women, except for the special form known as *kleptomania,* sexual excitement produced by stealing unneeded goods.
- *Transvestism* means sexual arousal achieved through wearing clothing of the opposite sex. Transvestism is closely linked to fetishism, because the transvestite uses clothing as an object of sexual excitement.

So, perhaps, *variant sexuality* is a better term than deviant sexuality. Variant forms of sex do not have to be unhealthy, evil, or sick; but they are preferences with appeal to a minority. Some people who engage in variant sex acts use them for the sake of variety; some can be sexually aroused in this way and in this way only.

Public Attitudes and the Law

Many people condemn forms of sex that seem unusual to them. They do not see how many of these, like masochism and sadism, are mixed into almost everyone's sex life. And they distort the real behavior of people whose sexual behavior they fear or dislike; homosexuals, for example, are often regarded "sex maniacs" and as attackers of young boys. Social suspicions of this kind create anxiety in homosexuals, as well as withdrawal and illness. These suspicions also deny them many of the rights of U.S. citizenship. In fact, homosexuality is not legal in some states.

In the 1970s many homosexuals "came out of the closet" and publicly proclaimed themselves. They, and many who were not homosexuals, began to say that homosexuality should be neither a crime nor a cause for shame. They started to campaign for the repeal of the laws against homosexuality, and for the passage of laws that guarantee homosexuals the protection of their rights as Americans.

In 1973, the American Bar Association passed a resolution urging the states to repeal all laws against homosexuality, as well as against all private sexual acts between consenting adults. Few states have so far complied either wholly or in part.

SUMMARY

Sexuality consists of all those ways in which women experience themselves as women and men experience themselves as men. Sexuality unites our physical to our social lives. It includes sex roles—the tasks, rights, and duties assigned to men and to women—and it also includes physical sexuality. Sex roles in most cultures give to women the "maintenance" functions and to men the "provider" functions. This division of duties tends to develop nurturing and dependent behavior in women and dominant behavior in men.

Sex roles are mostly learned, not inherited biologically. Both men and women possess traits that were considered male or female by tradition. Accepting both the male and female aspects of our nature—forming an androgynous personality—can help people avoid the sense of anxiety and failure often produced by sex roles.

Sexuality takes two forms: an *intra*personal form, confined to sexuality within, and an *inter*personal form, directed toward shared sexuality. Intrapersonal sexuality includes masturbation and fantasy, both of which can also be part of interpersonal sexuality.

Although interpersonal sexuality may be either heterosexual or homosexual in nature, homosexuality is often regarded as "deviant." It is the culture, not the act, that makes it so.

Cultures have, by tradition, condoned certain kinds of sexual behavior and not others. Today, though, many people claim the right to sexual freedom and privacy. Although our culture continues to frown on some sex acts, the law is starting to recognize that right.

Suggested Readings

Boggan, E. C., et al. *The Rights of Gay People.* New York: Avon, 1975. The American Civil Liberties Union's review of laws on homosexuality and other sexual behaviors.

Chafetz, Janet. *Masculine-Feminine or Human? An Overview of the Sociology of Sex Roles,* 2nd ed. Itasca, Ill. Peacock, 1978. An account of the socialization of males and females.

Hyde, Janet. *Understanding Human Sexuality.* New York: McGraw-Hill, 1979. An overview of all aspects of human sexuality, presented in an informative and readable style.

Money, John, and Erhardt, Anke A. *Man and Woman, Boy and Girl.* Baltimore: Johns Hopkins, 1973. A fine summary of Money's important research on hermaphrodites and sex-role assignment. Insights are offered into the development of sexuality.

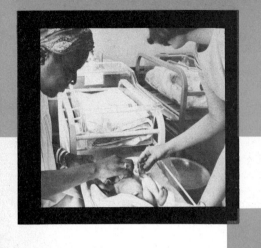

The Biology of Sex

chapter objectives

When you have finished reading this chapter you should be able to:

1. Discuss the working of the male and female sex organs
2. Explain conception and the trimesters of pregnancy
3. Describe the three stages of labor
4. Discuss the ideas and approaches to modern childbirth

It is hardly news that the *genitals,* or sex organs, of men differ from those of women. Indeed the concept of "man" versus that of "woman" is based on their differences. Despite the physical differences between the sexes, the sex organs of men and women function both for reproduction and for pleasure.

The Biological Man

Some parts of the sex organs of both sexes are *external,* on the outside of the body, and some parts are *internal,* within the body.

External Sex Organs

The external male genitals—the penis and the scrotum—are in full view on the front of the male body. The *penis* is a tubular structure at the groin; it is suspended over the *scrotum,* a sac that contains the two egg-shaped *testes,* which are internal sex organs. In a relaxed state the penis is about 3½–4 inches long and, in an erect state, about 6 inches long, but the overall dimensions vary from man to man.

The erection of the penis occurs when sexual excitement increases the amounts of blood that are sent into the genital area. This causes the penile blood vessels to become engorged, and the organ stiffens upward from the body. Men commonly suffer anxiety about the size of their penises as compared with those of other men. Most women, however, think that the size of the penis is not a major aspect of sexual relations.

At birth, the head of the penis (or *glans*) is surrounded by a fold of skin called the *foreskin* or *prepuce.* This foreskin (or part of it) is often removed right after birth in a procedure known as *circumcision,* which has ancient religious roots. Today it is chiefly performed for reasons of hygiene, although some physicians think that circumcision is not really necessary.

Internal Sex Organs

The internal sex organs of men have two chief functions. One is to produce *sperm cells* and to carry them out of the man's body. The other is to produce *testosterone,* the male sex hormone. Testosterone is produced in the testes and is discharged directly into the bloodstream. It is this hormone, along with others, that deepens the voices of adolescent boys, stimulates the growth of their face and body hair, and starts up all the other maturation traits. These male *secondary sex characteristics,* once established, need very little testosterone to be maintained.

Testosterone is produced within the testes, but only the first stage of sperm production begins there, in a complex system of canals called the *seminiferous tubules.* At puberty, the *germinal tissues* that line the walls of the seminiferous tubules produce sperm cells in great numbers. As millions of sperm cells are shed from the tubule walls, millions more

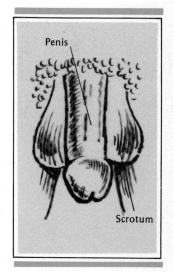

Figure 13–1.   External view of the male genitals.

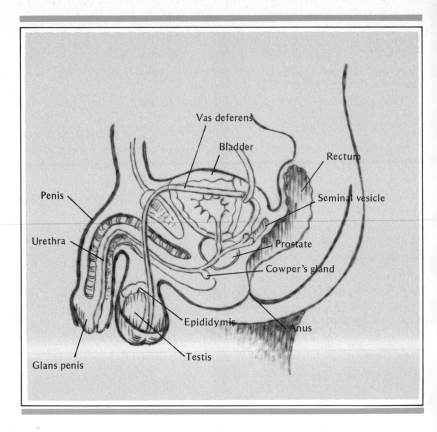

Figure 13–2. Cross section of the male organs.

are produced, without depleting the reserves. Packed into the head of each sperm cell is its cargo of genes (see below). The sperm's whip-like tail gives it the power of *motility*, or mobility, to swim the distance needed to meet up with the ovum.

The testes are first located in the abdomen of a male fetus. Before his birth, in the seventh month of pregnancy, they descend into the scrotum. In about 1 boy in 50 the descent of one or both testes is delayed. If both remain within the torso and do not descend after puberty, they degenerate; sperm production stops and feminine traits may appear.

The Sperm Is Made Ready.   When the sperm leaves the germinal tissues of the seminiferous tubules it is not completely ready for its mission of uniting with the ovum. The actions of a connected group of internal sex organs make it ready. First, the sperm travels from the seminiferous tubules to the *epididymus*, a complex system of storage canals coiled at the back of the testes. For 2 to 6 weeks, the epididymus acts as a maturation chamber, a screening point, and a waiting room, so that the healthy sperm develop and grow stronger while the defective sperm degenerate. When the sperm leave the epididymus, they travel through the *vas deferens*. At this point, the sperm cannot propel themselves, so they are moved along largely by muscular contractions in the vas deferens, and also by the sweeping action of the tiny *cilia*, or hairs, that line it.

The sperm move up the vas deferens to a point below and behind the urinary bladder (the sac-like structure that stores urine before it is voided from the body). Here the vas is joined by another duct from a structure called the seminal vesicle (a gland that supplies a sugar called fructose that provides nourishment and stimulates sperm movement). The combined ducts (vas deferens and seminal vesicles) are called the ejaculatory duct (a misnomer since it has little to do with ejaculation). The ejaculatory duct enters the prostate gland, where secretions fortify and protect the sperm by providing them with an alkaline coating. This alkaline coating is needed to neutralize the acidity in both the male and female bodies. Within the prostate gland, the ejaculatory duct joins the urethra (a tube from the bladder that voids urine). The urethra serves double duty: It conveys urine during urination and it conveys semen during the sex act.

The *Cowper's glands,* two pea-sized structures located at the base of the penis, are the last of the major male internal sex organs. They secrete *pre-ejaculatory fluid,* which both counters the acidity of the urethra and cleans it.

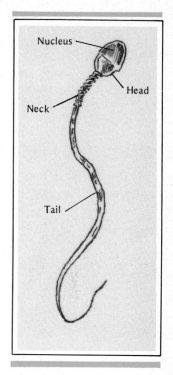

Figure 13–3. A sperm cell.

The Biological Woman

As with men, some parts of the female sex organs are external, others are internal. But even the outer female sex organs are largely hidden from view—quite unlike men's external sex organs.

External Sex Organs

The external sex organs of women are grouped in the *vulva*, which includes the *labia majora* and the *labia minora*, the *vestibule*, the *vaginal opening* and the *hymen*, the *urethra*, and the *clitóris*. All are in the genital (or pubic) area, between the legs. The labia are the lips of skin, fatty tissue, and delicate membranes that protect the genital area. The *labia majora*, or outer lips, are, after puberty, covered with pubic hair. The inner lips, or *labia minora*, located just inside the labia majora, are composed of delicate mucous membrane tissue. They are more sensitive than the outer lips, although both have a dense network of nerve endings. When stimulated, the labia become engorged with blood.

The labia minora surround the vestibule, the recessed area that contains the vaginal opening and hymen, the urethra, and the clitoris. The vestibule's tissues are delicate, with moist, pink, slippery skin.

The hymen is a membrane located at or across the vaginal opening.

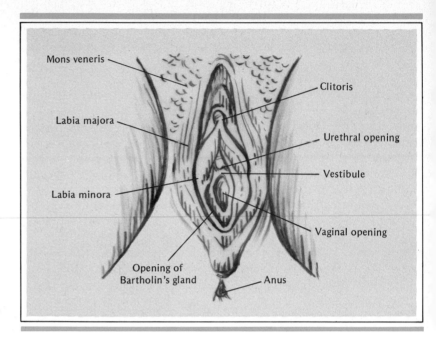

Figure 13–4. External view of the female genitals.

In young girls it protects the vagina from the entry of harmful microbes. (After puberty, the vaginal lining takes over this protective function.) Many cultures have considered an intact hymen as the sign of a virgin, and some even require it for marriage. But the hymen does not bar some forms of sex activity, and it can in fact be broken by accident.

The clitoris is centrally located at the upper end of the labia minora. It behaves like a tiny penis; and in fact the two structures develop in the embryo stage (see below) from the same tissues. Like the penis, the clitoris is rich in nerve tissue and blood vessels, and during sexual excitement it becomes full of blood, and throbs. The clitoris is composed of a glans and a shaft, and it is covered by its hood. When a woman is sexually excited the clitoris may become enlarged to twice its relaxed size and protrude beyond the sensitive folds of the hood.

Internal Sex Organs

The major female internal sex organs are the *vagina;* the *uterus* (or *womb*); the *fallopian tubes;* and the *ovaries.*

The vagina—sometimes called the birth canal—is a tubular opening some 3-4 inches long. It leads to the uterus, a hollow organ the size and shape of a pear, with thick muscular walls. The uterus is located in the center of the pelvic cavity, and its narrow end, the *cervix,* is at a sharp angle to the top of the vagina. The cervix has an opening through which menstrual fluids leave and sperm may enter.

The two *ovaries* are nestled one at each side of the dome, or *fundus*, of the uterus. Only about 1½ inches long, the ovaries are made up of gland tissue and egg sacs, or *follicles*. Each month, during *ovulation*, an egg cell, or *ovum*, leaves one of the ovaries and travels down its fallopian tube to the uterus.

Ovulation and Menstruation: Hormonal Cycles.   The follicles within the ovaries hold the ova, or egg cells. Each month the follicles in each ovary are stimulated by the follicle-stimulating hormone (FSH) from the pituitary gland. Hormones are chemicals, produced by the endocrine glands, that have a profound effect on all the body's functions. As the follicles grow they release *estrogen*, a hormone that helps to make the layer within the uterus called the endometrium ready to receive the fertilized egg, or *zygote*. Each month, one follicle grows more quickly than all the others. Then a second pituitary hormone called the lutenizing hormone (LH) causes it to burst, thus sending the ovum toward its fallopian tube. This takes place about midway through the

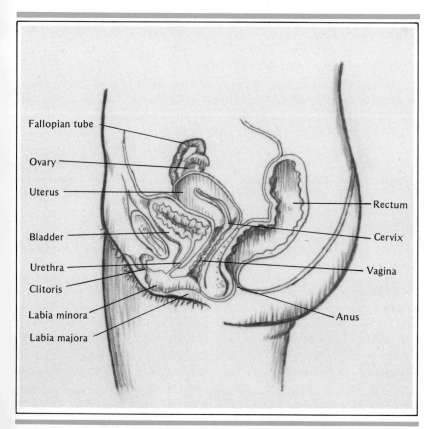

Figure 13–5.   Cross section of the female organs.

Fallopian tube

Ovary

Uterus

Bladder

Urethra

Clitoris

Labia minora

Labia majora

Rectum

Cervix

Vagina

Anus

monthly, or menstrual, cycle. In a cycle of 28 days, ovulation would occur about the 14th day.

The LH then causes the empty follicle to close and slightly increases its size. This closed follicle, now called the *corpus luteum,* along with the ovum itself, begins to produce another hormone, *progesterone.* Together with estrogen, this progesterone will cause the endometrium to become engorged with blood and nutrients.

If the ovum is not fertilized in about 48 hours, it breaks down. Later in the cycle the production of progesterone by the corpus luteum ceases, and the endometrium begins to dissolve and pass out of the body through the cervix and down the vagina.

The cycle of events that begins with the ripening of the ovum and ends with the passing of the endometrium from the body is called the *menstrual cycle.* The actual flow of the endometrium (the *menstrual fluid*) is called *menstruation.* The time during which this takes place is called a *menstrual period.* The average cycle lasts about 28 to 30 days, and it may vary somewhat from month to month. Usually it is slightly longer in young women than in older ones. The cycle often produces mood changes—anxiety, irritability, and depression—that may stem from the hormonal changes. But many women notice no mood changes at all.

Secondary Sex Characteristics

Hormones promote the development of secondary sex characteristics in women, as they do in men, beginning at about 11 years of age. At this time, a biological time clock in the genes increases the level of hormone activity, and this increase results in great physical changes. Female secondary sex characteristics include the widening of the hips, the growth of pubic and underarm hair, and the development of the *breasts,* which hold the *mammary glands.* The breasts, composed of fat and gland tissue, produce milk after the birth of a child. Breast growth is stimulated by hormones from the ovaries, so they are considered part of the female reproductive system.

Sexual Intercourse

The great number of people who throng sex counseling centers and psychiatrists' offices, and the popularity of "how to" sex handbooks, suggest that many people in the United States are troubled about sex, know little about it, or are not secure about what they do know. Yet there is not all that much to be known: The basic positions of sexual intercourse—the penetration of a woman's vagina by a man's penis—are few: man-on-top, woman-on-top, side-by-side, and rear entry. But these basic positions can be varied. And, of course, many positions may be

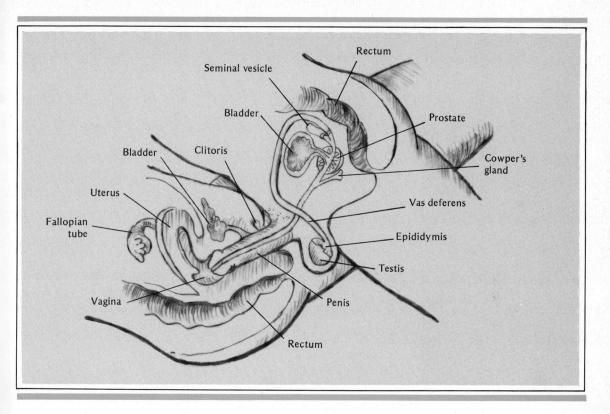

Figure 13–6. A cross-sectional view of sexual intercourse.

used during any one sex act; with experience, people learn to move from one position to another. Above all, there is no one "right" way to make love; there are only ways that give sexual pleasure to you and your partner, and ways that do not.

Positions

Man-on-Top. The most often used position for the sex act is the man-on-top, or the "missionary" position (called so because missionaries discouraged people in other cultures from making love with too much variety or zest). This position allows the man great freedom of movement and lets the partners kiss and caress each other's mouths and faces, whisper in each other's ears, and look at each other. It also allows the deepest penetration.

Woman-on-Top. This position gives the woman the greatest freedom of movement and provides her with some amount of clitoral contact. It is often used to allow the man to rest while the woman continues the movement.

Side-by-Side. The side-by-side position has several positive features: The partners are face-to-face; intercourse is restful and leisurely and can be prolonged; the penis does not enter the vagina deeply; and movement is somewhat restricted. This is a useful position for middle pregnancy. By late pregnancy only rear entry will allow the penis any access.

Rear Entry. In all the positions discussed so far the partners face each other. In the rear-entry position the man enters the woman from behind. In the standard rear-entry position the woman kneels and rests on her chest and arms while the man kneels behind her. This allows him great freedom of movement. The rear-entry position can also be used sitting or standing. Rear entry enables the man to stimulate the woman's breasts or clitoris, or the woman can stimulate her own clitoris. Rear-entry positions provide a mental and physical stimulation that differs from that of face-to-face intercourse. To many lovers variety is very desirable.

Sitting. In the sitting position the man sits on a chair or a bed. The woman sits over him and, either facing him (face-to-face) or away from him (rear entry), lowers herself onto his penis.

Standing. In the standing position the man stands before the woman (face-to-face) or behind her (rear-entry) and inserts his penis.

Lovemaking

There is a lot more to making love than positions. Making love is a complex and lovely act, one that often begins with kissing and caressing (or petting). The lovers sigh and whisper "sweet nothings" to each other. With words and with glances and with touch they make each other feel desired.

The lovemaking that leads up to intercourse sometimes includes *oral sex,* and sometimes oral sex is sought for itself. In oral sex, the mouth and tongue are used on the sex organs of the partner: *Cunnilingus* is the licking of the vulva and clitoris and *fellatio* is the sucking of the penis. Another technique that some enjoy is *anal intercourse,* the penetration of the anus by the penis.

Stages of Sexual Response

Every act of love has a story: It begins with a look or a word or a motion, progresses through several stages, then ends; and then a new act of love may begin. Two researchers named William Masters and Virginia Johnson have studied sexual response and divided it into four phases: excitement, plateau, orgasm, and resolution. In addition, men go through a refractory phase.

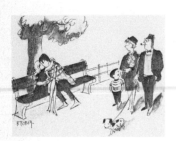

"We had that in school last week."

Drawing by B. Tobey; © *1969 The New Yorker Magazine, Inc.*

The excitement phase is the first response to sexual stimulation—either direct physical stimulation, as in long, deep kissing; or mental stimulation, as in reading a sexually explicit book. The man's first response is erection; the woman's is vaginal lubrication. Other typical signs of this phase include rapid breathing and pulse rate, an increased blood pressure that gives a "heady" feeling, and a flush on the back, neck, stomach, or chest.

During *the plateau phase*, sexual pleasure and tensions increase. Blood vessels swell in the sexual organs and throughout the body; awareness of sights and sounds is reduced. In women, the labia minora swell and turn bright pink; the inner two-thirds of the vagina expand; and the entrance to the vagina tightens by as much as 50 percent to form an *orgasmic platform* that "grasps" the penis as it moves. In men, the increased tension causes the erect penis to thicken and the testes to swell. The plateau phase tends to lead to *orgasm*.

The orgasmic phase is the height of sexual response. Orgasm (or climax) occurs as a powerful reaction, a release, which includes rapid pelvic-muscle contractions in both men and women. Sometimes the climax is described as an explosion that relieves the wound-up tension that built throughout the body, but mainly in the genitals, during the excitement and plateau phases. Orgasms differ from person to person and from time to time. Unlike most men, women can have *multiple orgasms*, that is, several within about half an hour, if the sex act or other stimulation is continued, with only slight pauses between each one.

The orgasm of a man consists of a series of powerful, rapid thrusts and contractions of the pelvic area, the penis, the prostate, seminal vesicles, rectum, and deep perineal muscles. Orgasm commonly (but not always) leads to ejaculation, in which semen is propelled through the urethra and out the head of the penis. The ejaculatory phase, or orgasm, lasts about 10 seconds.

The orgasm of a woman has been described as a more and more intense tingling sensation that explodes, pulsates, then descends into a warm glow, leaving feelings of satisfaction and contentment.

During *the resolution phase* the physical signs of excitement gently subside; the tension is gone, the sex organs shrink down in size, and the body feels very relaxed. Men go through a *refractory phase*; in other words, after orgasm they cannot quickly return to erection. Most women, if stimulated sexually just after orgasm, may re-enter the plateau phase right away and build to climax again.

Sexual Dysfunction

Most problems with sex, called sexual dysfunction, are rooted in the mind or the emotions, not the body. The idea that sex is sinful or dirty; feelings of low self-esteem, or of anger, lack of trust, or hostility for the partner—all can affect sexual response and performance for the worse.

Men.   Sexual prowess has always been regarded as a major part of manliness. This has always made it very hard for men to admit to having any kind of sexual problem without a great deal of emotional pain and shame.

Erectile Inhibition. Not getting an erection is called *erectile inhibition* (or *impotence*). Primary erectile inhibition is the failure ever to achieve an erection; secondary erectile inhibition occurs when a man who has not ever had a problem getting and keeping an erection develops such a problem.

Primary erectile inhibition sometimes has a physical cause—illnesses like diabetes, any radical surgery, and some heart disease (see Chapter 10), as well as the use of addictive drugs and alcohol. Secondary erectile inhibition is almost always caused by emotional problems.

It is misleading and harmful to "label" as impotence the failure to get an erection from time to time, since this occurs in almost all men at some time. It may be provoked by many of life's most commonplace hardships, including lack of money, marital strife, fear, or anxiety. Stress is the cause of many sex problems, and only the relief from stress may allow the soothing release that sex can bring to our lives.

Problems with Ejaculation. Two kinds of problems occur with ejaculation: These are *premature ejaculation* and *retarded ejaculation.* Men who ejaculate prematurely climax before, or within seconds of, entering the vagina. They cannot keep themselves from having quick and uncontrolled orgasms and so they do not stay erect long enough to satisfy their partner at least half of the time. Retarded ejaculation, which is a much more rare condition, involves a problem in ejaculating during intercourse, sometimes or all the time. Both of these problems with ejaculation often stem from emotional difficulties.

Women.   In our culture, until this century, women were not expected to enjoy sex, only to endure it. The idea that women might even have problems related to sex was realized only after it was known that they might enjoy sex at all.

Problems with Orgasm. Like the sexual problems of men, those of women are mostly emotional in origin. The most common sexual problem of women is a difficulty in achieving orgasm. Some women can climax in some conditions—through masturbation or oral sex—but not through intercourse. Perhaps as few as 20 percent of women can reach orgasm through intercourse alone—that is, without any direct stimulation of the clitoris. *Anorgasmia* (or frigidity) is a complete inability to reach a climax.

Problems with Intercourse. Vaginismus and *dyspareunia* often co-exist and have similar causes. Dyspareunia means painful intercourse. In vaginismus, tightly contracted muscles of the outer third of the vagina and the pelvic muscles prevent the penis from entering the vagina.

Treatment. Whether they are emotional or physical in origin, sexual disorders are treatable. Emotional problems are often dealt with through psychotherapy (see Chapter 3). Recently some treatment programs have achieved much success in treating sexual disorders by using the partly behavioral techniques developed by Masters and Johnson, who studied the human sexual response cycle. One of the cornerstones of the Masters and Johnson method is the treatment of couples, rather than individuals, with a team of sex therapists that has both men and women on it.

Older People

Until recently, older people were thought not to have a sex drive. Many people find the idea that their parents and grandparents make love distasteful, comic, or beyond belief. Physical changes, hormonal changes, and mental states that occur in middle age may reduce sex drive and desire. But they rarely destroy them to the point where people will not want to try again, if their partners do.

Menopause. In women, menopause is the permanent ending of the monthly menstrual cycle, an end that sometimes occurs suddenly, but more often over a few years. Sometimes the end is so gradual that a woman can get pregnant for 2 years after her periods become less frequent. In fact, several years should pass without a period before a woman stops using birth control if she is not willing to conceive at that time of her life.

A woman's feelings about herself and her general outlook on life greatly affect the way that she handles menopause. If she fears, quite needlessly, that her femaleness is defined by her ability to have children, or if she fears losing her sex appeal, a woman's adjustment to what is often called the "change of life" will be much more difficult than it need be. In any case, women entering menopause might need some understanding, since it is a reminder that time is passing and that their bodies are aging.

Climacteric. A man's production of androgen tends to drop in middle age, although this does not have to cause changes in sexual response and desire. The climacteric—a feeling in older men that they are less potent, less manly, or less desirable—seems to be mainly a state of mind.

Pregnancy: A New Life Begins

Sexual intercourse is nature's way to begin a new human life, one that is similar to each parent yet unique. The sperm cell contains the man's donation to this new life, and the ovum contains the woman's.

Heredity

Each cell of the human body contains genes, which are inherited "blueprints" that direct the course of the body's for growth. Genes are arranged on chromosomes, and in humans 23 pairs exist within the nucleus of each *body cell.* One chromosome of each pair comes from the mother's ovum; the other from the father's sperm cell. The sperm and the ovum have only 23 chromosomes each, one half the number in the body cells. When the two *germ cells* unite, they form a zygote, a fertilized ovum with the full number of 46 chromosomes. (For diseases of heredity see Chapter 10.)

Fertilization

At the midpoint of a woman's menstrual cycle an ovum is released by one of the ovaries, and it moves down its fallopian tube for several days. If a woman has intercourse at this time, hundreds of millions of sperm would be moving up her vaginal tract toward the ovum.

Their whip-like tails move the sperm toward the ovum at the rate of about an inch an hour. As they move they must overcome the force of gravity (which may draw them out of the vagina), the vagina's acidity, and sometimes hostile mucous in the uterus. Of the hundreds of mil-

Test-tube Babies

Once a fantasy of science fiction, test-tube babies became a reality in 1978, when an English woman gave birth to a baby girl who was conceived in a laboratory. The physicians who presided over the event extracted a ripe ovum from its follicle and placed it in a warm lab dish with drops of her husband's sperm. When cell division reached the 8-cell stage, the embryo was inserted into her womb.

This technique has opened up possible motherhood to women who could not conceive because of blocked fallopian tubes. But it has also stirred up a debate in medical ethics. Some think that this technique is interference with nature. Others think that this is a costly technique that may be sought by millions. What guidelines, they ask, should be used in deciding who receives such treatment?

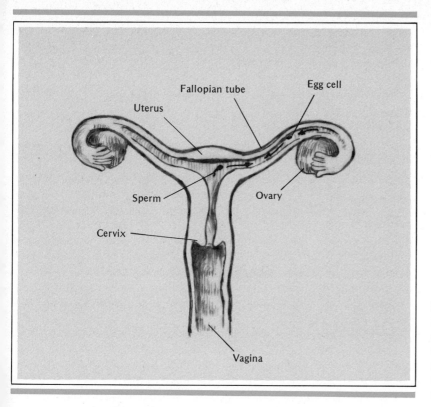

Uterus

Fallopian tube

Egg cell

Sperm

Ovary

Cervix

Vagina

Figure 13-7. Fertilization. Released by one of the ovaries, the egg cell moves down the fallopian tube. If sperm move up the vaginal tract and into the fallopian tube, fertilization occurs.

lions of sperm ejaculated into the vagina only a small number make it to the fallopian tube that bears the ovum. And only after several sperm enter the cell wall of the ovum does one fertilize it.

Fertility.   The sperm of all men is not equal; and sperm cells of the same man are not all equal. Some men have more sperm than others do in a given amount of semen; some sperm cells swim faster than others do. Sperm that can reach the ovum and fertilize it are called "viable" sperm. Recent evidence suggests that the viability of a man's sperm can be affected for the worse by the use of alcohol and by contact with certain industrial solvents and herbicides. The viability of the sperm is not the only thing that allows a couple to conceive a child. At times even quite viable sperm may not be able to reach the fallopian tubes unless they are deposited deep in the vagina. The vagina's acidity varies from woman to woman and from time to time. At times, too much acidity may prevent sperm from reaching the ovum.

About 1 of 10 couples cannot conceive, and for no physical reason. Often, this is caused by stress.

Pregnancy Tests.   A woman can often detect some signs of pregnancy. Of course, the best known of these signs is a missed period. Tingling and swelling of the breasts, frequent urination, darkening of the nipples, fatigue, and nausea ("morning sickness") are other signs of pregnancy.

Urine tests have become a way to detect pregnancy. Some of these tests indicate the presence (or absence) of HCG (human chorionic gonadotropin), a hormone produced by placental tissue. Kits that test for HCG can be bought in drug stores and used at home. A trip to the gynecologist, obstetrician, or family physician might result in an examination and a urine test that is sent to a lab.

The Three Trimesters of Pregnancy

The First Trimester.   By the time a pregnancy has begun the expectant mother will often begin to notice some changes in the workings of her body. During the first trimester (first 3 months) of pregnancy, hormones swell the breasts, darken the nipples, and cause bowel problems and "morning sickness" (nausea and revulsion against certain foods). Pressure on the bladder and the holding of body fluids make the woman urinate often.

Depression and fatigue seem common. A woman's reaction to pregnancy depends, first, on whether or not she wants a baby, and, second, on her overall mental state. Become pregnant by choice; a new life should not be a burden to bear with pain and doubt.

Zygote to Fetus.   From the moment of fertilization to the moment of birth, the fertilized ovum is called the *conceptus*. The conceptus passes through several stages of growth, each with its own name. Just after fertilization and before it begins to grow (through cell division), it is called a *zygote*. After a few days, when the conceptus has arrived at the uterus and planted itself in the endometrium, it is called a *blastocyst*. From the end of the 1st week of pregnancy to the end of the first 2 months, the conceptus is called the *embryo*. After the 4th week, it has a distinct backbone. By the 7th week, internal organs, like the liver, the lungs, and the intestines, begin to function in a limited way. After the 8th week, the conceptus is called the *fetus*. By the 10th week it has external features and organs, like arms, legs, eyes, and ears. At the end of the first trimester (the first 12 weeks), the fetus looks like a tiny infant. It is about 4 inches long and weighs less than an ounce.

Dangers. The first trimester is a time of danger for the fetus. Because of its simple structure and fast growth, it may be greatly changed or harmed by things that would be far less dangerous later in the pregnancy. Maternal illnesses like *rubella* (three-day, or German measles) may cause a number of deformities, including cataracts in the eyes of

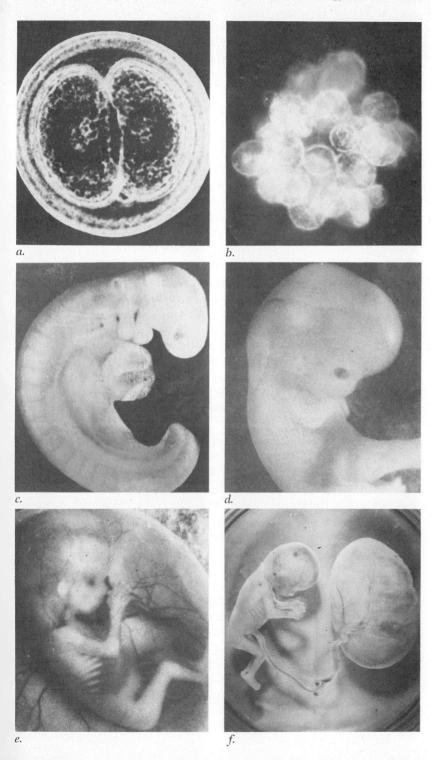

Intrauterine Development: a. the 2-cell stage; b. the blastocyst; c. the embryo at 28 days; d. the embryo at 8 weeks; e. the fetus in the 14th week; f. the fetus in the 16th week.

Courtesy of Dr. Landrum B. Shettles

the fetus; viral infections, like *herpes simplex* (both the oral and genital strains), can blind or abort it.

Pregnant woman must be careful about taking drugs at this time, since many drugs can hurt or even abort the fetus at this stage. Antibiotics like tetracycline can deform its bones and teeth. Even drugs as common as cold pills and aspirin can cause defects. Less common—and less well understood—drugs are more dangerous still. Thalidomide was once a widely prescribed tranquilizer, in the early 1960s. Its use caused thousands of children in the United States and Europe to be born with many defects. More recently, some daughters of mothers who took DES (diethyl stilbestrol) were found to have cancer of the genitals 16 to 20 years after birth. X-rays, too, are extremely harmful.

Remember that tobacco and alcohol are drugs, and that they, like other drugs, threaten the health of the fetus. Smoking and even moderate use of alcohol by pregnant women (see Chapter 5) can result in birth defects and lower birth weights. The baby of a pregnant woman who uses addictive drugs, like Heroin and barbiturates, will be "addicted" at birth and will require treatment for withdrawal symptoms (see Chapter 4). For a healthy birth, no drugs is the best policy.

Miscarriage. Even if a woman avoids using drugs or doing anything that might harm the fetus, there is still a risk of *miscarriage* (spontaneous abortion) during the first trimester. Miscarriages are quite common; they end about one-fifth of all pregnancies. Most miscarriages are caused by birth defects due to genetic problems that cause errors in fetal growth.

Abnormal bleeding or cramps sometimes mean that a miscarriage is about to happen. Any woman who fears a miscarriage should try to get to a physician, clinic, or hospital. Treatment may be required to prevent miscarriage or to make sure that it has been complete. Any fetal tissue that remains in the uterus might cause infection in the woman. After a miscarriage, there is a natural feeling of loss. Physical tests and genetic counseling (see Chapter 10) may then be in order if another pregnancy is wanted.

The Second Trimester.   In the second trimester (months 4 to 6) many changes occur in the pregnant woman, for the breasts and abdomen expand steadily. Nausea becomes less frequent, but other discomforts, like swelling of the legs, may occur. Most women, however, achieve a sort of calm and peace now.

In the 19th week the fetus begins to kick against the womb and, so, the parents, often for the first time, begin to regard the fetus as a new human being. As the fetus announces its life to its parents, it is also sending out signals to the physician: An audible heartbeat develops by the 18th week.

By the 20th week the fetus can open its eyes, and soon becomes sensitive to light and to sound. Periods of sleep alternate with periods of exercise.

The Third Trimester.   In the final 3 months (months 7 to 9), the uterus grows very large and tight, putting pressure on the woman's lungs, stomach, and bowels. Her navel (belly button) protrudes. She gains weight and may find this very hard to control. Since most of the weight is added to the front of her body, her new posture may cause her back to ache. Mild contractions may ripple through the uterus, strengthening the muscles for childbirth.

Both parents may talk about the baby's looks and about the pain and danger of labor. They wonder if the fetus will be born alive and healthy. Most couples—husband and wife—look forward very much now to the start of the new life that they have joined to create.

Like the mother, the fetus is gaining weight, and in the last 2 months, it gains 3 to 4 pounds. In the 7th month, the fetus normally turns so that it faces the birth canal head down.

Diet and Pregnancy

In the past pregnant women were often asked to consume great amounts of food. "You're eating for two, so eat a lot." Often the result of this advice was weight gains of 50 pounds or more during the pregnancy. The extra pounds not only caused discomfort and fatigue but also caused labor and delivery problems—not to mention the problems that the mother had losing the extra weight. Just how should a pregnant woman arrange her diet?

First she must eat a diet adequate for her own needs—1,200 to 2,800 calories. Then to this she should increase her calories by 15 percent, eat 65 percent more protein, 100 percent more folacin (a vitamin of the "B" complex), and 15 to 33 percent more of the other vitamins. Mineral intake should also be increased: 50 percent more of calcium, phosphorus, and magnesium, plus 25 percent more of iodine and zinc. Iron intake should remain about the same. Obstetricians often prescribe vitamin and mineral pills for women since it is hard to eat the needed amounts in the foods that are sold during any given season. If the woman began her pregnancy at her ideal weight, she should give birth weighing no more than 25 pounds more. This may seem like a lot, but the weight gain is due to the growth of the placenta, uterus, blood, vessels, and breasts of the woman, who may carry a 7½ pound fetus.

The pregnant woman should *avoid* alcohol; aspirin; acetaminophen; tranquilizers; antidepressants; antihistamines; antibiotics (Tetracycline, Kanamycin, and Streptomycin especially); hormones; antinausea drugs that contain Meclizine, Chlorocyclizine, and Cyclizine; and too much vitamin C or B_6 (pyridoxine). These may be included in drugs in the home medicine chest, so check the labels before taking any drug. If there seems to be a need for any drug, contact a pharmacist, a clinic, or a physician.

The best rule to follow is to eat sensibly, get enough rest, get some exercise, and avoid drugs of all kinds.

Birth

The Three Stages of Labor

Figure 13–8.   The three stages of labor. 1) The cervix dilates to permit the passage of the child. 2) The baby's head moves through the cervix and into the birth canal. The baby moves down to the opening and becomes visible. 3) The placenta and fetal membranes are expelled.

Labor and delivery follow a very distinct pattern of three stages in most women. Variations occur in all three, of course, and many of them are quite normal and pose no hazard to mother or child.

The onset of labor is announced by the discharge of the cervical plug—mucous that prevents bacteria from entering the uterus and infecting the child. True labor then begins by the breaking of the *amniotic sac,* or bag of water, that surrounds and protects the child while in the uterus.

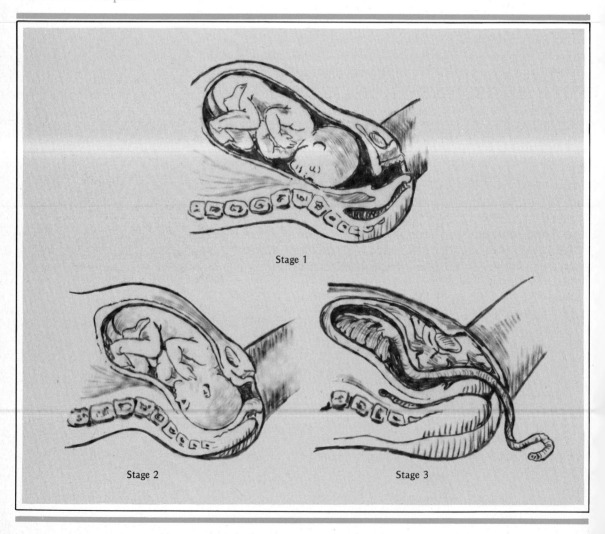

Stage 1

Stage 2

Stage 3

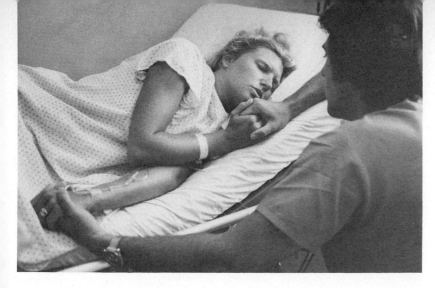

Hella Hammid/Photo Researchers

The First Stage.   The first stage of labor may last 2 hours or 24 or more. Active labor can begin right after the breaking of the water or be delayed a day or so. True labor starts with regular, painful, and rhythmic contractions of the uterus, 15 to 20 minutes apart, at first. These contractions then become more frequent and more intense. The cervix dilates (opens up) to permit the passage of the baby.

The Second Stage.   When the baby's head moves through the cervix and down into the birth canal, the second stage has begun. As the baby moves down to the opening it becomes visible. This event is called *crowning.* The mother often feels an intense urge to push and expel, and if properly guided she may speed delivery.

   The infant's head is delivered first, and gradually the rest of the body slides out. The *umbilical cord* still attaches the child to its mother as the baby begins to breathe on its own. The umbilical cord is then cut. The second stage of labor is shorter than the first, lasting about an hour or more.

The Third Stage.   The *placenta* and fetal membranes are expelled in the third and final stage of labor, often within an hour after delivery.

Fetal Positions

Ed Lettau/Photo Researchers

Most babies—96 percent—are born head first. Of the remaining births, most are the *breech presentations,* buttocks first, which involves a risk of broken limbs and other problems. A *transverse* presentation, with the baby lying crosswise in the uterus, occurs in 1 birth out of 200. In this case, the physician may use a tool called a forceps to turn the fetus in the uterus, or deliver the child by surgery called a *Caesarian section.* This operation is named after Julius Caesar who according to legend was delivered through an incision in the abdomen of his mother.

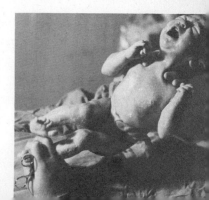

Anesthesia during Labor: Pros and Cons

The use of anesthesia, or painkilling drugs, during childbirth became standard practice in the mid-19th century, after chloroform, an anesthetic, was used on Queen Victoria. Among the drugs now used during labor are tranquilizers, to induce relaxation; barbiturates, to induce sleep; and general and local anesthetics. General anesthetics cause loss of consciousness. The woman is not an active participant in labor. Local anesthetics numb sensation only in part of the body.

The use of anesthetics in delivery is debated today. On the one hand, they eliminate the mother's physical pain. But on the other, they prevent her from actively assisting in delivery and from fully experiencing an important life event.

The effect of anesthetics on the fetus may also be harmful. Anesthetics can pass through the placenta to the fetus and depress its breathing—or cause even more serious harm. The best bet is to prepare for natural childbirth (see below) and try to go through with it. But if the pain of labor is too tiring, anesthetics should be ready—and then given with caution. The choice should always be the mother's.

Education for Childbirth

Parents face the birth of their first child with great excitement and little practice. So the months of pregnancy are a key learning time for both the mother and the father. Today, parents must make many more choices than ever before—about themselves and for their child.

Where Should the Baby Be Born?

Obstetricians, physicians who specialize in childbirth, want hospital deliveries, where Caesarian sections can be performed if needed and where intensive-care units and other resources are ready at hand. Major insurance carriers do not pay benefits for home births.

A new mother with a midwife, a nurse trained to deliver babies.

Robert Goldstein/Photo Researchers

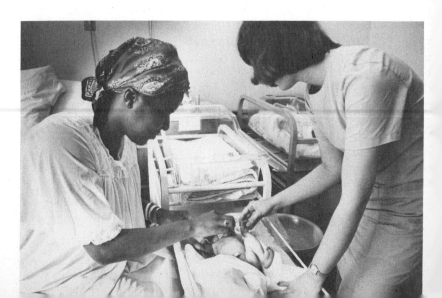

In many primitive cultures, the husbands of pregnant women go into a form of "mock labor" known as the *couvade,* which gives the new father an active outlet in the process of birth. In Western countries, however, control over childbirth has been given to physicians. In our culture the father's part in delivery declined through the years, just as his role in child care declined. Until recently, he mainly provided a model of authority, pride, competence, and strength. Traditional sex roles did not encourage child care and nurturing in men.

Yet even in Western countries men undergo mental changes during pregnancy that prepare them for fatherhood. They begin to think quite seriously about *family* obligations and often work hard to make extra money. They must come to grips with the fact that their partner will soon spend a great deal of time and energy caring for a helpless baby.

The more interested and involved in both pregnancy and labor the father becomes, the closer will be the bonds between all three members of the new family unit. All of the newer methods of childbirth emphasize the father's role in pregnancy and labor. The father's presence is good for many reasons: It gives the couple strength and often reduces the woman's need for painkilling drugs. It reduces the woman's sense of isolation. It helps to promote earlier *bonding,* the creation of intimacy, sensitivity, and responsiveness between parent and child. Men who are present at a child's birth are more likely to become deeply involved in their child's care.

The father's participation in delivery is still, in a number of states, restricted by law.

Many women are now resisting hospital births, choosing to have their children at home, often by a midwife. What is the advantage? Among other things, home births are not frightening; they permit eating, drinking, chatting, and free movement during labor. The parents can invite anyone they want. The mother can choose her own delivery posture—lying, sitting, or squatting. (The lying-down position used in most hospitals means pushing the baby upward, against the force of gravity.) In the home setting, the woman is not treated like a sick patient, but like the mother-to-be.

Some parents-to-be choose a birthing center. They are staffed by midwives, with back-up obstetricians, and they offer a good and fulfilling birth experience. Hospital birthing rooms, which are furnished in a homey sort of way and where the father and other relatives are welcome, are another option. In these birthing rooms mother and child are not separated right after birth, as they are with most hospital deliveries.

New Methods of Delivery

Home delivery, birthing centers, and birthing rooms are alternative places for babies to be delivered; midwives are alternative *health professionals* to deliver them. There are also alternative *methods* of delivery—alternatives, that is, to the idea of knocking out the mother-to-be to deliver the baby while she is asleep. These methods can be grouped under what is called *natural childbirth.* The pioneer of natural childbirth was an English physician, Grantly Dick-Read. Dick-Read believed that pregnant women approach labor in tension and fear because of all the frightening things that they have heard. This fear creates muscle tension, including tightening of the very muscles that must be flexible and yielding for a safe delivery. Dick-Read offered the idea of teaching women to focus on relaxing and pleasant images.

Dick-Read's approach was altered and popularized by a French physician, Fernand Lamaze. The Lamaze method teaches both parents how to take part in the process of delivery. In the months before childbirth, with the husband acting as "coach," the wife learns how to respond to the contractions of labor with breathing patterns and muscle-control exercises. Learning the Lamaze technique means that the couple attends a series of weekly classes.

Another method, the *gentle birthing* of Frederic F. LeBoyer, strives to minimize the trauma of delivery for the infant. LeBoyer wants lights

Learning the Lamaze technique.

Robert Goldstein/Photo Researchers

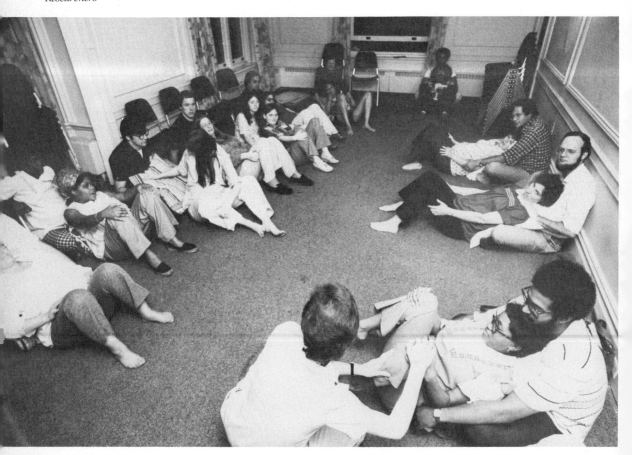

and voices kept low in the delivery room. The woman is assisted and supported during delivery, and the baby, still attached by the umbilical cord, is placed on her belly to sustain contact. The baby is kept warm, given a warm bath, and returned to its mother. The conditions of birth are meant to be as warm and dark as the womb, so that the child is not shocked into its new life.

The long-term effects of gentle birthing are not yet known, but developmental psychologists await them with interest.

The First Few Months of Life

The first few days and hours of life are the most critical of all, for the world outside the mother's womb is full of threats to life, and a baby is not equipped to deal with them.

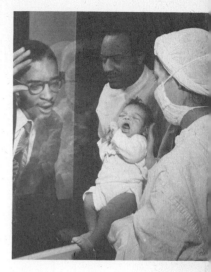

"Hi, Dad!"

Photo Researchers

Breast Feeding

One thing that can greatly help the well-being of a newborn child is breast feeding. Mother's milk is the ideal and natural food for a baby. Breast feeding gives the mother great benefits, too. The uterus shrinks more quickly to its normal size; the mother's sexual feelings return sooner; and the chances of a new pregnancy are decreased for the first few months. Remember, though, that a woman *can* become pregnant again soon after giving birth—even before the return of her first period.

Most mothers in our culture choose not to breastfeed and receive a drug that stops the production of milk. Two-thirds of all babies in the United States are bottle fed; only one-third are fed on mother's milk. Women who do choose to breastfeed should remember that a mother can transmit chemicals to her baby through her milk, so she must be very careful about diet and use of alcohol and other drugs.

Post Partum Depression

Many mothers go through a period of depression after the birth of their babies, usually within 2 weeks of the birth. They may have brief "crying spells" that seem to occur without reason, or they may feel annoyed with people.

The exact causes of post partum depression are unknown. The changing hormone levels of the new mother may be a physical basis for it. And the social relations between family members, friends, and co-workers may be greatly changed by the birth of a child. A new baby needs a great deal of attention, and this may wear out the mother or keep her from doing things or going places—other possible causes of the "after baby blues."

Whatever the causes, new mothers should know that it is quite a normal state and that it does not mean that they are "bad" mothers. And the father, other family, and friends should know this too.

SUMMARY

Sex organs distinguish men from women. The external sex organs are those directly involved in the sex act—the penis and scrotum in men, and the labia, vagina, and clitoris in women. The internal sex organs of men, of which the testes are the most important, produce the male sex cell, the sperm. The testes also produce the male hormone, testosterone, which maintains the secondary sex characteristics, like body hair, slim hips, and a deep voice. The internal sex organs of women, of which the uterus, fallopian tubes, and ovaries are the most important, produce the female sex cell, the ovum, or egg. They also produce the female sex hormone, estrogen, which maintains the secondary sex characteristics, like breasts and rounded hips.

During sexual intercourse the penis enters the vagina. The stages of sexual response—arousal, plateau, climax, and resolution—are similar in men and women. After men climax, however, they pass through a refractory period, a time when they cannot have an erection or an orgasm.

Ejaculation during the sex act places sperm inside the vagina. This may result in the fertilization of the ovum by the sperm, usually in the fallopian tubes, and thus a pregnancy. The course of pregnancy is divided into three trimesters, or periods of 12 weeks each. During the first trimester the fertilized ovum, or zygote, develops into an embryo, which after the 8th week is called a fetus. The woman may have some discomfort at this time, including nausea. By the time of the second trimester, these discomforts are gone, and there are more obvious signs of pregnancy: The breasts enlarge and the belly swells. The fetus announces itself to its parents by kicking. In the third trimester, the mother's breasts and abdomen enlarge even more as the baby grows and adds weight.

Labor is divided into three stages: a lengthy first stage, lasting from 2 to 24 hours, marked by regular contractions; a second stage, lasting a few hours, that begins with the baby's head entering the birth canal and ends with delivery; and a third stage, the expulsion of the placenta.

Parents today have a wide range of choices for delivery. These include home births; the use of midwives, birthing centers, and the techniques of Dick-Read, LeBoyer, and Lamaze—as well as traditional hospital care. The father's role has become very important to the mother's peace of mind during childbirth.

Early infancy is a period of complete dependence. The first hours, days, and months of life are the most dangerous, so infants need attention and concern from all around them.

Suggested Readings

Hyde, Janet Shibley. *Understanding Human Sexuality.* New York: McGraw-Hill, 1979. This book provides an overview of human sexuality—biological, psychological, and social. Practical information is presented in a very readable style. The book also contains guidelines for the critical review of sex research.

Masters, W. H., and Johnson, Virginia. *Human Sexual Response.* Boston: Little, Brown, 1966. This now classic study explores the way humans respond during sexual arousal and orgasm, and the mechanism involved in their responses. The results are based upon observation of sexual behavior.

Stewart, Felicia, et al. *My Body, My Health—The Concerned Woman's Book of Gynecology.* New York: Bantam Books, 1981. A thorough, scientific, and understandable book that focuses on self-care and informed choice. Conveys aspects of the female reproductive system and reproductive behavior.

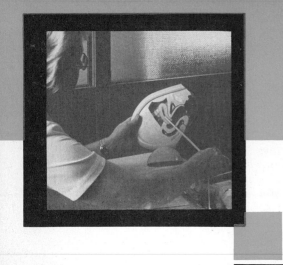

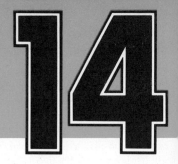

Birth Control, Sterilization, and Abortion

chapter objectives

When you have finished reading this chapter you should be able to:

1. Define contraception and discuss the biological basis for contraception
2. Participate in a discussion on "Contraception: Who is Responsible?"
3. Describe the methods of contraception
4. Respond to ideas for future contraceptive techniques
5. Discuss sterilization for men and for women
6. Discuss abortion, the pros and cons

Most people make love because it is fun and it feels good. This fun and the emotions that go along with it are nature's way of seeing that the *other* function of sexual intercourse—the propagation of the species—will be ensured. For thousands on thousands of years the good feeling of sex could not be separated from childbearing—even if people realized that it could be and wanted to do so—except by some not very effective methods of contraception, like *coitus interruptus* (see below). Gradually, other methods of *birth control*—preventing unwanted births—were devised. Most methods of birth control are also methods of *contraception,* or preventing conception (the fertilization of the ovum by a sperm cell). Birth control is a short-term method. A long-term method for achieving the same effect is *sterilization,* by cutting or tying the fallopian tubes in women or the vas deferens in men.

Birth control and sterilization are both preventive measures; to be effective, they must be done *before* sexual intercourse. *After* sexual intercourse has led to pregnancy, unwanted births can still be prevented, by *abortion,* or the removal of the products of conception. Abortion is one way to deal with an unwanted pregnancy; it is a response to pregnancy, not a way to prevent it.

Birth Control

Although fairly effective methods of birth control have existed for about a century, the subject is still debated in some quarters. Many people are against it. The Roman Catholic Church, for instance, teaches that sex is for creating new life; so interference ("contraception") is held to violate "natural law," since it destroys life or the potential for life. Outside of Church teaching, some feel that the use of contraceptives makes the sex act less natural or spontaneous. Others argue that contraception is a form of "genocide," designed to limit Third World peoples. Finally, research shows that birth control can create certain health risks, and that some methods are more dangerous than others.

For the most part the risks of birth control are not as great as those of pregnancy, so this is one of the chief arguments in *favor* of birth control. Although modern medicine has made pregnancy and childbirth reasonably safe, both still threaten the health of many women—and claim the lives of some. Women with diabetes, for example, may find their problems worsened by pregnancy. Women with weak hearts or lungs find labor to be life threatening. For these women, contraception can be viewed as an important form of preventive health care. Moreover, many women who do desire children still need to space them over time, to ensure their own health and the health of their families. Other families just do not have enough money to add another child. Many women in these circumstances feel that they must use birth control.

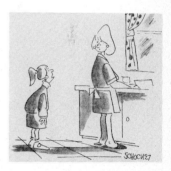

"Mom, will you tell me about the birds, and the bees, and the pill, the diaphragm and the coil?"

Reprinted by courtesy of New Woman. *Copyright © 1981 by* New Woman. *All rights reserved throughout the world.*

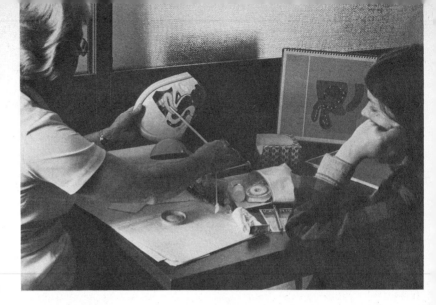

Birth control counseling.
Lynn McLaren/Photo Researchers

Responsibility

The bible says, "He that increaseth knowledge increaseth grief." In the days before birth control, people did not have to weigh the arguments for it and against it. Now we do. In the days before birth control, no one had to decide whether to practice it or not to bother. Now we do. In this, as in so many other matters, the fruit of knowledge is responsibility. But whose: the man's, the woman's, or both?

Since women bear the children and women in our culture usually raise them, American men often feel that birth control should be the concern of women. But since men are just as involved in *conception* as women, they should have a part in *contraception.* Later in this chapter we will see how this responsibility can be shared.

In every couple, both the man and the woman—in practice as well as in theory—must share the burden of decision. They owe it to each other to examine the methods of birth control that we now have. They should be aware of the differences between the *theoretical effectiveness* of any one method and its *use effectiveness.* A method's theoretical effectiveness is the effectiveness when used perfectly, without error. Actual (or use) effectiveness is the average level of effectiveness, the effectiveness in the real world, when all the users are taken into account—including careless users and those who ignore instructions. Whenever you consult charts or ask about a particular method you should always be sure to look for the statistics of use effectiveness.

The Biological Basis of Contraception

Contraceptive devices work by interfering with the process in which a sperm cell fertilizes an ovum, with the production of ova, or with the implantation of a fertilized ovum. To understand these devices, let us take another look at the life cycles of ova and sperm.

When a woman with a 28-day menstrual cycle is about half way into it, an ovum is released from one of the two ovaries and begins its 3-day trip down the fallopian tube to the uterus. When the ovum reaches the fallopian tube conception becomes possible. Sperm swim up a woman's genital tract at a rate of about 1 inch an hour, but some sperm may reach the ovum in only 1 to 1½ hours after ejaculation. Sperm have been found to live inside a woman's body for about 48 hours, and recent reports show that some survive for as long as 5 to 10 days. The ovum though, can be fertilized only within the first 12 to 24 hours after ovulation.

If a woman were to have intercourse 2 days before ovulation, there is a good chance that sperm would still be alive at the release of the ovum, and conception could occur. If a woman were to have intercourse 2 days after ovulation, some fast-moving sperm assisted by uterine contractions might reach the ovum while it was still viable, and conception could also occur. The best chance for conception would be intercourse on the day of ovulation or 1 or 2 days before.

Birth Control Methods

Some methods of birth control are, in theory, more effective than others—more effective, that is, if used perfectly. Some are easier to use and may have a higher level of actual, or use, effectiveness. Some methods, too, are safer than others. Let us now take a look at these methods.

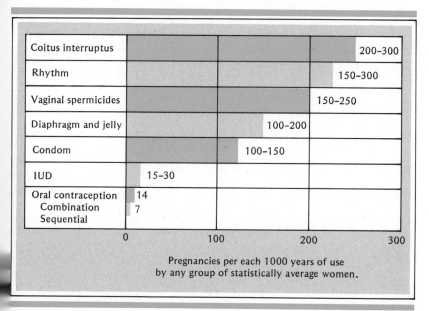

	0	100	200	300
Coitus interruptus				200–300
Rhythm				150–300
Vaginal spermicides				150–250
Diaphragm and jelly			100–200	
Condom			100–150	
IUD	15–30			

Oral contraception
  Combination
  Sequential
	14
	7			

Pregnancies per each 1000 years of use
by any group of statistically average women.

Figure 14–1. Nonsurgical methods of birth control. The effectiveness increases as you read down the chart.

Natural Methods

Fertility Awareness.   These methods attempt to pinpoint the time of ovulation so that a couple may refrain from sexual intercourse when the woman is most fertile. This would be the point at which an ovum is moving from the ovary into the fallopian tube. This point has to be determined by careful record keeping, so these methods may be the most difficult of all to use. Since the cycles of the majority of women are irregular (87%), the theoretical effectiveness of the fertility awareness methods is lower than the effectiveness of some other methods. But—the fertility awareness methods are safe, free or very cheap, and acceptable to religious groups that oppose other methods of birth control.

Rhythm (Calendar) Method. The rhythm method requires that a woman determine the time during which a viable ovum can be fertilized, by recording the length of her menstrual cycles over a 12-month span. The first day of each cycle is the first day of menstrual bleeding.

The earliest day in the cycle on which a woman is likely to be fertile is calculated by subtracting 18 days from the length of her shortest cycle. The last day in the cycle on which a woman is likely to be fertile can be calculated by subtracting 11 days from the length of her longest cycle. Of course, using the rhythm method for determining the time of

Figure 14–2.   For the rhythm method of contraception you need a chart to calculate the "safe" and the "unsafe" days for sex.

Length of Shortest Cycle	First "Unsafe" Day after Start of Any Menstrual Period	Length of Longest Cycle	Last "Unsafe" Day after Start of Any Menstrual Period
20 days	2nd day	20 days	9th day
21 days	3rd day	21 days	10th day
22 days	4th day	22 days	11th day
23 days	5th day	23 days	12th day
24 days	6th day	24 days	13th day
25 days	7th day	25 days	14th day
26 days	8th day	26 days	15th day
27 days	9th day	27 days	16th day
28 days	10th day	28 days	17th day
29 days	11th day	29 days	18th day
30 days	12th day	30 days	19th day
31 days	13th day	31 days	20th day
32 days	14th day	32 days	21st day
33 days	15th day	33 days	22nd day
34 days	16th day	34 days	23rd day
35 days	17th day	35 days	24th day
36 days	18th day	36 days	25th day
37 days	19th day	37 days	26th day
38 days	20th day	38 days	27th day
39 days	21st day	39 days	28th day
40 days	22nd day	40 days	29th day

fertility is most effective if a woman's menstrual cycle is regular. The cycles of women, young and old, are mostly irregular. Women who use the rhythm method can now make a safer determination of their fertile time if they supplement it with the two methods discussed below: the *basal body temperature method* and the *cervical mucus method*.

Basal Body Temperature Method. The lowest temperature of a healthy person during waking hours is called the basal body temperature (BBT). If taken upon waking, the temperature of most women may be seen to drop a bit just before ovulation. Then, from 24 to 72 hours after ovulation the basal body temperature may be seen to rise. A woman who takes her temperature and charts her BBT daily for 3 to 4 months in a row may determine her time of ovulation by noting any consistent temperature drops and rises during the middle of her cycle. Though the changes in each woman's BBT will differ, each woman's chart can be seen to be somewhat consistent from month to month.

The BBT should be taken and recorded each morning, just after waking, with special basal-temperature thermometers that come packaged with extensive instructions on how to read them and interpret the chart. The most effective way to use the BBT method is to avoid intercourse, or use a back-up method, during the first half of the cycle. To stay on the safe side, a woman should assume that her fertile period is over only when her BBT has remained high for three full days.

Changes in a daily schedule, illness, electric blankets, even nightmares, can cause changes in the BBT. Infections, irregular sleeping hours, and failure to record a truly basal temperature—the lowest on any given day—can confuse the BBT record. If the BBT record is not clear, it cannot be used as a basis for birth control. The BBT method requires careful record keeping.

Cervical Mucus Method. This technique is designed to help women estimate the time of ovulation by teaching them to note fairly regular changes in the amount and nature of cervical mucus. It is a matter of reaching into the vagina to collect some on a finger tip. The cervical mucus that is produced during ovulation is clear, slippery, and abundant. It stretches out into a 1-inch strand between two finger tips. Before and after ovulation, the mucus is opaque—white to yellow in color—and there is less of it. It is very easy for a woman to confuse her midcycle secretions with other substances in her vagina—semen, lubricants, spermicides, or discharges caused by infections. Some counselors advise that there be no sex or other disturbances within the vagina through the first cycle that is charted, to reduce the chances for confusion. Of course, women who douche regularly (see below) cannot use the cervical mucus method, because they are washing away the secretions that need to be examined.

Effectiveness of Fertility Awareness. A 1978 World Health Organization study concluded that the cervical mucus method, even when combined with the BBT method, is "relatively ineffective for preventing pregnancy." The researchers who conducted the study suggested that the "accidental" pregnancies they recorded were caused not by theoretical defects in these two methods, but by a practical problem—the tendency of couples to risk intercourse during the fertile phase *before ovulation.* These conclusions are reinforced by research that indicates that some sperm may survive in the female tract for 5 days or more. To use fertility awareness effectively, a couple may have to endure a good deal of sexual frustration or find alternate forms of sexual pleasuring.

The fertility awareness methods require another kind of self-discipline, too: the keeping of extensive records. Women who do not have that sort of patience should not rely on fertility awareness methods. And even women who are willing to keep records should bear in mind that about 85 percent of all women may find their records unclear and, therefore, not usable.

Coitus Interruptus.   Another natural method, one that works on principles very different from those of fertility awareness, is *coitus interruptus.* Using this technique, the man withdraws his penis from the woman's vagina before his ejaculation. This technique does not involve the use of any devices, costs nothing, is always possible, and needs no record keeping or extensive instruction. Just before the point of ejaculation the man must withdraw his penis completely from the vagina and ejaculate away from it and the other external sex organs of the woman.

The important disadvantage of this method is that it is ineffective. Its theoretical effectiveness is between 9 and 15 pregnancies for each 100 women involved in its use during 1 year; its actual effectiveness during that period is 20–25 pregnancies. Most people do not realize that some semen escapes from the penis in the lubricating fluid before ejaculation and, therefore, before withdrawal. Semen stored in the Cowper's glands (see Chapter 13) contains an increased sperm count after a recent ejaculation, so that the rate of failure for this method tends to increase if a man has had several orgasms in a short span of time. Coitus interruptus requires great self-control on the man's part—a degree of self-control that many men lack all of the time and all men lack some of the time. Finally, coitus interruptus can markedly reduce a couple's pleasure, since during the plateau phase of intercourse, when both people may be caught up in what they are doing, the man has to focus his attention on the timing of withdrawal.

Abstinence from Sexual Intercourse.   It is sexual intercourse—the insertion of the penis into the vagina—that creates the chance of pregnancy, not sexual expression itself. There are many forms of sexual intimacy that do not involve the penetration of the vagina by the penis but that do lead to orgasm for both sexes (see Chapter 13). Abstinence is not, strictly speaking, a form of birth control, since if no sperm are deposited in the vagina there is no chance of pregnancy, but like birth control it does prevent pregnancy. And unlike birth control it is completely effective.

Mechanical Methods

Mechanical methods of contraception block the sperm from gaining access to the ovum. They are barriers, devices that must be inserted in the vagina or placed over the penis before or during the sex act. People who use them have complained that using them correctly interrupts the flow of feeling that inspires the sex act. One way to prevent this is to make the positioning of the devices a part of precoital foreplay. This is also a positive and a fair way to share in using contraception.

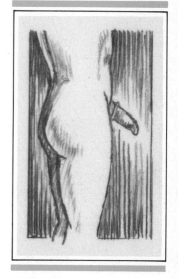

Figure 14–3. A condom in place—note that about ½ inch of space is left at the tip to collect the semen.

Condom (men).   The condom covers the penis during the sex act and collects the semen after it is ejaculated. The condom prevents direct genital contact and is the only form of birth control that provides real protection for both partners against venereal disease. To be effective the condom should be rolled all the way along the erect penis before it ever enters the vagina, with about a half inch space at the tip to collect semen. After ejaculation, the penis must be carefully withdrawn *before* it relaxes fully. Care must be taken to keep the condom from slipping and thereby spilling semen into the vagina. The condom is quite a reliable contraceptive, especially when used with a spermicide (see below).

Although condoms are inexpensive, lightweight, compact, and disposable, some men resent the loss of feeling that occurs. Otherwise, they have no real side effects and require no prescription (see Chapter 13) or medical supervision. Condoms can break if handled carelessly or during the thrusts of intercourse. They also tend to be undermined by age or by exposure to light or heat. Look for the expiration date to be sure you buy and use freshly packaged ones. Then handle them carefully since they are made of very thin materials. Most condoms are made of rubber, and these cannot be reused. Condoms made of animal skins are the most expensive, and they are reusable if they are washed, dried, powdered with cornstarch and tested before re-use.

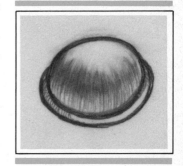

Figure 14–4.
A diaphragm.

The Diaphragm (women).   The diaphragm is a simple effective device that has been used for more than 100 years. It is a small disc of thin rubber stretched across a frame that is fitted in the vagina to cover the cervix (the opening into the uterus). When used with contraceptive cream or gel (a spermicide) a properly fitted diaphragm has a theoretical effectiveness of about 93 percent. But because many women do

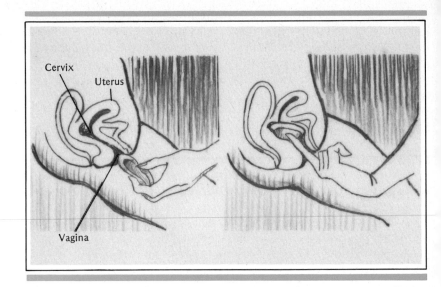

Figure 14–5. Inserting a diaphragm to cover the cervix. Note that the cervix fits within the rubber dome.

not always use it, or use it in an incorrect way, its use effectiveness is about 83 percent.

There are three keys to using the diaphragm successfully. The first is to have one that fits and to know how to insert it and how to remove it—carefully. The size or type of diaphragm needed may change, mainly after surgery or childbirth, so it should be fitted by a gynecologist or at a birth control clinic, and it should be refitted during periodic visits. The second key is to use some spermicide on initial insertion and to add some for each sex act that occurs while the diaphragm remains in place. The third is to keep the diaphragm in place in the vagina for 8 hours after the last act of intercourse.

Cervical Cap (women).   The cervical cap is another barrier device that prevents the sperm from moving from the vagina into the uterus. It is of thicker material than the diaphragm, shaped like a thimble, and fits tightly around the cervix, where it is held in place by suction and the surrounding tissue. The cap's advantage over the diaphragm is that a woman can leave it in place for several days, instead of hours, making possible greater sexual spontancity. But it can be hard to put in place and remove for women with deep vaginas. In the United States, cervical caps are still being tested.

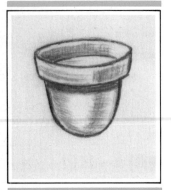

Figure 14–6.   A cervical cap.

Spermicidal Agents (women).   Diaphragms are devices that are used with spermicidal agents; these contain a chemical that kills sperm. Spermicidal creams and gels should *always* be used with a diaphragm, not alone. Spermicidal foams, though, are used alone. Foam's theoretical effectiveness rate used alone is quite high—97 percent—and this has misled some women, for its use effectiveness—78 percent—is much lower. Foam fails this often because it is hard to place and because it is often placed carelessly. Some women use too little foam, or they fail to shake the dispenser with vigor, or they fail to realize that the container is empty, or they simply refuse to interrupt the sex act to use it at all. When foam is used correctly and when, at the same time, the man uses a condom, their combined effectiveness is very high.

Suppositories (women).   Contraceptive suppositories are small solid pellets that contain a spermicide. In the vagina, with the presence of warmth and moisture, they melt to form a thick chemical barrier around the cervix, blocking the passage of sperm and killing them. The effectiveness of these suppositories and any adverse effects have yet to be determined, but suppositories are small and convenient, and they are available without prescription. Like foam, they may be used for fail-safe protection when the man uses a condom. They may also be used when a diaphragm must be left in place for 8 hours and more spermicide should be added for another sex act (see above).

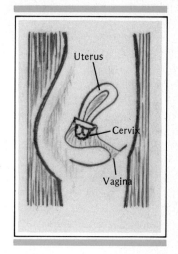

Figure 14-7.   A cervical cap in place.

Hormonal Methods

The fertility awareness methods of birth control are used to keep sperm from making contact with the ovum when a woman is fertile. Mechanical methods are used to prevent sperm from making contact with the ovum at all. But hormonal methods do not work by keeping the sperm away from the ovum. Instead they "fool" a woman's body into thinking it is pregnant, so it does not produce ova at all. Fertilization does not occur when hormonal contraceptives are used because there just is nothing to fertilize.

The Pill (women).   The best known hormonal contraceptive is the famous Pill, which is available only by prescription. A few companies make various versions of it. Women "on the Pill" take one every day for a set number of days each month. The Pill fools the body into thinking a woman is pregnant by releasing two chemicals that are closely related to the female hormones estrogen and progesterone (see Chapter 13). Menstruation still occurs regularly because when each month's Pill supply ends the estrogen and progesterone are withdrawn. Then the lining of the uterus breaks down in normal fashion and bleeding takes place. The next month's Pill supply is then started on a set day.

Some women who take the Pill have mild symptoms of pregnancy, such as tenderness in the breasts, mild nausea, headaches, and weight gain. Switching to another kind or brand of Pill may end some or all of these symptoms, but at times the use of the Pill must be discontinued.

The Pill may cause serious problems in a small number of women

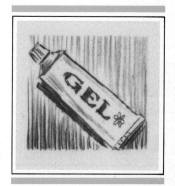

Figure 14-8.   A tube of spermicidal gel. Some are designed for use with a diaphragm, but some spermicides can be used alone. Read the package instructions carefully to tell one from the other.

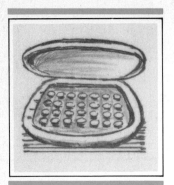

Figure 14–9. Birth control pills and dispenser. The Pill is taken one each day in a set order. The Pill is sold only by prescription because a physician must take your physical fitness into account before deciding which type might be best for you.

who take it. For some there seems to be an increased risk of getting heart attacks or strokes (due to the increase in blood clotting in the users). This is a problem for women older than 40 who smoke. The Pill may also aggravate an existing cancer's growth (see Chapter 10). Women who have had a history of blood clots or vein inflammations, serious liver disease, or cancer of the breast or uterus should *avoid* the Pill. Women who have heart disease, kidney disease, high blood pressure, diabetes, epilepsy, fibroids of the uterus, migraines, vaginal bleeding, sickle cell anemia, gall bladder disease, or asthma should avoid it unless a physician determines that their condition will not be aggravated by the Pill. Yet when all is said and done, the Food and Drug Administration (FDA) declares it safe for most women. The cost is about $2 per month and it is very effective.

The Pill's side effects are not all bad. Some women find that their menstrual periods are shorter and less painful and that their menstrual flow is reduced. The size of the breasts may increase or decrease, and some women's acne clears.

Minipill. Among the many Pills is the so-called Minipill, which contains only one hormone: progesterone. (There have been a number of so-called Minipills so this term is really a misnomer when applied to the progesterone-only type.) The Minipill does not stop the production of ova, so it is less likely to cause side effects. It is a bit less effective than the Pill as a contraceptive, though.

"Morning-after" Pill (women).   A series of pills containing a massive dose of estrogen can be taken the morning after unprotected intercourse. It can also be taken as a series of injections (see below). The morning-after pill makes women very sick, unfortunately, and its side effects are not really known. At the moment the FDA has approved it only for special situations, such as rape.

Hormonal Injections (women). The Pill resembles the fertility awareness methods of birth control in requiring women to keep track of things—at any rate, to remember to take one and only one pill in a set pattern of days. If a woman forgets to take the pill for a day or two, there are some countermeasures. An every three months injection is available to women who do not want to have to remember to take a pill at all. The injection contains progesterone in a long-lasting form that is effective in preventing both the release of the ovum and also pregnancy. Some women who have used it have had difficulty in getting pregnant later, when they wanted to do so. But the risks of long-term use are not yet clear, so the injection is still being tested by the FDA.

IUDs

An IUD is a coil (made of plastic or copper and sometimes hormones) that is placed in the uterus by a physician. A string that leads from the IUD into the vagina enables a woman to check that it is in place. It is not yet known how they work, but since IUDs require a woman to do nothing beyond getting a pelvic exam, their use effectiveness is close to their theoretical effectiveness—about 96 percent. In fact, most of the pregnancies that surprise women who have been fitted with IUDs occur because the device is no longer in place and was not checked.

Some women have no problems adjusting to their IUDs. Others may experience some bleeding, backache, or cramping after the insertion. Some women develop heavier menstrual flows after insertion with small blood losses between periods. Women who use IUDs are more likely to develop pelvic infections (which can lead to sterility). If they should become pregnant, the risk of miscarriage is great. Women with acute pelvic infections, including gonorrhea, should not use IUDs under any circumstances. Women with acute cervicitis, a history of ectopic pregnancy, or valvular heart disease, heavy menstrual flow, or abnormal Pap smears should not consider them. The most serious side effect is perforation of the uterus. Some women expel the IUD.

The initial cost of an IUD may be high, but it is a one-time-only cost. Some family planning centers or clinics insert the device for a minimal fee.

Birth Control in the Future

About 150 years ago, there were no really effective methods of birth control. Today there are many to choose among and in the future there will likely be even more. Let us take a look into a crystal ball.

You will recall that hormone injections are much easier for some women than the Pill. A lot of work is being done to improve those injectable contraceptives. One of them, now being tested, contains small amounts of different types of synthetic progestin in a time-released dose only one-tenth that of the Pill. It is reported to be highly effective and has few side effects.

Another approach is vaginal rings that release hormones to inhibit ovulation, fertilization, or implantation. One kind of ring can be inserted once each month by the woman herself; some are reusable and can last as long as 2 years. Though the ring does not use synthetic estrogen, it is quite as effective as the Pill and has fewer side effects.

Along other lines, vaginal sponges are being developed to block and absorb the semen; the spermicide in the sponge then kills the sperm. Contraceptive tampons with spermicide are similar to the sponges.

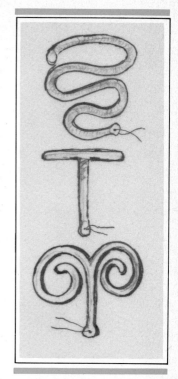

Figure 14–10. Three types of IUD. All IUDs must be inserted carefully into the uterus—then monitored for several months to be sure they are positioned correctly and not causing undue bleeding.

One method now being tested might work for both women and men. Both the testes (male) and ovaries (female) are controlled by two hormones from the pituitary gland. This gland gets its signals from a part of the brain called the hypothalamus via substances called peptides. A chemical has been developed that "overloads" the pituitary gland to inhibit ovulation and sperm generation. These chemicals can be taken in the form of a nasal spray.

The idea of a male contraceptive has intrigued many researchers. Some contraceptives use synthetic male hormones to suppress sperm production. The best-known effort to develop a "male Pill" used an antifertility agent (derived from the cottonseed plant) called gossypol. In China, this drug is reported to induce infertility in men after 2 months of use. Its side effects may include weakness at first, changes in appetite, and minor digestive discomfort.

Surgical Sterilization

Birth control is temporary. If a man does not use a condom properly, or if a woman stops taking the Pill, has her IUD removed, or has unprotected sex during her fertile period, she can become pregnant. Surgical sterilization is a long-term way to control fertility—in fact, it is rarely reversible. That is why some people call it "permanent birth control." Both men and women can be sterilized, and for both the technique is really the same: It consists of the surgical cutting and tying of parts of the internal sex organs (the vas deferens in men, the fallopian tubes in women). The sperm and the ovum cannot unite, since their union is blocked by the cut tubes. As a result, those who have this surgery are said to be sterile; the women cannot get pregnant and the men cannot make women pregnant.

Sterility can also be caused by removing the testes (castration), the ovaries (ovarectomy), or the uterus (hysterectomy). When testes or ovaries are removed, the loss of the hormones produced by them has in profound effects on the body—and hysterectomies are not without surgical risk. For these and other reasons, such procedures are not commonly used for sterilization. By the early 1980s more than 11.5 million adults had been sterilized in the United States, and this option is becoming more and more popular.

Men

Vasectomy.   In a vasectomy (male sterilization), the vas deferens is cut and tied so that sperm cannot pass that point and mix into the semen. The surgery is simple and brief, and it can be done in about half an hour in a physician's office or in a clinic. The man can leave that day, and sex may be resumed within 2 to 3 days if he feels no discomfort. Men do not become sterile the day of the surgery, but several weeks later, since sperm has been stored in the semen beyond the point

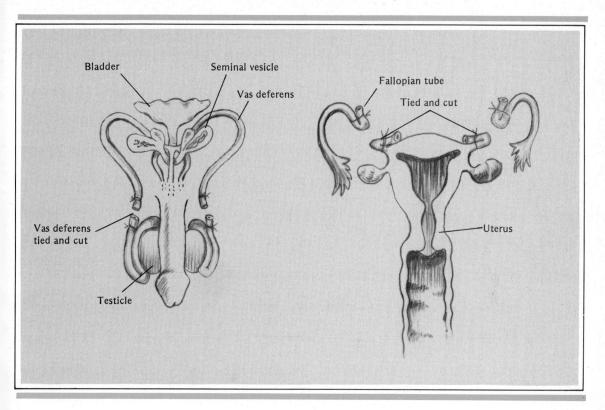

Figure 14–11.   Sterilization. (*Left*) A vasectomy showing the cut and tied vas deferens. (*Right*) A tubal ligation showing the cut and tied fallopian tubes.

of the tied tubes. Until a sperm count shows that no sperm are present in the semen, another birth control method must be used. Sperm production does continue in the testes, but the new sperm are absorbed by the body since they cannot pass the barrier and reach the rest of the semen source. Men with vasectomies do continue to ejaculate semen, but successful surgery means semen without sperm.

Of all the techniques of sterilization, vasectomy is the easiest to perform and the one most free of complications. Some men have wanted to become fertile again, but this step is rarely successful. Those who choose vasectomy should consider it permanent.

Women

Tubal Ligation.   There are two surgical approaches to tubal ligation, which is the cutting and tying of the fallopian tubes to keep the ovum from reaching the sperm. The vaginal route is considered the "classical," or standard, one, and it has been endorsed by many experts because it is effective and relatively safe. The operation is simple and the patient can go home by the next day.

Abdominal tubal ligation has become very popular in Europe and, more recently, in the United States. The safety, minimal discomfort, speed, and cheapness of the abdominal route make it attractive to many women. Since the operation requires only a small incision in each side of the abdomen, it is considered relatively risk-free. One of the variations of the abdominal tubal ligation, laparotomy, needs a special device and a skilled surgeon. It may, however, be reversible.

Hysterectomy.   A hysterectomy, the surgical removal of the uterus (and often the ovaries and fallopian tubes), is much more dangerous than a tubal ligation. Hysterectomies are commonly done to remove damaged or cancerous organs, but once they are removed pregnancy cannot occur.

Abortion

Contraception and sterilization both prevent conception. *Abortion* is the removal of the product of conception from a woman's body.

There are two major types of abortion. "Induced" abortions are brought about through free choice—to end a pregnancy. "Spontaneous" abortions (or miscarriages) include all the other pregnancies that end before term. In this chapter we shall discuss only induced abortions. The legal status of induced abortion varies from country to country. Most countries permit abortions on medical grounds, and most countries that permit abortion limit it to the first trimester of pregnancy, when it is safest for the woman. It is hard to determine the incidence of abortion worldwide, since the countries that probably have the largest numbers of them—China, the U.S.S.R., and Japan—do not publish figures on the subject. In the rest of the world, about 2 million legal abortions occur each year.

Methods

An abortion can be induced in three ways. During the first trimester, vaginal aspiration (suction curettage) is the preferred way of ending a pregnancy. The contents of the uterus are removed by suction with an electric pump. Menstrual regulation, limited to the first two weeks after a missed menstrual period, is a variation of the suction procedure. Here the uterus is emptied with a large syringe. The uterus can also be scraped with a curette (known then as a D and C, for dilation and curettage). Since a D and C is done by hand, it takes longer than the suction method and may create more complications.

Abortions in the second trimester of pregnancy are often done by induced labor. First, a saline (salt-water) solution is injected through the abdomen into the uterus, and within hours the fetal heartbeat stops, labor begins, and the fetus and then the placenta are expelled. The entire procedure takes about 72 hours.

Surgery is the third way to abort a fetus. A hysterotomy is the removal of the fetus by surgery before it can survive on its own outside the mother's body.

Legal abortions do not often result in serious physical complications. During the procedure the uterus has, on occasion, been perforated by a surgical instrument; the intestines or other nearby organs may be injured. Other, but even less frequent, risks include major hemorrhage, laceration of the cervix, and severe disturbances of blood coagulation. After the procedure there may be complications, like bleeding or infection, should fragments of the fetus or placenta be retained in the uterus. A greater danger, perhaps, is the impact of abortion on the mind, and this can vary from intense guilt to feelings of great relief. Some psy-

Figure 14–12. The most common abortion method for the first trimester is vacuum, or suction, aspiration. It takes about 10 minutes in many clinics and hospitals where abortions are routine.

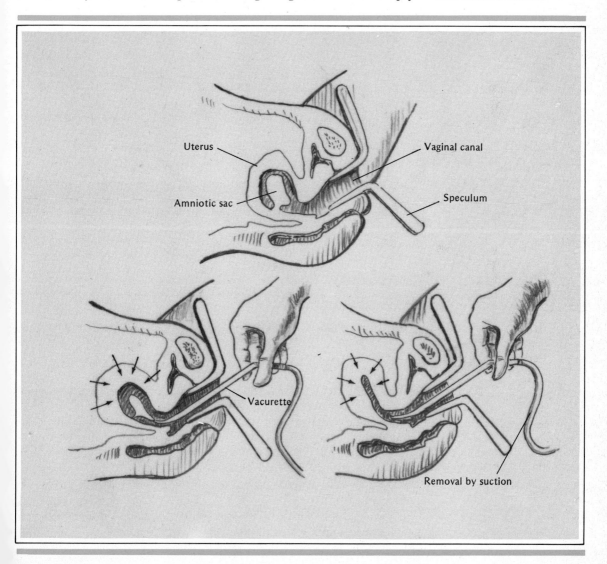

Uterus

Vaginal canal

Amniotic sac

Speculum

Vacurette

Removal by suction

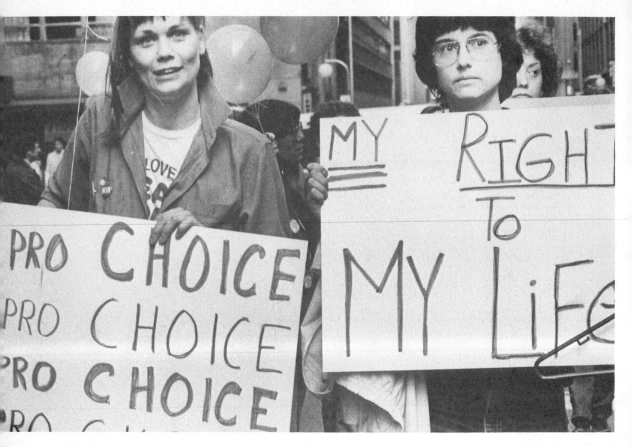

Bettye Lane/Photo Researchers

chiatrists argue that every abortion is a very stressful event in a woman's life. Others point out that having an unwanted child can be more stressful—and damaging. Illegal abortions are far more dangerous than legal ones, because conditions may not be clean, suitable, or safe.

Debate over Abortion

In 1973, the U.S. Supreme Court ruled that abortion during the first 24 weeks of pregnancy is a private matter between a woman and her physician; then the states could not interfere with federal law. Public opinion seems to agree with the high court's decision. A majority of Americans feel abortion is justified if a mother's health is in danger, if her child is likely to be born deformed, and in cases of rape and incest. About 50 percent approve if the woman is not married, if the family cannot afford more children, or if the mother does not want the child. Opponents of abortion, who are also numerous, believe that a fetus is a new human being with the right to life and to protection by society and

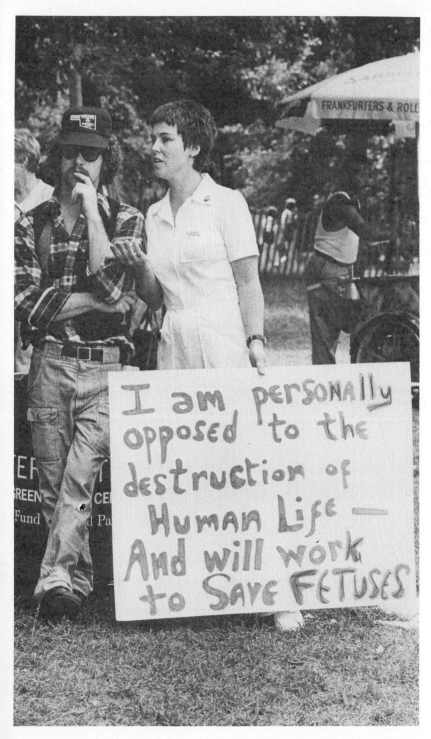

the government. Members of the Right-to-Life movement argue that human life is sacred, that it begins with fertilization, and that abortion is therefore a form of killing. Of course, some counter that the mother is equally human and as a living member of society, she has legal rights to life as well.

Abortion is now a political issue, since the Right-to-Life movement is seeking to overturn the Supreme Court's 1973 decision.

SUMMARY

The existing methods of birth control fall mostly into three groupings: natural, mechanical, and hormonal. Natural methods include "fertility awareness" techniques, which require that a woman study her menstrual cycle, basal body temperature, and cervical mucus over a period of time. Once it is possible that a woman might be fertile, she must refrain from intercourse during that period. Another natural method of birth control—an ineffective one—is coitus interruptus, in which the man must withdraw from the vagina before he ejaculates.

Mechanical methods of birth control—for men, the condom; for women, such devices as the diaphragm, the cervical cap, and spermicidal agents—block the access of sperm to the ovum. Women often use spermicidal agents along with other devices to increase their effectiveness.

Hormonal forms of birth control "fool" the body into thinking it is already pregnant. Some increase the body's production of certain hormones. Some interrupt the process of conception by preventing the production of ova. Hormonal methods include the "Pill" and various hormonal injections.

Birth control creates only a temporary barrier to conception. Sterilization is considered permanent. Men can be sterilized by surgery called a vasectomy and women by surgery called a tubal ligation.

Both sterilization and birth control are used to prevent conception. Once conception occurs, the birth of a child can be prevented by abortion, either spontaneous (miscarriage) or artificial. Artificial abortion, which has been legal throughout the United States since 1973, is now the focus of a political and moral debate.

Everyone who engages in sexual intercourse should know its consequences and how they might be prevented. The responsibility should be a shared one, borne by both men and women, for the sex act and its pleasures are shared.

Suggested Readings

Bardshaw, Barbara R., et al. *Counseling on Family Planning and Human Sexuality.* New York: Family Service Association of America, 1977. This work was designed to provide social workers with up-to-date information about reproductive biology, sexual behavior, and birth control technology. All contraceptive techniques are explained in detail, including the pros and cons for each method.

Hatcher, Robert A., et al. *Contraceptive Technology 1880-1981.* New York: Irvington, 1980. A complete and up-to-date account of contraceptive technology.

Hawkins, D. F., and Edler, M. G. *Human Fertility Control.* Boston: Butterworth, 1979. This volume is intended for use as a textbook for those involved in clinical fertility-control practice.

Hubbard, Charles William. *Family Planning Education.* St. Louis: C. V. Mosby Company, 1973. This book offers information in four areas concerning the sexual aspect of living: contraception, abortion, sterilization, and the venereal diseases. It is written for every student but mainly for those whose major interests will be with the health-oriented professions.

Life Cycles

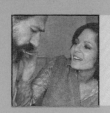

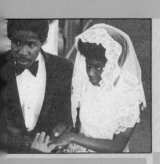

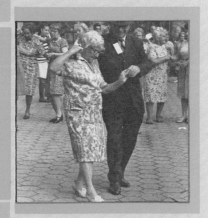

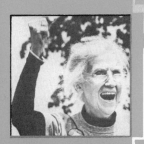

UNIT FIVE

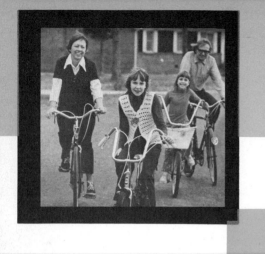

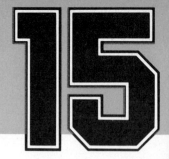

The Family

chapter objectives

When you have finished reading this chapter you should be able to:

1. Communicate techniques of "getting along with a roommate"
2. Discuss the advantages and disadvantages of being single
3. Consider the value of choosing a good marriage
4. Discuss the idea of parenthood
5. Recognize the symptoms that lead to separation and divorce
6. Discuss alternatives to the traditional family

These days, people tend to regard the family as an endangered institution. It is true that today's couples can make choices that couples in the past could not consider—choices about whether to have children and about the nature of marriage itself. Some choose to "live together"— called by older generations "living in sin." Others opt for marriage, for serial monogamy, or for common-law marriage. None of these choices is really new. In the past divorce was expensive and hard to get, while living together without a formal marriage contract was not respectable, and it was often illegal. Yet even in the face of today's freedom of choice, most people get married and have children. If anything, that freedom seems to show that the family is far from endangered.

The College Years

In some cultures, the transition from childhood to adulthood and adult choices is made very quickly. Ours is not one of them; on the contrary, in the United States a whole period of life, adolescence, is devoted to this transition. Adolescents make choices that look forward to and lead to the choices of adulthood. Let us take a look at some of those choices.

College students can decide to live in private dorm rooms, to share a dorm room with someone else, to join a fraternity or sorority, or to take an off-campus place. If they choose to live off-campus, they can live alone or with people of the same sex, with people of both sexes or with someone of the opposite sex. Each of these choices requires certain adjustments and offers certain benefits. Living alone, for example, gives you control over many day-to-day decisions: How to decorate your room, what kind of food to eat, when to turn off the stereo or the lights, and how much housekeeping to do, among others. Besides, without a roommate you may have more time for concentrated study or other activities.

Students who live by themselves, though, may become lonely and insecure. Without anyone close at hand to talk with or to turn to for advice and sympathy, they may feel overwhelmed by the pressures of college life. Also, there are reasons to think that students with roommates mature faster than those who live alone. Intense exposure to a fellow student forces a person to rethink many ideas that were taken for granted. Challenging discussions force roommates to listen, to communicate, and to learn tolerance. This dialogue can help bring the person out of the self-centeredness of adolescence. Thoughts and fears that were once "too personal" to expose become raw material for confessions, honest examinations, and even self-mocking humor. Roommates learn to accept themselves and to make and fulfill personal commitments to others.

Living with roommates can also generate stress—even when there is

Unmarried Couples in the United States

These figures show the tremendous growth in the number of unmarried couples—with or without children—sharing the same household.

	1970	1979
All unmarried couples (1,000)	523	1,346
Percent of all couple arrangements	1.1	2.7
No children present (1,000)	327	985
Children present (1,000)	196	360

Source: U.S. Bureau of the Census, *Statistical Abstract of the United States, 1980* (101st ed.), table 60, p. 44.

A Roommate Self-starter Kit

Getting to know a new person can be one of life's most enjoyable experiences, but it can also be one of the most awkward. New roommates, like other people who meet for the first time, have to deal with this awkwardness. This exercise (for an hour-long conversation) can help pinpoint potential problems and set up strategies for solving future problems.

First quarter hour: Your personal history

1. The important things about your family.
2. The important things about your friends back home.
3. The most important facts about your hometown.
4. The way you would sum up your neighborhood and town, and their people.
5. Your major activities in high school.
6. What you will miss most and least about home.
7. The most hilarious moment of high school.

Second quarter hour: Your special likes and pet peeves

1. The activities you are most likely to pursue in college.
2. Your study habits.
3. Your academic goals.
4. Your sleep patterns.
5. Your general health.
6. Your attitudes toward drugs, including alcohol.
7. Your favorite way to get exercise.

8. Your standards of neatness.
9. Your degree of possessiveness about books, clothes, and other personal belongings.
10. Your hopes for dating and other social activities.
11. Your feelings about a guest of the opposite sex in the room.
12. Your ability to make friends.
13. Your religious convictions.
14. Your musical tastes.
15. Your spare-time activities.

Third quarter hour: Your emotional style

1. How you show it when you are upset.
2. Your ability to communicate your feelings.
3. What brings you out of the blues.
4. What you are like when you are really happy.
5. When you need to be alone.
6. Your normal mood.
7. What puts you on edge.
8. How you act under pressure.
9. What really gets your goat.
10. How you like to release tension and relax.

Last quarter hour: Feedback

1. Views you both share.
2. Things you don't agree on.
3. Areas for compromise.
4. What I can learn from you.
5. What I learned about myself from this discussion.

---

no sexual relationship to complicate matters. Roommates have to learn a lot about themselves and each other at a time when each faces new academic and social pressures. But mainly, roommates must learn how to share physical and psychological space.

These good points and bad points, as you will soon see, are in some ways similar to those of marriage. That is why living with roommates, of either sex, is one way to prepare for married life. Coping with roommates provides the chance to learn to deal with the daily needs of other people—new, nonfamily people—as well as your own needs, and that is one of life's hardest and most rewarding lessons.

Marriage

Advantages of Marriage

We hear on every side that marriage, as an institution, has just about had it. As we will see a little further on, that idea does not really have a firm statistical base. And more, it ignores a key fact: that since the earliest known times most people have married—and most people still do. Marriage, despite today's divorce rates, is the most hardy of all social institutions. It is found in every kind of culture and among every kind of people. Why?

In the first place, marriage is one of the ways in which children, of whatever age, are turned into adults, and adults into mature adults. For adults do not stop growing; as we saw in Chapter 1, the ego changes and grows throughout life. Marriage promotes this change and growth, and in a number of ways.

First, marriage permits the husband and wife to indulge freely and regularly in one of life's greatest pleasures: sex. Despite what you may have heard about divorcees and bachelors, it is clear that married people have much more sex than the unmarried. And their sex lives are extensions of their daily lives; so the caring and the sharing that can grow within marriage enhances their sex lives too.

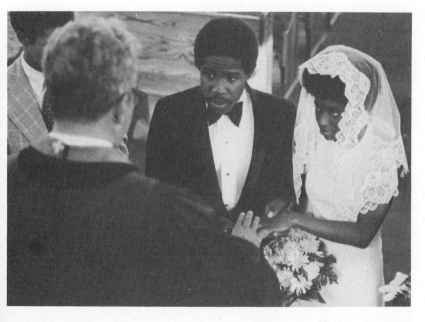

"Till death us do part."
Chester Higgins, Jr. / Photo Researchers

Second, marriage (like having a roommate, at an earlier stage of development) compels us to abandon the self-centeredness of childhood. People who are married can no longer think first of their own needs, because they are concerned each about the other. The benefits of intimacy result from their attitude.

Third, marriage helps us to separate ourselves from our parents mentally. This process that begins in childhood is confirmed by the selection of a partner in marriage and the formation of a new family unit.

Fourth, we have a paradox: Personal independence increases in marriage, but so does intimacy. This is because intimacy nurtures self-esteem and personal confidence, maximizing personal fulfillment.

Finally, marriage presents new chances for character change. As children, we admired and imitated certain features of our parents' personalities—that is, we "identified" with them. We continue to identify as adults, but with more conscious control. In living with those we love, we identify with them, but in a more selective way than the way in which we identified with parents.

Of course, not everyone derives from marriage all the benefits it has to offer. Some married people do not know that all these benefits even exist. For to benefit from marriage, or from any friendship, we must know what is possible, be able to compromise, and be able to respond to the common humanity of the other person. To respond in these ways we must first discover the humanity within ourselves.

Why People Marry

Of course, most people do not decide to marry for the sake of mental growth or mental health. They marry for "love," to enjoy a stable and permanent arrangement based on affection (and sometimes on lust), and to raise a family. Many people marry for status, to raise their social or economic level. Others, mainly women, marry for economic security, though this is less common than it used to be. Can you think of other reasons for which people marry?

Preparation for Marriage

It is very easy to get married in this country; in fact, it might be too easy. In most states when we attain the lawful age we can marry a few days after filing a marriage certificate. Quite a few marriages are made in a way that is quite casual. Two people meet at a party and like each other a lot. They see each other every evening for a month. Then they decide to marry, and they do so without really knowing very much about each other's attitudes, preferences, and problems. They do not sit down and discuss money, where to live, whether to have children.

After a few weeks of marriage, reality sets in. The man, it seems, is not the strong, cheerful person he seemed to be during courtship; on the

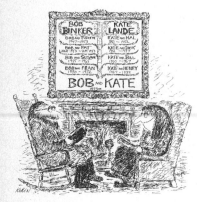

Drawing by Koren; © 1978 The New Yorker Magazine, Inc.

SELF-ASSESSMENT DEVICE 15-1: ARE YOU READY FOR MARRIAGE?

The following questions should stimulate thought about readiness for marriage. There are no right or wrong answers. Answer by drawing a circle around the "?," the "Yes," or the "No." Use the question mark only when you are uncertain. After you are through think about the meaning of your answers, and if possible discuss them with someone. The questionnaire assumes you are now considering some specific person as a possible marriage partner.

Yes No ? 1. Even though you may accept advice from your parents, do you make important decisions for yourself?

Yes No ? 2. Are you often homesick when you are away from home?

Yes No ? 3. Do you ever feel embarrassed or uneasy in giving or receiving affection?

Yes No ? 4. Are your feelings easily hurt by criticism?

Yes No ? 5. Do you enjoy playing or working with small children?

Yes No ? 6. Do you feel embarrassed or uneasy in conversations about sex with older persons or members of the other sex?

Yes No ? 7. Do you have a clear understanding of the physiology of sexual intercourse and reproduction?

Yes No ? 8. Do you understand the psychological factors determining good sexual adjustment?

Yes No ? 9. Have you had the experience of using some of your earnings to help meet the expenses of others?

Yes No ? 10. In an argument, do you lose your temper easily?

Yes No ? 11. Have you and your fiance(e) ever worked through disagreements to a definite conclusion agreeable to both of you?

Yes No ? 12. Can you postpone something you w want for the sake of later enjoyment?

Yes No ? 13. Are you normally free from jealousy?

Yes No ? 14. Have you thought carefully about the goals you will strive for in your marriage?

Yes No ? 15. Do you sometimes feel rebellious toward facing the responsibilities of marriage, occupational or family life?

Yes No ? 16. Have you been able to give up gracefully something you wanted very much?

Yes No ? 17. Do you think of sexual intercourse chiefly as a pleasure experience?

Yes No ? 18. Do you find it difficult to differ from others on matters of conduct or dress, even though you disagree with what they think?

Yes No ? 19. Do you often have to fight to get your way?

Yes No ? 20. Do you often find yourself making biting remarks, or using sarcasm toward others?

Yes No ? 21. Do you find yourself strongly emphasizing the glamor aspects of marriage, e.g., the announcement, congratulations, showers, the wedding?

Yes No ? 22. Have you and your fiance(e) associated with each other in a variety of non-amusement situations, e.g., caring for children, in a work project, in time of stress?

Yes No ? 23. Have you and your fiance(e) discussed matters which might cause marital conflict? For example: (Underline those you have discussed) religious differences; plans for having children; attitudes toward sex; differences in family background; financial arrangement in marriage; basic values in life.

Source: From Kirkendall, Lester A., and Wesley J. Adams, *The Students' Guide to Marriage and Family Life Literature: An Aid to Individualized Study and Instruction*, 8th ed. © 1971, 1974, November 1976, 1980 Wm. C. Brown Company Publishers, Dubuque, Iowa. Reprinted by permission.

contrary, he is dependent and often depressed. The woman, who had seemed to be happy and self-reliant during courtship, is equally dependent and depressed. Neither gives the other the sense of comfort and reassurance that each had sought. Battles are fought over many trivial problems that had been ignored before the marriage. The couple is soon headed for divorce.

Marriages in the past were probably subjected to the same kinds of disappointed illusions. What has changed is that divorce is now easier to get (but not as easy as marriage) and that most people now consider happiness a constitutional right. Of course, happiness cannot be guaranteed, not even in marriage. But you can prolong courtship long enough to get to know, to really know, the person you want to marry—weaknesses as well as strengths. In that time you can learn something more about yourself—and why successful marriages are successful, and why failed marriages fail.

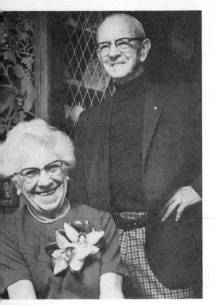

The first 50 years.
Michael C. Hayman/Photo Researchers

Even if you are not married, you can use these questions to evaluate any romantic relationship in which you may be involved.

SELF-ASSESSMENT DEVICE 15-2: DO YOU HAVE A VITAL MARRIAGE?

Indicate the degree to which you agree with each of the following statements about your marriage relationship by circling the appropriate response. The code is as follows: SA = Strongly Agree; A = Agree; U = Undecided; D = Disagree; SD = Strongly Disagree. Complete the test, and then read how to score it below:

1. My spouse and I enjoy doing many things together. SA A U SD
2. I enjoy most of the activities I participate in more if my spouse is also involved. SA A U SD
3. I receive more satisfaction from my marriage relationship than from most other areas of life. SA A U SD
4. My spouse and I have a positive, strong emotional involvement with each other. SA A U SD
5. The companionship of my spouse is more enjoyable to me than most anything else in life. SA A U SD
6. I would not hesitate to sacrifice an important goal in life if achievement of that goal would cause my marriage relationship to suffer. SA A U SD
7. My spouse and I take an active interest in each other's work and hobbies. SA A U SD

To calculate your score: Give yourself 5 points for SA, 4 for A, 3 for U, 2 for D, and 1 for SD.

Source: By permission of Paul Ammons.
Note: This test can be taken by couples who are not married as well as by married couples.

Successful Marriages

What makes a marriage successful? The causes of divorce have been studied and studied again. But successful marriages have received far less attention. Yet the study of successful marriages might well be more useful, for as the great Russian novelist Tolstoy said, each unhappy marriage is unhappy in its own special way, while happy marriages resemble each other.

Two social scientists, each happily married, decided to find out what kinds of people are likely to be happily married. They found that these people tended to be generous, committed to their marriages, optimistic, spiritual, or moral (though not necessarily religious), sensitive to the feelings of others, and thankful for their good fortune. They were, as well, people of strong opinions, full of sexual energy, and well able to express their feelings and ideas in words. Of course, merely reading this list of traits will not of itself enable anyone to have a successful marriage. But it is useful to know that successful marriage is not an illusion; it has definable qualities that we can all strive to cultivate and achieve.

Marriage demands patience, tolerance, and compromise. Above all it demands openness and honesty. Every couple has problems. But some couples confront their problems with love and truth, and those are the couples whose marriages are happy and satisfying.

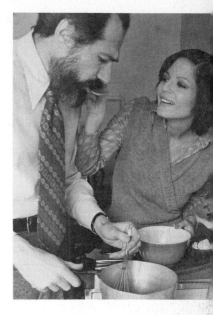

"I think it needs more salt."
Alice Kandell/Photo Researchers

Equal Marriage

"Equal marriage" is not a specific institution, like monogamy (see below), but a state of mind, an attitude. Its essence is the equal sharing of work and rewards. The husband and the wife do those tasks that they enjoy and are good at, not the ones their culture says that they should do to be "real" husbands and "real" wives. Of course, they must compromise on tasks that neither wants to do—or such tasks will never get done. In the process, both wives and husbands stand to lose certain things. Men may lose a full-time cook, housekeeper, governess, and personal assistant. Women may lose a full-time provider. But these losses are more than balanced by great emotional freedom and chances for personal, as well as mutual, growth. Husbands gain a real feeling of partnership with their wives and create a warm, nurturing role with their children. They are free to cook, if they like, and to perform other domestic arts. Women are free to do these same things and so both people can create the best situation for themselves and each other. All they have to do is talk it over and agree on how to proceed.

Sexuality does not suffer in an equal marriage; in fact, sex and all other kinds of intimacy flourish freely in a partnership of equals. But remember, this type of marriage works only for those who want to have it and agree to work at it.

SELF-ASSESSMENT DEVICE 15-3:

1. What is the most common marriage complaint heard by both psychiatrists and marital therapists? Lack of (a) sex; (b) money; (c) communication.

2. Can too much honesty between a couple create major difficulties? (a) yes; (b) no.

3. Is the woman who stays home and takes care of the children (a) more likely or (b) less likely to have marital problems than the working wife?

4. The more money you make, the longer your marriage is likely to last (a) true; (b) false.

5. Are more women who get divorced (a) under age 30; (b) between 30 and 40; (c) over 40?

6. Which emotion is most likely to drive a husband or wife into an affair? (a) jealousy; (b) anger; (c) hate.

7. Is your spouse likely to have at least one extra-marital affair? (a) yes; (b) no.

8. If you have had an affair and feel guilty, confessing will clear your conscience. (a) true; (b) false.

9. The marriage of a couple who have an excellent sex life will last considerably longer than that of a couple with an ordinary or bad sex life. (a) true; (b) false.

10. Nearly 40 percent of all first marriages end in divorce. Is the percentage larger on second marriages? (a) yes; (b) no.

11. A close friend is having serious difficulties with his or her marriage, and wants to talk to you about it. You should: (a) encourage your friend to get any hidden feelings into the open; (b) give direction when you feel your friend is unable to cope; (c) just be available as a sounding board.

Test Answers

1. (c) Lack of communication. People have problems communicating, says Dr. Helen Singer Kaplan, if they are unable to talk about their own feelings or to sense those of their partner. Suppose a woman finds her husband too fast or mechanical in their sexual relationship. She might be afraid to speak out and may express her frustration by demanding new furniture when she knows her husband is anxious about money. So, instead of saying something constructive such as "Sweetheart, let's try to make love in a better way," she'll say she needs a new dining-room set, and they will end up fighting.

2. (a) Yes. Too much frankness sometimes shows a lack of consideration, says Dr. William Appleton. You don't have to state *everything* that's on your mind—there's a big difference between a tactful and loving sharing of thoughts and a continual broadcasting of one's feelings and criticisms. While candor is often commendable, too much of it can be cruel. Try to avoid hurting your partner unnecessarily. That never accomplishes anything.

3. (a) More likely. According to Dr. Harold I. Lief, studies show that—surprisingly—the housewife is subject to more mental and physical illness than the working wife. The reason: a housewife often is unable to fulfill herself and gain status in her own eyes; the weight of the marriage thus falls unevenly upon her.

The woman who stays home needs outside group contact with church, recreational or other kinds of organizations that will give her some sense of support and community. Her husband also has to recognize the serious problem she faces.

Source: Condensed from a WNBC-TV Program. Written, produced, and directed by Don Luftig © Don Luftig.

Parenthood

Should You Be a Parent?

We have already discussed the fact that couples now have a choice of whether or not to have children. But how should they use that choice? Parenting can be one of life's most joyous choices. It can also lead to frustration, irritation, and—sometimes—heartbreak. The decision to have a child is one of the most serious that any couple makes. It should be made with thought and care, and for the right reasons.

A child is not simply a little "bundle of joy," it is a new person. It may start out as a bundle, but it soon becomes a toddler, a school-age kid, a teenager, and, then, an adult. All couples will not find each of

THE MARRIAGE TEST

4. (a) True. According to a U.S. Department of Commerce survey, people who earn more than $20,000 a year are more likely to stay married longer than people who make less.

5. (a) Under age 30. Statistics show that almost two-thirds of all first marriages ending in divorce do so before the wife reaches 30.

6. (b) Anger. But this emotion is only an indication of other feelings, warns Dr. Sidney Lecker. It is important to recognize what motivates the anger. An unfaithful person is often saying, "I'll show him [or her] that I can't be treated this way." Behind that anger there's usually loneliness and a desire to be loved. Seeking that love elsewhere causes pain to both partners. But they can use the lesson of an affair to help strengthen their marriage, by trying to find what's wrong with their communication and thus improve the quality of the relationship.

7. Unfortunately, (a) yes. Studies indicate that 80 percent of men and 60 percent of women have extra-marital affairs. However, Dr. Kaplan stresses, an affair need not be the end of a marriage. At some point, virtually every relationship faces this or some other crisis, and this is both a hazard and an opportunity to deepen a couple's understanding and commitment.

The danger signal to look for is a change of feelings. Are you happy to hear his key in the door? Do you schedule a hundred chores for Saturday, just to get away from her? Change of feeling means that your marriage is not what it used to be and that it's time to look at it and at yourself. Admitting a problem is the first step toward solving it.

8. (a) True. Confessing will clear your conscience—but also ask yourself *why* you're confessing, advises Dr. Appleton. Is it so your spouse will stop you from doing it again? No one can stop you but yourself. Is it to be forgiven? The problem is forgiving yourself. The other person will be hurt by your confession—and for a long time. So it's usually best not to compound the problem unnecessarily by confessing it.

9. (b) False. There's no guarantee that a good sex life will save a marriage, let alone add years to it, explains Dr. Lief. Besides, a good sex life doesn't necessarily last throughout a marriage. The sexual excitement that people experience early in marriage may weaken and be replaced by boredom. A couple have to work at keeping their marriage—and sex life—exciting.

10. (a) Yes; 44 percent end in divorce. Newly divorced people usually rush right out to get married again, notes Dr. Lecker. You need to update your identity after leaving a marriage. And you can do that only by being single for a while.

11. (c) Just be available. Dr. Lecker explains that it's important to recognize what you *shouldn't* do as well as what you should do. Probing, unless done by a professional, can lead to more harm than good. And if you take over, you'll be denying your friend the opportunity to develop mastery over the situation. A crisis is a chance for growth. So let your friend learn to master the situation on his or her own.

THIS QUIZ HAS NO SCORE. But it does have wiinners—those people who have learned how to make their marriage work a little better.

these stages to their liking. Adolescents are often rebellious; and if the idea of putting up with that frightens you, consider not having children.

Couples who are thinking about having children should consider the purely practical problems of having children. Being a parent involves drastic changes in a couple's life style. Let us start with the fact that having to feed, clothe, and shelter another human being (or more?) for 18 years, or even longer, costs a tremendous amount of money. At the same time that the family's need for money grows, its income may not—since someone may have to stay home to care for the child or the children. And children restrict their parents in numerous ways, for a child's needs often have to be met before any others.

Potential parents should evaluate the strength of their own relationships before including children in them. Many people suppose that babies bring couples together and can even help some troubled marriages—but they are wrong. Children often have the opposite effect. Constant care for a small child or children can make both parents tired and annoyed. They may become too busy to spend much time alone together, too busy to talk things over and share and smile and relax together. New fathers often feel left out because their wives become involved in their new mothering roles. New mothers sometimes feel cut off from adult company and, therefore, stifled.

Before you decide to have children you should understand your feelings about children and your own childhood. People who were unhappy as children may decide, perhaps correctly, that they would not make good parents. But some will surely want to try to be the parents they wish that they had had. No one should decide to have children in order to "get" something from the child—a companion for the twilight years, for example, or a source of income, or a substitute to achieve the parents' failed ambitions. Of course, many children have been and are born to parents who never "decided" to have them—and they too must grow up to make decisions about having children of their own.

Protecting a Relationship

Children, as we have seen, can enrich the feelings between a man and a woman, but they can hurt them too. One way to deal with this is to share the duties of childrearing. If the father feeds and cares for the infant and toddler, he is less likely to feel left out and jealous—and the mother will get some relief. New mothers must spend some time away from their babies, so that they will not be isolated from adult company. As the children grow older parents can take the opportunity to share many life experiences with them. Remember that for all the problems of parenthood, many—perhaps most—people are suited to it. Along with all the problems children bring into their parents' lives, they also bring joy, happiness, and fulfillment.

Adoption

Childbirth is not the only way to build a family. The other way is adoption, a choice not only for couples who cannot have children but also for couples who just want to open up their homes to children who have no family.

Adoption is a legal process that makes children members of the family that takes them in. It differs from foster care, the temporary placement of children in private homes. During the 1970s, about 170,000 families, annually, chose to adopt children in the United States, both privately and through social-work agencies. Private adoptions are arranged with the person or the family wishing to give up the child or

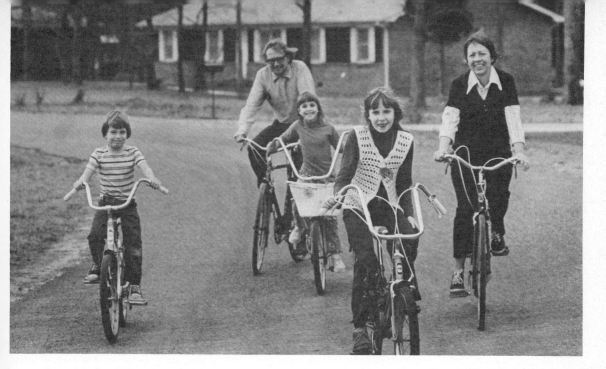

Bruce Roberts/Rapho/Photo Researchers

Ken Karp

through a go-between (often a lawyer). Some of these private adoptions amount to the sale of babies by their parents. The reason for this is that, due to birth control and legalized abortions, fairly few white babies— the kind most people want to adopt—are offered for adoption, so those that are offered fetch high prices. Older children, nonwhite children, and handicapped children are much harder to place for adoption, but not as hard as in the past, for the supply of white babies has fallen drastically.

Like children for adoption, would-be adopters used to be viewed, and to some extent still are viewed, as more and less desirable by such standards as class, background, age, and education. But these standards may not be important. What is more important are the adoptors' attitudes toward parenting and their understanding of the special needs of their child. Adopted children should be told that they are adopted and helped to develop a clear sense of identity, of who they are. With the right kind of help from their parents and from the social agencies that deal with adopted children, they can achieve their own identities and live happy lives.

Divorce

We have already spoken of marriage as "the most durable of all social institutions." But sometimes it almost seems as if divorce is now just as much of an institution. Certainly divorce is no longer rare, and it is no longer a shameful secret; the divorces of celebrities are the daily

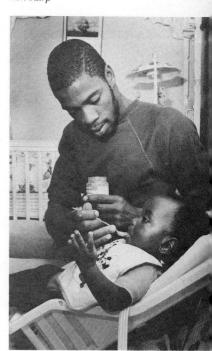

fare of the popular press. Newspapers print these stories because people like to read them, and people read them because they reflect a reality in the lives of all Americans, not just in the lives of celebrities.

Each year, 1 million Americans are divorced. Sometimes, that figure of 1 million divorcees annually is compared to the number of people getting married during the same year—say, 2.2 million—so that the divorce "rate" appears to be a whopping 45 percent. The reality is somewhat less depressing; for only a small number of the divorces obtained in any year come from marriages begun in that same year. Linked to this so-called rate of failure is the common idea that marriages ending in divorce last but a short time. True, many marriages collapse after the first couple of years. But most marriages, even those that do collapse, last at least 6½ years; and at least 50 percent of all divorced couples had been married 7 years or more.

A much more meaningful way to compute a divorce rate would be to figure how many of the total number of marriages break up in any 1 year. If there are 51 million married couples in a year, and 1 million divorces, the rate shrinks down to a little under 2 percent. If this rate held constant for 25 years, almost half of all married couples would *eventually*—not in any 1 year—be divorced. But divorce rates do not hold constant. Some periods, like the late 1940s (just after World War II) and the 1970s, were marked by very high divorce rates. But over the past 50 years the divorce rate, although rising overall, has not changed much.

A great part of the current divorce "epidemic" is probably temporary, brought about by affluence, rising expectations, and the improved status of women. Despite the present very high rates of divorce, a majority of married couples will stay together.

There is another way of looking at the statistics, however: Even if today's *very* high rates of divorce are temporary, the long-term rate of divorce for Americans is *fairly* high. Many people have been, are being, and will be divorced.

Mickey Rooney and four of his eight wives.

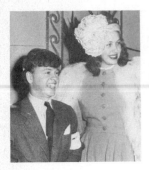

Number 1.
UPI

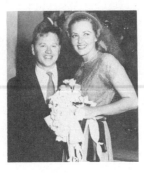

Number 3.
UPI

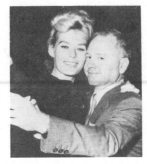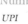

Number 5.
UPI

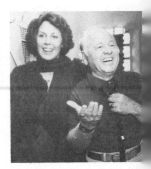

Number 8.
UPI

Table 15–1. Marriage and Divorce Rates for Selected Years

Year	Number (1,000)		Rate per 1,000 population	
	Marriages	*Divorces*	*Marriages*	*Divorces*
1930	1,127	196	9.2	1.6
1940	1,596	264	12.1	2.0
1950	1,667	385	11.1	2.6
1960	1,523	393	8.5	2.2
1970	2,159	708	10.6	3.5
1975	2,153	1,036	10.1	4.9
1976	2,155	1,083	10.0	5.0
1977	2,178	1,091	10.1	5.0
1978	2,282	1,130	10.5	5.2
1979	2,359	1,170	10.7	5.3

Source: U.S. Bureau of the Census, *Statistical Abstract of the United States, 1980* (101st ed.), table 85, p. 61.

"Splitsville"

The events that lead up to a divorce often begin with arguments about problems like sex and money. But sex and money are almost never the real causes of a divorce. The real cause is almost always a failure to communicate, especially to communicate anger. This failure shows itself in arguments about problem issues, like sex and money. As a husband and wife fight more intensely, they withhold their feelings from each other and grow farther apart. Then they create a distance that results in "just not caring."

Paul Bohannon, a family sociologist, has written that with each divorce there are, so to speak, six different divorces—six kinds of adjustment for the divorcing couple and for their family and friends. The first is the "emotional divorce," the concealment by the husband and wife of their true feelings. They each feel trapped, unloved, and unable to tolerate the other. When their relationship has collapsed they begin to seek a "legal divorce." Now others, mainly lawyers and judges, make decisions the divorcing couple cannot make for itself, and the legal bond of marriage is dissolved. This legal divorce makes the former husband and wife legally—but not, perhaps, emotionally—able to remarry. The "economic divorce" divides the household and its goods and assets into two separate sets, one for the husband, one for the wife. Besides coping with property and tax law, the former husband and wife must also cope with their mistrust of each other and their feelings of being deprived.

If the couple had children, a *coparental divorce* must be arranged to provide care for them. The divorcing couple's friends must take up an attitude toward the divorce and deal with any conflict of loyalties they have toward the former husband and wife; while the divorcees must accept their new social status as single people. These adjustments make

Table 15–2.   Persons under 18 Years—with Whom Do They Live?

| Year | Persons under 18 years old (1,000) | Percent living with both parents | Percent Living with Mother Only Who Is— | | | | Percent living with father only | Percent living with neither parent |
			Married, spouse absent	Widowed	Divorced	*Single (never married)*		
1968	70,617	85.0	4.9	2.3	2.9	0.7	1.1	3.2
1970	69,458	84.9	4.7	2.0	3.3	0.8	1.1	3.3
1975	66,087	80.3	5.8	2.4	5.5	1.8	1.5	2.7
1979	62,389	77.4	5.6	2.0	6.8	2.5	1.6	3.4

Source: U.S. Bureau of the Census, *Statistical Abstract of the United States, 1980* (101st ed.), table 75, p. 52.

up the *community divorce.* Finally, and perhaps most painful, is the *psychic divorce.* The former husband and wife must stop expecting help and support from each other and attempt to meet new challenges by themselves.

Social Trends Encouraging Divorce

Divorce used to be a matter for shame, and it was expensive and hard to get. Today, the legal divorce is usually quick and fairly cheap. Most people, too, now regard divorce as the best way out of an unhappy marriage—an attitude that is encouraged by the current emphasis on self-fulfillment and the lesser importance attached to values like dis-

A single-parent family.

Ray Ellis / Rapho / Photo Researchers

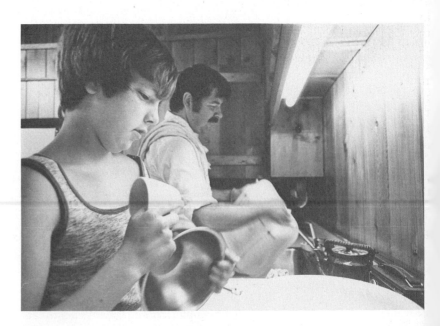

cipline and commitment, home, and children. These attitudes, in turn, have been encouraged by the weakening of traditional authorities.

Women have been affected by these changes more profoundly than men have. In the past it was, above all, women who were expected to sacrifice themselves and their ambitions for the good of their husbands and children. And women were, for the most part, economically dependent on men. The rejection by many women of these roles has helped to dissolve the foundations of traditional marriage and to raise divorce rates.

At the same time that many women refuse to make the sacrifices formerly demanded of them, both men and women are placing new demands on marriage—demands for intimacy, companionship, and creative sex. Not all marriages can fulfill all these needs.

The Family Regroups

One-parent Families

Did you know that in the United States 22 percent of those 18 years or younger live in households with only one parent? Of all these young people, less than 2 percent live with their fathers.

Children in these households face special problems. They may feel self-conscious about not having both parents. After a divorce, these children have to cope with the new state of affairs. They may grieve for the absent parent. And they must work out a tremendous amount of anger at one parent or both. Some children feel deeply anxious that they were themselves responsible for their parents' divorces.

The parents, meanwhile, have their own problems. Mothers who raise their children without a husband's help have an especially hard time. In the first place, women earn on average 40 percent less than men do. They are also discriminated against by employers who suspect that family duties will interfere with work. As if these were not problems enough, childcare is expensive, and good childcare is hard to find at any price.

Single fathers who raise children without the help of wives also have problems balancing work and family. Men are expected to commit themselves to work; employers do not like it when men stay home with sick children or ask for time off to meet their children's other needs.

Remarriage

Until recently, couples married "until death us do part"—that, at any rate, was what they expected or pretended to expect. But the high rate of divorce in the United States has created new expectations about marriage—and even new *kinds* of marriage. Marriages (at least legal ones)

"I'd Like to Introduce My . . . Uh . . ."

When a man introduces his wife he says, "I'd like you to meet my wife. . . ." How do unmarried people who live together describe each other? Here is a real problem for the English language. Some people say, "I'd like you to meet my 'friend,' or roommate, or *ami*, or (rather stilted, this) 'con-vivant'." Awkward attempts at coyness include "sin-law," "unlywed," and "attache." "Partner" captures the democratic spirit of contemporary roles, but could be misleading. "Lover" is the traditional term and it is also the most accurate, but it tends to embarrass people by its honesty. Many people avoid the issue by simply introducing their lovers without description: "This is Pete."

are still *monogamous*, that is, between one man and one woman. But many people now enter into one short-lived monogamous marriage after another. Specialists call this *serial monogamy*. As a result of it, the members of families are regrouped and shuffled as single parents remarry and acquire stepchildren. Children may be exposed to a wide variety of adults, without enough continuity for sound emotional growth. They may not be able to attach themselves to anyone deeply. Adults may have so many family ties of one sort or another that they cannot really meet all their obligations.

Remarriage creates economic problems, too. Supporting or sharing in the support of more than one household is expensive. Yet people continue to pay this heavy price in the hope of having better luck next time around.

"Without Benefit of Clergy"

Although serial monogamy is new, it is traditional in at least two respects: First, each marriage is monogamous and, second, each marriage is entered into legally. Some kinds of relationships between men and women dispense with one or both of these elements. A *common-law marriage* is one entered into without legal formalities, though in some states such a marriage becomes legal after 7 years of living together. A *trial marriage* involves living together before making a final decision; the line between trial marriage and "living together" is unclear. What is quite clear is that "living together," common-law marriages, and trial marriages are becoming more and more common; in 1970, 650,000 people were living in this way, but by the end of the decade that number had grown to about 1.5 million.

Staying Single

Most people, as we have already noted, still get married. But more and more they do so by choice, not by necessity. In the past, men got married because that was just about the only way of getting their clothes washed and their meals cooked, women got married because there were very few ways for them to earn a living, and both men and women got married to be considered "normal." Today people are not quite so sure about what is "normal" and what is not. More and more people are delaying marriage, or choosing not to marry at all, and they are not feeling like rejects. About 16 percent of the adult women over 18 years of age in the United States (1978) have never married, and approximately 23 percent of the men of the same age have never married.

Freedom of choice is not the only reason that so many people are staying single. Another is the fact that more men and, especially, more women are pursuing professional careers. Such a career is very difficult to combine with long-lasting emotional commitments.

SUMMARY

The college years are a link between the dependency of childhood and the independence of adulthood. Learning to live peacefully with roommates, whether of the same sex or the opposite one, is an important part of this transition. Another part of it, for many young people, is "living together," either as a preparation for marriage or as an alternative to it.

The intimacy of marriage or of a long-term relationship has great advantages for most people. It promotes personal growth and completes our separation from our parents. Romantic love has always been only one of several motives for getting married; others include the desire for economic security and for social status, and the fear of having to take care of oneself alone.

No one should get married hastily or without considering the benefits and problems of marriage. The dangers of getting married before you are ready—and the fact that many Americans do get married without much thought—are shown clearly enough by this country's high rate of divorce.

One of the most important decisions any couple has to make is whether or not to have children. The raising of children costs a good deal in time, energy, and money, and this can threaten the parents' marriage. But raising children can also be one of the great joys of life.

As a result of divorce, among other causes, many children are now raised by single parents. If divorced people marry others, they must cope with such delicate problems as stepchildren and former husbands or wives, as well as with the financial pressures of paying for more than one household at a time.

More and more people are choosing to remain single, either permanently or for a long period of adulthood. Remaining single allows great freedom and no longer carries much of a social stigma. But marriage still is the statistical norm.

Suggested Readings

Belkin, Gary S., and Goodman, Norman. *Marriage, Family, and Intimate Relationships.* Chicago: Rand McNally, 1980. This book is concerned with the functioning of marriage and family life.

Clayton, Richard R. *The Family: Marriage and Social Change.* Lexington, Mass.: D.C. Heath, 1975. The family is discussed as a social institution and as an intimate environment for developing human potential.

Goldenberg, Irene, and Goldenberg, Herbert. *Family Therapy: An Overview.* Monerey, Cal.: Brooks/Cole, 1980. Although geared toward counseling, this is an excellent resource on the interaction and the dysfunction within families.

Satir, V. *Peoplemaking.* Palo Alto, Cal.: Science & Behavior Books, 1972.

Satir, V., et al. *Helping Families to Change.* New York: Jason Aronson, 1975. Both of Satir's books discuss the family's importance to personal development. Both are geared to counseling, but have excellent information of the structure of the family.

Stinnett, Nick, et al. *Building Family Strengths.* Lincoln: University of Nebraska Press, 1979. This book includes readings by educators in the field of family life. The focus is on the power within a family to enhance the quality of family relationships.

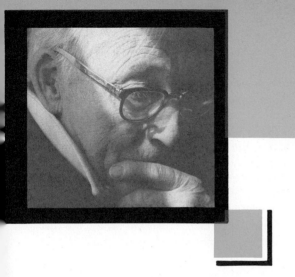

16

Aging, Dying, and Death

chapter objectives

When you have finished reading this chapter you should be able to:
1. Discuss the situation of the aged in America
2. Explain the physical, emotional, and social changes that go with aging
3. Recognize aspects of modern life that lead toward denial of death
4. Apply Kübler-Ross' stages of grief to the terminal patient
5. Describe the development of the hospice movement
6. Discuss the problem of euthanasia

In almost every culture, the great milestones of life are birth, childhood, adulthood, middle age, old age, and, finally, death. In the United States, the final stages of life—old age and death—are milestones with little honor and seem to take place almost in secret. Some cultures revere the elderly, and in many of them older people live with their children. But in the United States youth has the place of honor, and many older people live behind closed doors—in city apartments, in decaying houses, in institutions, and even in towns limited to the elderly. As for death, it mostly takes place in hospitals, out of sight and out of mind.

Each of us who lives long enough must grow old, and everyone without exception must die. Many people now think that American values should be modified to reflect these realities, and to reflect the fact that people can find old age to be a happy and productive time of life.

Trends

The population of the United States has grown from about 4 million in 1790 to 226 million in 1980. In this country's youth, almost all of its people were young, for the birth rate was then very high—higher, probably, than at any other time or place in human history. As industrialization spread, the birth rate began to fall, but the population increased because more people were living longer and more of the newly born survived. Following World War II, we had a "baby boom," but the birth rate has never returned to the sustained rate of increase that occurred during the early 1800s.

As the birth rate began to fall, medical and nutritional improvements, better sanitation, and a higher standard of living kept people

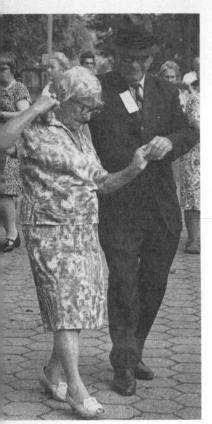

Hanna W. Schreiber/Rapho/Photo Researchers

Table 16–1. Birth and Death Rates for Selected Years

| Year | Number (1,000) | | | Rate Per 1,000 Population | | |
| | Births[1] | Deaths | | Births[1] | Deaths | |
		Total	Infant[2]		Total	Infant[2]
1930	2,618	1,327	142	21.3	11.3	64.6
1940	2,559	1,417	111	19.4	10.8	47.0
1950	3,632	1,452	104	24.1	9.6	29.2
1960	4,258	1,712	111	23.7	9.5	26.0
1970	3,731	1,921	75	18.4	9.5	20.0
1975	3,144	1,893	51	14.8	8.8	16.1
1976	3,168	1,909	48	14.8	8.9	15.2
1977	3,327	1,900	47	15.4	8.8	14.1
1978	3,333	1,928	46	15.3	8.8	13.8
1979	3,473	1,906	45	15.8	8.7	13.0

[1] Through 1955, adjusted for underregistration. [2] Infants under 1 year, excluding fetal deaths; rates per 1,000 registered live births.

Source: U.S. Bureau of the Census, *Statistical Abstract of the United States, 1980* (101st ed.), table 85, p. 61.

Table 16–2.   Resident Population of the United States, by Age, 1979 (1,000)

Total	Under 5 years	5–13 years	14–17 years	18–24 years	25–44 years	45–64 years	65 years and over	Percent Under 5 years	5 to 17 years	65 years and over
220,099	15,644	30,647	16,275	29,029	59,938	43,903	24,658	7.1	21.3	11.2

Source: U.S. Bureau of the Census, *Statistical Abstract of the United States, 1980* (101st ed.), table 35, p. 32.

alive longer. The result is that the average age of the people of the United States has grown older and older—because older people have made up a larger and larger proportion of our total population. By 1979, over 11 percent—one out of eleven—of the people in this country were 65 years of age or over. That represents over a sevenfold increase in the *number* of elderly people—from 3 million to 25 million—between 1900 and 1979, and almost a tripling (from 4.1 percent to 11.2 percent) of the *proportion* of Americans who are old.

Because men tend to die at an earlier age than women do, this growing population of older people consists mainly of women. Many older women are widows living alone.

Population and Society

Changes in the proportion of a country's total population in any age group may well have important political and social consequences. The "youth culture" of the 1960s and 1970s is explained by many as a result of the rise in this country's birth rate between 1946 and 1960. This baby boom, for a short time, reversed the long-term increase in the proportion of Americans over 65. But the members of the baby-boom generation have also continued to age. Now that they have entered the job market, we find that too many people are looking for too few jobs. By the year 2010, the oldest members of the baby-boom generation will have begun to retire, and they will start collecting Social Security. The Social Security system is already under great stress, but nothing like the stress it will face after 2010, for the generation that followed the baby boom is much smaller than its predecessor. What exactly does this mean? It means that this much smaller generation of workers will be paying for the Social Security of the much larger baby-boom generation. You can bet that aging, and paying for it, will be one of the great political issues of the next 50 years—and you can bet, as well, that *you* will be profoundly affected by this issue. How do you think the growing numbers of elderly will affect you, personally? How do you think that growing old yourself will affect you?

Life Expectancies

There will be more old people tomorrow because there are more young people today. But the number of old people will also grow because many of us will just live longer. Trying to predict average *life expectancy* (the length of an average life) in the future is a tricky business. Natural disasters (floods, earthquakes, famines) and worldwide calamities (nuclear accidents or wars) could shorten average life expectancy at the same time that medical advances, better living conditions, and improved public health could lengthen it. In this country, right now, children born in 1974 can expect to live, on average, 72 years. Children born in 1900 lived, on average, only 47 years. The change in the average has been due mainly to better medical care for infants and to improved public health.

One final point about these statistics: They are misleading. Although more children reach the age of 20 today than in 1900, the average age of death for people who live past the age of 20 has not increased very much since 1800, and neither has the age of the oldest people among us. In other words, people who reach age 70 today cannot expect to live much longer than people who reached the age of 70 in 1950. In fact, for people who live to the age of 60, average life expectancy is only one year more than it was in the 18th century. As these startling facts indicate, the maximum life span of human beings seems to be quite fixed.

Table 16–3. Living Arrangements of Elderly Widowed Persons, Age 65 and over: 1968 to 1979

		Householder				Not a Householder	
			Percent nonfamily householder living—				
Widowed Persons	Total (1,000)	Percent house holder family	Alone	With non-relatives	Total (1,000)	Percent in families	Percent living with no relatives
1968: Total	4,902	24.5	71.8	3.7	2,047	91.2	8.8
Widow	3,948	24.5	72.2	3.3	1,613	92.2	7.8
Widower	954	24.3	69.8	6.0	434	87.6	12.4
1970: Total	5,296	22.3	74.6	3.1	1,984	89.4	10.5
Widow	4,344	22.2	75.0	2.9	1,519	92.2	7.7
Widower	952	22.9	73.0	4.1	465	80.0	19.8
1975: Total	6,117	18.6	78.9	2.5	1,588	92.3	7.7
Widow	5,110	18.8	78.7	2.4	1,407	93.5	6.5
Widower	1,007	17.3	79.4	3.2	181	82.9	17.1
1979: Total	6,886	16.5	81.1	2.4	1,575	90.7	9.3
Widow	5,833	16.7	81.0	2.4	1,277	93.3	6.7
Widower	1,053	15.5	81.8	2.6	298	79.2	20.8

Source: U.S. Bureau of the Census, *Statistical Abstract of the United States, 1980* (101st ed.), table 77, p. 52.

SELF-ASSESSMENT DEVICE 16-1: HOW LONG WILL YOU LIVE?

This is a rough guide for calculating your personal longevity. The basic life expectancy for males is age 67 and for females it is age 75. Write down your basic life expectancy. If you are in your 50s or 60s, you should add ten years to the basic figure because you have already proven yourself to be quite durable. If you are over age 60 and active, add another two years.

Basic Life Expectancy _____

Decide how each item below applies to you and add or subtract the appropriate number of years from your basic life expectancy.

1. Family history
   Add 5 years if 2 or more of your grandparents lived to 80 or beyond. _____
   Subtract 4 years if any parent, grandparent, sister, or brother died of heart attack or stroke before 50. Subtract 2 years if anyone died from these diseases before 60. _____
   Subtract 3 years for each case of diabetes, thyroid disorders, breast cancer, cancer of the digestive system, asthma, or chronic bronchitis among parents or grandparents. _____

2. Marital status
   If you are married, add 4 years. _____
   If you are over 25 and not married, subtract 1 year for every unwedded decade. _____

3. Economic status
   Subtract 2 years if your family income is over $40,000 per year. _____
   Subtract 3 years if you have been poor for greater part of life. _____

4. Physique
   Subtract one year for every 10 pounds you are overweight. _____
   For each inch your girth measurement exceeds your chest measurement deduct two years. _____
   Add 3 years if you are over 40 and not overweight. _____

5. Exercise
   Regular and moderate (jogging 3 times a week), add 3 years. _____
   Regular and vigorous (long distance running 3 times a week), add 5 years. _____
   Subtract 3 years if your job is sedentary. _____
   Add 3 years if it is active. _____

6. Alcohol
   Add 2 years if you are a light drinker (1-3 drinks a day). _____

   Subtract 5 to 10 years if you are a heavy drinker (more than 4 drinks per day). _____
   Subtract 1 year if you are a teetotler. _____

7. Smoking
   Two or more packs of cigarettes per day, subtract 8 years. _____
   One to two packs per day, subtract 4 years. _____
   Less than one pack, subtract 2 years. _____
   Subtract 2 years if you regularly smoke a pipe or cigars. _____

8. Disposition
   Add 2 years if you are a reasoned, practical person. _____
   Subtract 2 years if you are aggressive, intense and competitive. _____
   Add 1-5 years if you are basically happy and content with life. _____
   Subtract 1-5 years if you are often unhappy, worried, and often feel guilty. _____

9. Education
   Less than high school, subtract 2 years. _____
   Four years of school beyond high school, add 1 year. _____
   Five or more years beyond high school, add 3 years. _____

10. Environment
    If you have lived most of your life in a rural environment, add 4 years. _____
    Subtract 2 years if you have lived most of your life in an urban environment. _____

11. Sleep
    More than 9 hours a day, subtract 5 years. _____

12. Temperature
    Add 2 years if your home's thermostat is set at no more than 68°F. _____

13. Health Care
    Regular medical checkup and regular dental care, add 3 years. _____
    Frequently ill, subtract 2 years. _____

Source: Richard Schultz, *The Psychology of Death, Dying, and Bereavement* (Reading, Mass.: Addison-Wesley, 1978), pp. 97-98. Table 5.1 © 1978. Reprinted with permission.

The increase in the length of an average life—a statistic, pure and simple, has been due mainly to the increased survival of infants.

Aging

Despite the fact that most adults do not really live much longer than they ever lived in recent centuries, more people survive to old age. So more people experience the changes, challenges, and discomforts of old age. Old people as a group cannot be described as sick or healthy, depressed or happy, productive or unproductive. Like people of other ages, older people are older individuals—all of them are different. Nonetheless, certain physical and social changes are very common among the elderly. What are these changes?

From age 50 to 65, anyone who has had children can expect to see them grow to adulthood and leave the family home. By the age of 75, most working people are retired and this often means a loss of income and prestige. At this time, too, many older people become widows or widowers—usually widows—and they lose their old friends to moves, illness, and death. Then physical energy gradually declines.

Even greater physical losses can be expected in the years from 75 to 85. The senses of taste, vision, and hearing decline markedly. This, and the loss of physical mobility and independence, leads to less physical and social activity. Many people at this age find that they cannot maintain their houses or apartments and move into institutions.

In the years after 85, a serious decline in health is common, and many old people must accept a further loss of independence and mobility. At this stage, illness or lack of mobility often cut older people off from social activities. The continuing decline of the senses of hearing and vision prevents other social activities, such as talking on the telephone, going to plays and movies, watching television, and reading. Their world becomes an inner world, filled with thoughts and memories and insights.

Diseases of Old Age

Older people are really not, by and large, the physical wrecks that many people think they are. Only about 5 percent of them, for example, live in nursing homes and mental hospitals. Each person responds to the changes of aging as an individual. Some people age quickly and are ridden with sickness and depression. Others are quite healthy but have problems with particular organ systems—the respiratory system or the cardiovascular system. Still others stay completely healthy well into old age.

Despite these variations, aging bodies are less able to respond well to biological and emotional stresses. Organs and systems work less ef-

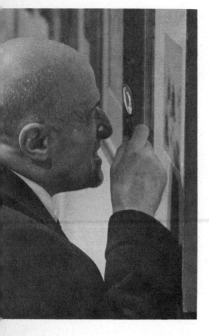

Some older people, like this one, find that their vision declines, but the vision of some others improves with age.

F. B. Grunzweig/Photo Researchers

ficiently. Disease strikes more often and with greater and more deadly effect. Heart disease, strokes, and cancer are the three most common killers in our society. Most of their victims are older people.

The medical problems of old age are real, but they are often exaggerated. For instance, the idea that old age is a time of sexlessness is completely false. And so too is the idea that most older people suffer from senility, a state caused by hardened blood vessels in the brain, which leads to impairment of thought process—like lack of memory about recent events, loss of orientation, emotional disturbance, and decline of intellect and judgment. In fact, many older people who seem to be senile are really victims of a number of treatable problems, like anxiety, depression, malnutrition, alcoholism, or the overuse of prescription drugs.

Personality and Aging

Another myth of aging is that old age makes people depressed and dissatisfied. Some old people may be depressed and are dissatisfied, but most of them were this way even when they were younger. Old age does not change people's personalities; it subjects them to new challenges.

The *circumstances* in which people grow old affect their personalities more than old age itself. Older people who live alone, whose children rarely visit them, and whose health problems force them to withdraw from lifelong social ties feel lonely and unhappy. Those who stay in their own homes, close to family and friends, and those who move to stimulating retirement communities, tend to remain cheerful and optimistic. They also tend to stay healthier and live longer. One investigation of almost 5,000 adults found that older people who are married, have contacts with close friends and relatives, maintain church membership, and belong to informal or formal group associations have a much lower death rate than people without these ties. Older people with social ties also have less heart disease, cancer, stroke, and fewer circulatory problems.

Those older people who lose touch with friends and family and who struggle with serious diseases and social problems (poverty, for example) are sometimes depressed—and with good cause. As many as 25 percent of all suicides in the United States involve people over 65—and these are mostly men (see Chapter 3).

Older people do have a limited future. Some avoid facing this fact by living in the past or by denying the fear of their own mortality. Others are overwhelmed by hopelessness and give up on life, literally dying while waiting for death. Still others are able to look back on the past, resolve their conflicts and regrets, and enjoy the pleasures of the present.

Another Double Standard

In the matter of aging, as in so much else, women are the disadvantaged sex. Men with graying hair are said to be "distinguished"; women who show similar signs of aging are said to look "old." An old bachelor is often viewed as "attractive"; older single women are often pitied as unwanted "old maids." In fact, older men tend to avoid women of their own ages to date and marry younger women; traditionally, older women had "no chance" with younger men. But things seem to be changing.

Poverty and Old Age

Although many of the physical problems of old age are preventable, treatable, or reversible, older bodies do develop physical problems because they start to wear out. But the social problems of aging are not as inevitable. The greatest of these, in a word, is poverty. According to a 1977 report 28.5 percent of older women had incomes of less than $2,000 per year. One out of every five couples in which the husband is over 65 had (in 1974) incomes of under $4,000. Older people living alone or with nonrelatives had even lower incomes; half were below $3,000. Only one elderly couple in four received as much as $10,000 a year. Although there have been some rises in Social Security benefits, the fact remains that many elderly Americans are now economically deprived.

Despite their low incomes, older people in 1978 spent an average of $2,026 on health care, nearly three times more than the average $763 required by younger adults. Benefits from medical insurance (see Chapter 17) covered only 60 percent of older people's health-care bills. And since most older people are living on fixed incomes they are hit very hard by inflation. "Heat or eat" is a real and demoralizing choice in old age in places where large fuel bills must be met.

What Is to Be Done?   These social problems, as we have seen, are less inevitable than the diseases of old age. But the question of what, if anything, to do about them is a political one. Groups of old people, such as the Gray Panthers, have demanded more government action on behalf of the elderly—rent regulation, for example. But these demands went against the conservative political climate of the United States in the late 1970s and early 1980s and little was done about them. At that point, in fact, even the future of Social Security (created as long ago as 1935) seemed uncertain. No one proposed to abolish Social Security, but the system on which millions of older people rely for most of their income was short of money.

How to Live Forever

As we have seen, the natural limit of human life is about 100 years. So there may never be a time when people live long beyond that. Let us adopt a more limited but fully realistic goal: to live a long, healthy, and enjoyable life. The key to achieving that goal is clear and simple: *Prevent diseases instead of curing them.* The way to act on that principle is also clear and simple.

First, exercise regularly (see Chapter 7). This will help prevent heart disease, the most common health problem of old age. It is also good for increasing general circulation, strengthening musculature, improving

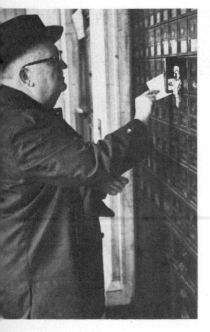

The monthly check arrives. Many older people depend on Social Security.

Michael Philip Manheim/Photo Researchers

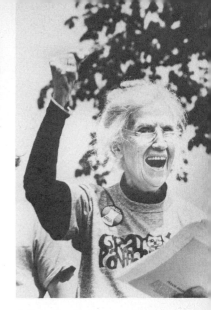

A Gray Panther.
Bettye Lane/Photo Researchers

Richard Frieman/Photo Researchers

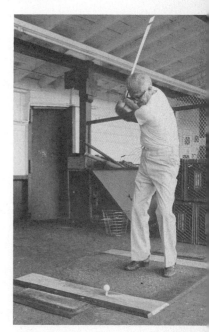

the digestive process, and providing an outlet for frustrations. Physical fitness also promotes self-esteem and, therefore, mental health.

Second, eat a balanced diet (see Chapter 8) in the proper amounts (see Chapter 9). Eating the right things helps to prevent such disorders as atherosclerosis, vitamin deficiency disease, high blood pressure, and bowel problems. Avoiding overweight is a good way of avoiding arthritis, cardiovascular disease, high blood pressure, and surgical risks. It also keeps you thin and, in our culture, this helps to promote self-esteem.

Third, don't smoke.

Finally, get regular checkups by a physician. Sometimes physicians can help prevent diseases, and sometimes they can help cure them. In any case you are better off knowing what is going on in your body.

Death

In some places and in some times, death was an everyday experience—and a public one. At the time of the Black Death, a plague that struck Europe in the 14th century, one-third of the total population died; and as recently as the mid-1970s the Vietnam war dramatized death daily, both to those on the scene and, on TV, to the U.S. home audience.

In our culture, death is not a public event. It taks place in private, and it is followed by restrained and guarded mourning. In the United States, death has been removed from the home, for the most part. It has been transferred to other places, and the dying are regarded with great dismay as discomforting freaks of nature. Because of these attitudes, the dying are isolated; most Americans die in private, almost in secret.

Table 16–4. Death Rates, by Cause, Sex, and Age, 1978

Sex and Age	Diseases of heart	Malignant neoplasms	Cerebrovascular diseases	Accidents	Pneumonia, flu	Diabetes mellitus	Cirrhosis of liver	Arteriosclerosis	Suicide	Early infancy diseases
Total	334.3	181.9	80.5	48.4	26.7	15.5	13.8	13.3	12.5	10.1
Male[1]	375.3	203.5	69.4	69.6	29.0	13.1	18.6	10.9	19.0	12.0
15–24 yr	3.2	7.7	1.2	100.5	1.6	.3	.3	–	20.0	(X)
25–44 yr	37.2	26.9	5.8	69.1	3.9	2.9	11.0	0.1	24.0	(X)
46–64 yr	527.6	345.7	55.0	64.2	22.4	18.3	51.7	3.7	25.3	(X)
65 yr. and over	2,812.6	1,357.0	612.3	129.6	239.8	93.4	57.0	109.6	38.0	(X)
Female[1]	295.5	161.4	91.0	28.3	24.6	17.8	9.3	15.5	6.3	8.3
15–24 yr	2.1	4.9	1.1	28.0	1.1	.4	.3	–	4.7	(X)
25–44 yr	12.0	31.0	5.5	17.9	2.4	2.2	5.2	–	8.9	(X)
45–64 yr	177.9	268.9	44.2	23.1	11.2	17.2	24.4	1.9	10.5	(X)
65 yr. and over	2,001.5	759.0	628.7	80.2	161.2	106.7	22.1	118.7	7.5	(X)

— Represents zero. X Not applicable. [1] Includes persons under 15 years old, not shown separately.
[Rates per 100,000. Causes of death classified according to eighth revision of the *International Classification of Diseases*]
Source: U.S. Bureau of the Census, *Statistical Abstract of the United States, 1980* (101st ed.), table 117, p. 79.

What Is Death?

Today, we are no longer quite sure what death even means. In fact, it has come to mean more than one thing.

Clinical Death.   Many victims of drowning who are pulled from the water are not breathing and their hearts have ceased to beat. Yet they revive after cardiopulmonary resuscitation. Have these people been raised from the dead? It is far from clear. When someone's body systems (such as the cardiovascular and respiratory systems) stop working, that person is said to be *functionally,* or *clinically,* dead. In some states, to be dead in this sense is to be legally dead. Nonetheless, if cardiopulmonary resuscitation is begun, clinical death can be reversed, life can sometimes be restored, and the patient can make a full recovery.

Brain Death.   If resuscitation is not successful, the body's cells quickly begin to suffer the effects of a lack of oxygen. Brain cells are the most sensitive to oxygen loss. The first body cells to die of *anoxia* (oxygen starvation) are those in the cerebral cortex, the brain area that controls sensation and voluntary action, stores memories, and directs complex thought and decision-making processes. If this area of the brain dies, the patient may continue to live, but only as what is called a vegetable.

If the anoxia continues, the midbrain, which controls emotion, alertness, and consciousness, proceeds to die. The victim then enters the unconscious state known as a *coma.* Since heart function and breathing continue, however, comatose patients are not considered to be dead. With prolonged anoxia, the lower area of the brain, known as the brain stem, will die. Since this area stimulates the action of the heart and lungs, clinical death follows if no further steps are taken.

Cellular Death.   Even at the point of total *brain death,* a patient may still remain "alive" if artificial machine systems are used to stimulate heart function and breathing. If artificial respiration stops and the patient does not resume independent breathing, cells in all organs of the body begin to die for lack of oxygen.

Medical Death.   The lack of any one accepted definition of death has forced the medical profession to develop guidelines to define the point at which a dying person is beyond all hope of revival. These guidelines stipulate that a person is well and truly dead if for 12 hours there has been no spontaneous voluntary movement (such as breathing), no brain-controlled reflexes (if, for example, the pupils of the eyes do not blink when light is shined into them), and no output of electrical energy from the brain.

Recently a technique (cerebral angiography) has been developed to test whether or not blood is being circulated to the vital centers of the brain. If blood is not being circulated, it is assumed that "brain death" has occurred.

Dying: Myths and Realities

Just as physicians, scientists, and lawyers disagree among themselves about the definition of death, different cultures disagree about its meaning. Some cultures glorify death as a release from the troubles of human existence. Others see it as a punishment for sin. Despite any differences (and there are many more of them), some people have argued that each person instinctively fears death. This fear, they claim, is inborn, and it serves the goal of self-preservation by inspiring in all of us a desire to stay alive.

Fear of death can also be explained as the direct result of learning. Children are born into a world full of living, loving, amusing, and caregiving relatives and friends. As they grow older, children realize that flowers in the garden fade and disappear, that pets die and are taken away, that this relative or that one has died. They begin to realize that each one of us must die. By 9 or 10 years of age, most children accept that death occurs, but they do not fully understand its impact on survivors. But, in time, the deaths of pets or close relatives teach them this final lesson.

Impact of Death on the Dying

In most cultures the great events of life and death occur in full public view. But not in American society. People who are close to death remain hidden from view today, mainly behind hospital doors, and dying people are now cared for chiefly by medical experts, not by their families. Death is not something that most of us have to deal with—not, that is, until someone who depends on us is dying, or we ourselves are.

Ignorance of death is one of those things that breed fear of it. The friends and the families of dying people try to avoid them. Death makes people "uncomfortable," because people do not know what to expect or how to handle their responses. Those who are themselves close to death may be even less able to cope with it, and the detachment and drawing back of friends and family may make the burden even more difficult to bear.

Stages of Death

Death is sometimes sudden and without warning, as in a car accident. But many people learn that they are dying some time before the actual moment of death. These people face life's final challenge: accepting the fact that they will soon die. Although death itself is sometimes sudden, the process of accepting it rarely is. Acceptance is rooted in one's past experiences. Many of the dying learn to accept their deaths by stages. These were described by Elisabeth Kübler-Ross in her well-known book *On Death and Dying* (1969).

Stage one is "denial," when one is not willing to admit that death is near. This stage gives patients time to think and, in time, to accept their fates.

Stage two is "anger"—envy of others who can still plan and act, while the dying person cannot. During this stage, patients are often hostile to their medical caretakers and to friends and family. Anger is a natural and understandable reaction, but it drives away the very people that patients need for support.

Stage three is "bargaining," when the dying person attempts to postpone the end by praying, seeking better medical treatment, promising to be a better person, and so on. Most often these attempts to stave off death by reforming do not work. New symptons and increased fatigue signal that death is now approaching.

In stage four, that of "depression," dying people give themselves over to worries about family and money, and they regret their past misdeeds and failures.

In stage five, "acceptance," death is at hand, and the dying person comes to terms with the end of life—realizing that anger, worry, and depression are futile.

Dying is a part of life, and people respond to it differently, as to all of life's challenges. Many people pass through all the stages of dying, just as Kübler-Ross described them. For others, the stages are less distinct, while some never emerge from the stage of depression.

Grief

Just as dying precedes death, so does the grief of a dying man or woman's survivors. Many physicians and death researchers have observed that grief is a distinctive medical syndrome with both physical and emotional symptoms: weeping and sighing, physical exhaustion, lack of appetite, stomach pains, colitis, thoughts fixed on the dead person, guilt about the past, restlessness, depression, agitation, and sleeplessness. Mourning begins when the friends and family of a dying person learn that death is approaching. Mourning develops through a series of stages that resemble Kübler-Ross's stages of dying.

Stages of Grief.   People sometimes know in advance that a friend or relative is dying. At this point they experience "anticipatory grief," with substages of "disbelief" and "denial" of the medical evidence. The close survivors pass through a stage of "anger" at the dying person for having failed to live a healthy life, thereby forcing them to face the future alone. Then comes the stage of "bargaining," when through prayer or other means they attempt to prolong the dying person's life. The stage of "depression" sets in when they realize that these efforts are futile. Finally, at the stage of "acceptance," the intimate survivors understand that death is a reality that will soon have to be faced.

As we have mentioned, each of us responds in our own way to the events of life. Grief is no exception. Some grief-stricken people exhibit severe physical and mental symptoms; they themselves actually run an increased risk of falling ill and dying, perhaps from the lowered resistance to disease that stresses produce. Some deny their grief; they hide or suppress it. Others change from day to day.

The death of someone you love is one of life's most shocking, and even shattering, experiences. Yet the grief that precedes death serves a very useful purpose for the survivors: It prepares them for the inevitable and makes the death easier to bear when it finally comes. In fact, survivors who pass through more grief before the death seem to suffer less as a result of the death itself.

Mourning.   Grief is sudden, brought on by the prospect or fact of death. It is only the beginning of the survivor's response, a response that over the long run is called *mourning.* As with dying and grief, each of us mourns in our own way, but mourning has its own somewhat distinctive phases.

The "immediate stage" is one of numbness, a dazed, stoic response that often goes with a collapse of feeling. In the second, or "post-immediate" stage (to the end of the funeral), the bereaved may be despondent and detached, and although the death may be accepted, it may be angrily protested. The "transitional stage," from funeral to re-entry into an active social role, is one of changing emotions and depression mixed with resolution to adjust and attention-getting behavior.

The "projective stage" takes place when social participation begins. There is a regaining of personal identity apart from the deceased and the memory of the deceased. Grief may also be tinged with guilt; the bereaved may "wish they had done more" and be disturbed by persistent dreams of the deceased.

Dealing with death requires that the bereaved relate to the deceased, not attempt to forget forcefully. Each of the survivors must place the deceased in perspective in their own lives—to reaffirm the life of the deceased within the survivor's. Until this occurs, the survivors will have great trouble even in speaking of the dead, social life will not be re-

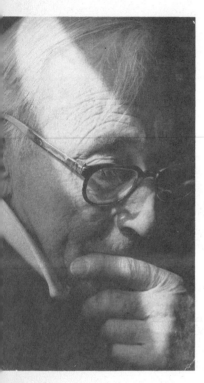

James Foote/Photo Researchers

The Dying Person's Bill of Rights

I have the right to be treated as a living human being until I die.

I have the right to maintain a sense of hopefulness however changing its focus may be.

I have the right to be cared for by those who can maintain a sense of hopefulness, however changing this might be.

I have the right to express my feelings and emotions about my approaching death in my own way.

I have the right to participate in decisions concerning my care.

I have the right to expect continuing medical and nursing attention even though "cure" goals must be changed to "comfort" goals.

I have the right not to die alone.

I have the right to be free from pain.

I have the right to have my questions answered honestly.

I have the right not to be deceived.

I have the right to have help from and for my family in accepting my death.

I have the right to die in peace and dignity.

I have the right to retain my individuality and not be judged for my decisions which may be contrary to beliefs of others.

I have the right to discuss and enlarge my religious and/or spiritual experiences, whatever these may mean to others.

I have the right to expect that the sanctity of the human body will be respected after death.

I have the right to be cared for by caring, sensitive, knowledgeable people who will attempt to understand my needs and will be able to gain some satisfaction in helping me face my death.

This Bill of Rights was created at a workshop on "The Terminally Ill Patient and the Helping Person," in Lansing, Mich., sponsored by the Southwestern Michigan Inservice Education Council and conducted by Amelia J. Barbus, associate professor of nursing, Wayne State University, Detroit.

Source: Andrea B. O'Connor, ed., *Dying and Grief: Nursing Interventions* (New York: The American Journal of Nursing, 1976), p. 9.

sumed, and hundreds of everyday reminders of the deceased may prevent the bereaved from performing the daily round. Old friendships may be neglected and the hobbies and pastimes, once shared, may be ignored because it may seem too painful to do them alone.

Help for Mourners. Time and encouragement are needed to help survivors pass through mourning and regain their mental, physical, and social strength. Yet our society seems unable to provide this in the right way.

Centuries ago, death released violent passions, and a funeral was an occasion for tears, sobs, and rage. These displays of sorrow had a useful purpose. Once the great torrent of emotion was let loose, the survivors were quickly able to resume their normal lives. This was vital when illness often led to death, when brothers and friends often fell in battle, when infants and wives often died in childbirth.

Today's social ideals do not encourage public displays of emotion, and modern funerals therefore lack the healing qualities of funerals in the past. Because each of the survivors wishes mainly to keep a "stiff upper lip," all are protected from each other and their own feelings about death, which is and ought to be a cause of sorrow.

Survivors ought to "talk out" their grief, not avoid it. Such talking helps release negative emotions, recover the self-image often lost with a death, break past ties or renew them, and let the bereaved rediscover meaning in life. Survivors should "feel out" and "act out" their grief as well. For many people crying and openly expressed anger are probably more valuable than psychotherapy (see Chapter 3) or drugs.

The Hospice. Physicians and nurses often deny an approaching death, even more than survivors do. For health-care workers are trained to preserve life, not to accept the coming of death. Rather than accept the "defeat" that is involved when a patient dies, many physicians will resort to "heroic" means of keeping patients alive, like artificial respirators, heart-lung machines, and machines to cleanse the blood. And hospitals often ignore the specific needs of dying patients, since these hospitals hate to admit that their services might be likely to fail.

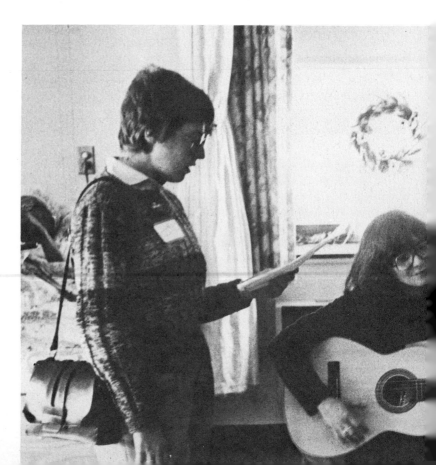

In the mid-1960s some physicians and nurses in England, people who felt that the traditional sort of hospital did not really serve the needs of the dying, developed a new kind of institution, called the *hospice*. The philosophy and services of hospices are designed to serve the needs of dying patients. Instead of fighting disease "actively" and hoping for a cure, hospices provide only "supportive" and comfort-producing treatment, like painkillers and special diets. Instead of removing patients from the company of relatives, hospices encourage them to spend as much time together as possible. Instead of working *against* death, hospices work *toward* it, encouraging grief, mourning, and acceptance. Hospice workers have found that the most effective therapy for dying people and their survivors is contact with other dying people and other survivors.

Euthanasia. For many dying people racked with pain and suffering the greatest comfort of all would seem to be death. But the law does not distinguish between murder and *euthanasia*—willfully putting people to death or allowing them to die to relieve their suffering. Should law distinguish between them? People disagree. Some believe that each person's body is his or her own personal property, to be used as its owner

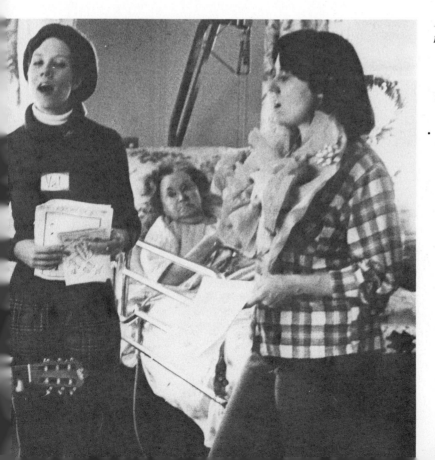

A hospice.
Bellina Cirone/Photo Researchers

sees fit. Others believe that the spark of life within each human is divine and does not belong to anyone. Whatever the rights and wrongs of the issue, *euthanasia is illegal,* even if it is inspired only by love for the dying.

SUMMARY

Aging and dying are normal parts of the life cycle. The elderly represent a large percentage of the population of the United States. As the "baby boom" generation ages, that percentage will rise even higher.

Although individuals respond to aging in their own way, aging produces many physical and social changes that are common to all older people. These changes include retirement from work, loss of loved ones and friends, physical disabilities, and chronic illness. The effects of aging are progressive, gradually altering every organ and system of the body, including the brain, the skin, the muscles, the bones, the joints, the heart, and the lungs, and the digestive, excretory, and sex organs. The personality, too, changes. Some older people respond to change and illness with calmness and hope, others with grief and depression. The previous development of the personality, the expectations, and the living conditions all play a role in shaping an elderly person's response to aging. The social problems of the elderly include limited income; the high cost of health care, housing, and energy; and crime.

All older people are faced with the nearness of death—their own and those of their friends and family. Death is not always clear-cut any more. It can be defined functionally, legally, and medically; and brain death is distinguished from cellular death.

Fear of death may be inborn, but the meaning attached to death differs from culture to culture. In the United States, death is often viewed as a medical "failure," and Americans are discouraged from reacting strongly to death. Yet the dying and those who survive them must pass through several stages in their attempts to cope with dying, on the one hand, and with grief, on the other.

Physicians have attempted to treat every illness as curable and have resisted dealing with the specific problems of the dying. New institutions, most notably hospices, recognize that their patients are in fact dying, and they provide purely supportive care even for those patients who are in great pain and despair.

Suggested Readings

Burger, Larry. *Death and Dying*. Dubuque, Iowa: Brown, 1979. This book is concerned with the impact that death has on society and on our own lives.

Hatton, Corrine L., et al. *Suicide: Assessment and Intervention*. New York: Appleton-Century-Crofts, 1977. This study is concerned with the prevention and treatment of suicide.

Klagsbrun, Francine. *Too Young to Die*. New York: Pocket Books, 1977. In this discussion of youth and suicide, the author offers myths and facts about the subject as well as tell-tail signs to help us aid a potential suicide victim.

Kubler-Ross, Elisabeth. *On Death and Dying*. New York: Macmillan, 1969. A classic study of the stages leading to death for the terminally ill.

Kubler-Ross, Elisabeth. *To Live until We Say Good-bye*. Englewood Cliffs, N.J.: Prentice-Hall, 1978. This book deals with the effect of the terminally ill on those around them and the effect that proper handling can make to all concerned.

Wilcox, Sandra G., and Sulton, Marilyn. *Understanding Death and Dying*. Sherman Oaks, Cal.: Alfred, 1981. The social implications of aging, medical ethics, and decisions about prolonging life.

Zarit, Steven H. *Aging and Mental Disorders*. New York: Free Press, 1980. An in-depth look at the aging process, with a psychological approach to the assessment and treatment of the mental disorders that sometimes occur as people age.

Social Health

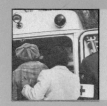

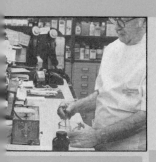

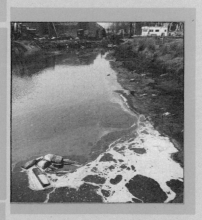

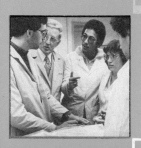

UNIT SIX

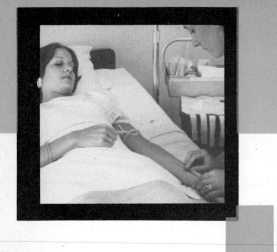

17

The Health-care Delivery System

chapter objectives

When you have finished reading this chapter you should be able to:

1. List the barriers to effective health care
2. Explain how consumers should go about choosing physicians, dentists, and other health-care specialists
3. Describe how the present health-care system might be improved

Our society's attitudes toward health care are full of paradoxes. On the one hand, most Americans view health care as a "public good," for a healthy society is a productive one. On the other hand, many Americans do not in fact get adequate health care, and the government takes only a limited role in providing for it. To a great extent, the people of the United States must pay for health care out of their own pockets or through payroll deductions for health insurance. It is true that some Americans are lucky enough to have employers or unions that help to pay the cost of that insurance. But other Americans, 30 to 40 million of them, must fend entirely for themselves in the health-care marketplace.

And they must do so at a time when health-care costs are skyrocketing. The plain fact is that our health-care delivery system is itself in very doubtful health.

Medical Care: A 20th-Century Revolution

Until the end of the 19th century, medical care was largely a matter of hit or miss, and there were many more misses than hits. Physicians had few effective medicines and few effective treatments of any kind; in fact, they probably made most of their patients more sick. Luckily, there were few such patients. Not until the early decades of the present century did large numbers of people begin to consult physicians, and not until then were they as likely to be helped as hurt by doing so. Before then, people tended to rely on "home remedies," like concoctions made from plants. Hospitals were mainly "charitable institutions," places where the poor and homeless came to die; and they were dangerous, more dangerous than staying at home.

Beginning around 1900, medical care underwent a revolution, one that has not yet stopped. This revolution was two-fold: First, physicians at last began to treat disease effectively; and, second, the services of physicians became available to the great mass of the people, and the people sought out those services eagerly, for they began to credit physicians with almost magical powers. The skepticism inspired by the physicians of old had vanished.

Medical Care Today: A Problem of Availability

Americans now believe in health care. But can we get it? The answer depends on how much you make and where you live. For health care is essentially a private enterprise, so that the rich have more of it. And people in certain parts of the United States have more of it, since physicians are not distributed equally throughout the nation. The result is that health care, especially high-quality health care, is simply not available to many Americans. How did this come about?

Until the 1940s, most physicians had a "general," or "family" practice. These general practitioners (or GPs) delivered babies at home, made house calls, and treated any kind of illness or injury. But today, nearly three-quarters of the physicians in the United States are "specialists"—they treat illnesses or injuries to only one part or system of the body, or treat only children or only women, and so on.

Fewer physicians today, and especially few specialists, work in rural areas and small towns. Instead, they work in cities and their suburbs. First of all, that is where people who can afford to pay for medical care tend to live. Second, that is where many of the largest and most prestigious hospitals are located, and many specialists work only in hospitals. Finally, some physicians are attracted to the bright lights simply because other physicians are attracted to them, too.

One part of this country's population has even less access to high-quality health care than rural people do: the members of minority groups, including Chicanos, native Americans, blacks, and Hispanics. The reason is simply that many of them are too poor to pay. Yet minorities tend to suffer more than most Americans do from violence, poor housing, poor nutrition, and unemployment; and this tends to make them more prone to injury and disease.

Can physicians be encouraged to practice where they are actually needed? Should they be? In the 1960s and 1970s, the National Health

Specialists and Subspecialists: What Do They Do?

Until the 1940s, general practitioners took care of most people's medical needs. Since then more and more physicians have become specialists—they treat only one system or function of the body (such as the heart) or only one kind of patient (children, for example, or women), or they perform some specialized function (like anesthesiologists, who make patients about to undergo surgery lose consciousness).

Perhaps you were not aware of it, but even your own "family doctor" may be a specialist too, the kind known as an internist. Internists practice "internal medicine"—medicine of the body as a whole—and they are specialists because they do not deliver babies and usually do not treat children. They should not be confused with interns, physicians just out of medical school. Four other types of specialists (besides internists) are "front-line" practitioners: surgeons, pediatricians (for children), gynecologists (who specialize in the reproductive system of women), and psychiatrists (for mental disorders).

The *subspecialists* work within each of the five primary-care specialties. Under internal medicine, in fact, almost every organ or system of the body has a subspecialist: cardiologists for the heart, dermatologists for the skin, neurologists for the nervous system, renal disease specialists for the kidneys, among others. Surgery, too, is divided into subspecialties, dealing with operations on the eyes, on the heart, on the brain, and so on. Some physicians, such as ophthalmologists (who treat the eyes) and ear-nose-and-throat specialists, practice both surgery and "medicine" (in this sense, the term refers to treatment other than surgery).

Table 17–1. Physicians, by Sex, Specialty, and
Major Professional Activity, 1978

Specialty	Percent
Total	100.0
Male	89.6
Female	10.4
General practice	12.8
Medical	25.1
Internal medicine	14.3
Pediatrics	5.6
Surgical	23.4
General surgery	7.3
Obstetrics, gynecology	5.5
Ophthalmology	2.7
Orthopedic	2.9
Other	24.6
Anesthesiology	3.3
Psychiatry	5.9
Pathology	2.9
Radiology	2.6

As of December 31. Includes Puerto Rico and outlying areas.
Source: U.S. Bureau of the Census, *Statistical Abstract of the United States, 1980* (101st ed.), table 168, p. 111.

Service Corps was set up to provide jobs for physicians in parts of the country without enough of them. Efforts have also been made to increase the number of minority-group students attending medical schools and to encourage medical schools to offer more courses in general (or family) practice. At the moment, however, the final choice of

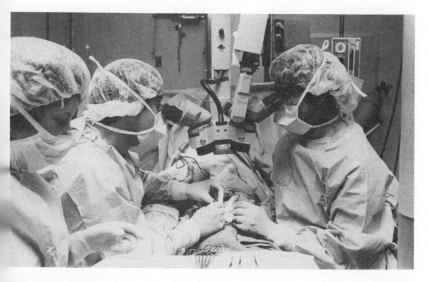

Surgery is a specialty that is divided into subspecialties.

Martin Rotker/Taurus

where to set up shop, and whether or not to become a specialist, is left to the physician, and the result is that some people do not get adequate medical care.

The High Cost of Health

Like all goods and services, health care costs money, and at a time of inflation you would expect it to be more and more expensive. But you would still be surprised to learn *how much* more expensive. Between 1965 and 1975, hospital costs increased by some *300* percent, while the cost of other goods and services rose by an average of merely 75 percent. What's behind this difference?

Third-party Payers

Although health care is mostly a private responsibility, a majority of Americans receive some of their health care free or at a reduced cost. If you have health insurance, for instance, you get part or all of your hospital bills paid either by an insurance company or by the government.

Table 17–2.   Public and Private Health-care Coverage by Family Income and Age, 1976

| Family Income in 1975 and Age | Percent Distribution | | | | |
| | | With coverage | | | |
	Without coverage	*Total*	*Private Only*	*Public Only*	*Public and Private*
Total	10.2	89.8	63.4	12.7	13.6
Under $5,000	17.4	82.6	18.9	42.7	20.8
$5,000-$9,999	16.6	83.5	41.6	20.0	21.8
$10,000-$14,999	9.2	90.8	65.2	7.3	18.2
$15,000 and over	5.7	94.3	85.0	3.4	5.7
Under 6 years	13.9	86.2	67.6	14.4	4.1
6-18 years	11.2	88.8	71.6	11.6	5.4
19-24 years	20.5	79.5	67.6	8.1	3.4
25-44 years	9.3	90.7	72.0	8.3	10.3
45-64 years	7.6	92.4	70.0	8.8	13.5
65 years and over	1.0	99.0	1.5	37.7	59.8

Source: U.S. Congress, Congressional Budget Office, *Profile of Health Care Coverage: The Haves and Have-Nots, 1979.*

Sometimes the cost of the health insurance itself is paid in full or in part by an employer, a union, or the government—not by the people who are insured.

Third-party payments for health care—that is, payment of its costs by insurance companies or by the government, rather than by patients themselves—now cover about 90 percent of hospital bills and 65 percent of all medical bills. The system benefits those who have private or government health insurance, of course. But there is a price for all desirable things. In this case, the price is the rising cost of health care, for many Americans are not concerned about medical bills they do not have to pay themselves.

Table 17–3. Gross National Product and National Health Expenditures: United States, Selected Years 1929–79

Year	Gross national product in billions	National health expenditures	
		Amount in billions	Percent of gross national product
1929	$ 103.4	$ 3.6	3.5
1935	72.2	2.9	4.0
1940	100.0	4.0	4.0
1950	286.2	12.7	4.4
1955	398.0	17.7	4.4
1960	506.0	26.9	5.3
1965	688.1	42.0	6.1
1970	982.4	74.9	7.6
1971	1,063.4	83.1	7.8
1972	1,171.1	93.5	8.0
1973	1,306.5	103.0	7.9
1974	1,412.9	116.3	8.2
1975	1,528.8	132.1	8.6
1976	1,702.2	148.9	8.7
1977	1,899.5	169.9	8.9
1978	2,127.6	188.6	8.9
1979	2,368.8	212.2	9.0

Source: Data are compiled by the Health Care Financing Administration (Washington, D.C.: U.S. Government Printing Office, 1980).

You might think, though, that hospitals would have an interest in keeping costs down. It is true that hospitals are to some extent forced to watch their pennies, especially in the larger cities. But hospitals know perfectly well that a certain percentage of their patients' bills will be largely or entirely paid by third parties. With the money they get from third-party payers, hospitals buy expensive equipment—in some cases, perhaps, more than they actually need—and hire high-priced specialists. Even employers that provide insurance for their workers don't care too much about its higher cost, since for them it is just another tax-deductible business expense.

As for physicians, they are freed by third-party payers from any pressure to give their patients more economical treatment. If there is any chance at all that an expensive treatment might help a patient, why not try it; after all, the patient probably will not be the one to pay, and doing everything possible, regardless of cost, may prevent malpractice suits.

Medical Technology

By the standards of the past, the modern physician is a maker of miracles. But modern miracles, unlike those of the past, are expensive, so technological advances in health care are continually driving up its costs.

Specialization among Physicians

By and large, a specialist charges more for a service than a general practitioner does, even if it is for the same service. For example, a dermatologist, who specializes in the disorders of the skin, would probably charge more for treating a rash than a family physician would. Since more and more physicians are becoming specialists, doctor bills are bound to increase more and more quickly.

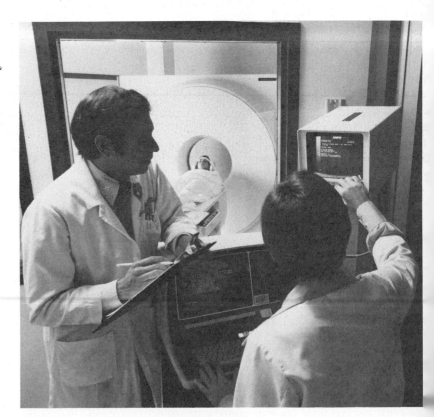

A CAT Scanner, one of the most expensive of medical miracles.

John Blaustein/Woodfin Camp & Associates

An "Imperfect" Market

In what economists call a "perfect market," supply and demand balance each other in the long run. If the demand for a service is high, its costs will be high; and in a perfect market, more people will then offer that service. Since more people are offering it, the supply of it will increase and its cost will fall.

Consumer demand for medical care has increased enormously since World War II. Now, the service of medical care is provided above all by physicians. In a perfect market the number of physicians would have risen as much as the demand for their services, or even more so. But the market for medical services is far from perfect—partly because the number of places in American medical schools is held down and partly because a medical education is so expensive and lengthy that few students can afford it.

Another reason for this imperfect market is the lack of information among consumers. A perfect market requires "perfect information"—in other words, consumers have to know what their choices are. But most of us do not know them, because we are completely dependent on the judgment of our physicians. We feel uncomfortable asking questions, and we do not know how to judge the answers if we do ask. But this ignorance and fear are beginning to change. For example, many patients today do not submit to surgery until they have gotten a "second opinion" from another physician. Second opinions have no doubt reduced the amount of needless surgery and thus health-care costs in general.

Still, people just do not shop around for medical care, so physicians do not have to compete with one another. They do not advertise their fees, so you often do not know how much you will have to pay until after you have been served. Sometimes, comparing fees would be useless anyway, since in many places fees are set by agreement among local physicians.

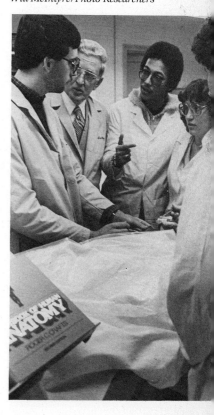

Students and faculty at a medical school.

Will McIntyre/Photo Researchers

The Consumption of Health Care

Stages of Care

Primary Care. When you first get sick and want help, you look for a general practitioner, a physician in family practice, or an internist (see below). This sort of help, which patients seek out on their own, is called primary care, and it is most often provided in a physician's office or a clinic.

Secondary Care. When primary-care physicians feel that they do not know enough about a medical problem, they refer their patients to specialists. This stage of treatment is called secondary care, and sometimes it involves a visit to a hospital for more extensive testing than you could get in an office or a clinic.

Tertiary Care.   On occasion, even secondary care is not enough, and the patient must be sent to get tertiary care, which involves advanced equipment and procedures—for example, kidney dialysis treatment, and intricate heart and brain surgery. Tertiary care is generally available only in the best-equipped hospitals.

Place of Care

Consuming health care can also be considered from another point of view—the *place* where you receive it: a doctor's office or a clinic, an institution, or your own home.

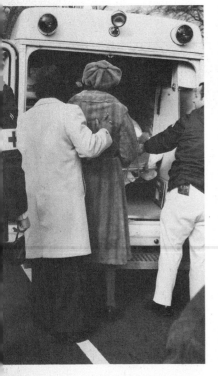

Marc Anderson

Ambulatory Care.   When patients are sick, but not so sick that they cannot travel under their own power to a physician's office, to a hospital emergency room, or to a clinic, they get what is called "ambulatory," or "outpatient" care. Clinics and physicians' offices provide nothing but ambulatory care. But only some patients get to a hospital emergency room under their own power: those without real emergencies. These are simply people who do not have a family physician. Some emergency rooms provide high-quality medical care, but emergency-room staffs have little time to devote to patients, and patients are not likely to see the same physician twice.

Institutional Care.   When you have a medical problem that prevents you from moving around freely, you must get "institutional" care. The institutions that provide this care include general hospitals, special hospitals (those for alcoholics or mental patients, for example), rehabilitation facilities (such as the places where accident victims are taught to walk again), and nursing homes (see Chapter 16) for the elderly.

At-home Care.   In the old days, GPs routinely went on house calls. Few physicians today think that house calls make good use of their time, for they can see many more patients at their own offices. But nurses, rehabilitation therapists, and other health-care professionals do go to the homes of patients too ill to leave home, especially elderly patients. This "at-home" care is usually suggested and supervised by a physician. Most of this country's urban areas have it in some form.

New Ideas in Health Care

Not long ago, people who got sick had four choices: to get no treatment at all; to be treated at home, in the doctor's office, or in a hospital. This set of choices gave little help to people whose doctors were out-of-town or to people who were afraid of hospitals; and it provided relatively few services. When the medical industry began to expand after World War II, it began to provide new services and to provide them in a more flexible way. Let us take a look at the institutions and arrangements that made this possible.

Solo Practice and Group Practice.   Have you ever called a physician's office and been told by the answering service, "Sorry, the doctor is not available. Please call back next week. If you need a physician before then, call Dr. So-and-so"?

These two physicians each have "solo practices"—they are the only physicians in their respective offices. But when they leave their offices, each asks the other to "cover"—to see the other's patients.

Some physicians have gone one step further by joining in a "group practice," in which two or more physicians share office space, nurses, and often patients, who don't necessarily see the same physician on each visit. Some group practices include different kinds of specialists; others consist of two or more physicians in the same specialty.

Group practices cut costs because they permit physicians to share rent, equipment, and staff. Second, the members of the group can consult with each other quickly and easily and enjoy the stimulus of working closely with colleagues. Third, patients always see one of their own doctors, and not just a fill-in.

Health Maintenance Organizations (HMOs).   When you go to a solo practitioner or to a group practice, you pay for their services each time you need them, much as you pay for a loaf of bread only when you need one. A health maintenance organization (HMO), on the other hand, requires you to pay a fee before you get any services. (In 1977 the family average fee was $87 a month.) The prepaid fee—often paid by the member's employer—entitles you to receive many medical services from the HMO at little or no cost beyond the membership fee.

How, you might ask, do HMOs provide so much health care for so little money? One reason is that they pay their physicians by salary, not by a fee for each service, so the physicians have little reason to suggest unneeded treatments. Another is the fact that HMOs stress preventive medicine—they try to prevent medical problems from developing in the first place, and therefore to prevent the need for expensive remedies. But there are disadvantages for HMO patients, too, mainly the fact that they usually cannot choose their own physicians. Some HMO patients complain about what they call an "assembly line" atmosphere; and others rightly or wrongly suspect that HMO physicians cut costs by shortchanging patients on services.

In 1978, there were about 165 HMOs in the United States, with some 6.3 million members. Right now, you can join only through a group—an employer, for example, or a union or professional group.

Health Insurance

In 1981, American hospitals charged their patients an average of about $170 a day. The average hospital stay, of 7½ days, came to about $1,192. Many medical treatments cost more than that, sometimes a lot more, and that is why third-party payments, or insurance payments, came into existence. Insurance is a device to help people reduce financial risk. In health insurance (as in fire, auto, and life insurance) the "subscribers"—those who are insured—regularly pay a "premium" (or fee) to the insurance company. (Sometimes it is the subscriber's employer or union that pays the premium.) The company agrees that if the subscriber suffers certain diseases or injuries, and has to seek out certain kinds of treatment, it will pay all or part of the costs of treatment. The conditions of the insurance are specified in a "policy," which usually covers the subscriber and the subscriber's spouse and children.

Types of Health Insurance

Many health-insurance policies come in two parts. One part, "hospital insurance," covers the cost of a hospital room and meals, and of general nursing care, for a specific number of days. The other part, "medical insurance," covers the cost of physicians' fees. Certain policies only cover physicians' services if they are performed in hospitals. And medical insurance sometimes pays only a set amount for these services; a policy might pay $400 for an appendectomy, for example, so if the surgeon who removes your appendix charges $600, you'll have to shell out the difference yourself. At least you would have to do so if you did not have additional insurance, such as a "major medical" policy.

A major-medical policy takes over where hospital and medical insurance leave off. Some major-medical plans also pay for services like visits to a psychiatrist, prescription drugs, and physical therapy and prosthetic appliances.

How to Shop for Insurance

Everyone needs some kind of health insurance coverage. Ask your parents if they have a policy and if you are covered by it. Should the answer be no, find out if your college health service provides health insurance. If it does not, talk with a health-service adviser about buying some.

When you shop for health insurance, the most important point to find out is just what a policy covers—and what it *excludes*. Many policies do *not* cover all kinds of medical problems or all kinds of treatments. The mail-order policies (those sold through the mail) are the most restrictive—you get the least coverage for your money. But other insurance policies, too, do not cover everything, or not until you have had the policy for a certain time or until you have paid out a certain amount of money. Read before you sign. But many policies are written in insurance jargon—a special lingo that confuses most people. If you cannot understand a policy, ask the insurance representative to explain it. If you are not satisfied with the answers, call your state or local department of consumer affairs, or your state insurance department or attorney-general's office.

Private Insurance Companies

Blue Cross and Blue Shield are private nonprofit organizations that offer complementary kinds of health insurance. Blue Cross pays the costs of hospital care; Blue Shield pays for medical care, including surgery. The two groups return to members some 87 percent of the money they collect in premiums, and they spend only 8.5 percent on the costs of administration. Other insurance companies sell policies that provide fewer benefits and cost more. A number of them pay in benefits less than 10 percent of the money they collect and keep the rest.

The Government's Role: Medicare and Medicaid

As we have already noted, the American people have never really decided if health care is a private matter or a public one. At the moment it is a little of both. The federal government has a role, not so much in *providing* medical care (though it does provide some for veterans) as in *paying* for it. Mostly, it pays for the medical care of those who are least able to deal with its rising costs and are most likely to need it: the poor and the elderly. The government helps pay their medical expenses through two programs: *Medicare*, primarily for those 65 and over, and *Medicaid*, for the poor of all ages, including those who are also on Medicare.

Medicare.   Medicare comprises both hospital insurance and medical insurance. Hospital insurance enrollment is free to people who paid Social Security taxes when they were employed. This includes the majority of workers, even those who are self-employed. Medicare hospital insurance covers most of the cost of the first 60 days of a hospital stay and part of the cost thereafter. It also pays for professional health services, either in the patient's home or in a skilled nursing facility, where nursing services are provided 24 hours a day. Medicare medical insurance is not free; it has to be purchased through a premium of about $10 a month (1981). The insurance pays part of the cost of physicians' fees (in the hospital and in the office) and of other medical items, such as ambulances and crutches. But the medical insurance and the hospital insurance do not, by a long shot, pay all the health-care bills of this country's older people.

Medicare was created for the elderly. But since the 1970s, people who need certain costly and specialized treatments, and people with injuries

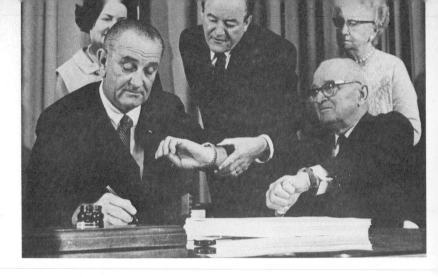

President Johnson (left) signs the Medicare Act in 1965, as former President Truman (right), Vice President Humphrey, Mrs. Johnson (left), and Mrs. Truman watch.

UPI

so serious that they have been receiving Social Security disability payments for 2 years, have also been eligible for Medicare.

Medicaid. Most people under 65 are not receiving disability payments and do not need highly specialized health care. But that does not mean that the only people under 65 who need help to pay their medical bills are the people in those two categories. For the blind, the disabled, and the aged poor (who often have bills medicare does not pay), and for desperately poor people of all ages, the federal government provides another kind of health-care payment program: Medicaid. Medicaid pays for hospital care, physicians' bills, at-home nursing care, and some other health-care services. It is financed partly by federal funds and partly by the 50 states, which would like Uncle Sam to pay for all of it because it is so expensive.

Reducing Health-care Costs

We have seen that the total cost of health care in the United States has risen, is rising, and will continue to rise even more rapidly than the cost of other goods and services. Much effort has been made to reduce the bill, and we will now look at three of the means: investor-owned hospitals, physician extenders, and governmental planning.

Investor-owned Hospitals: Benefits as Business

Hospitals have traditionally been regarded as institutions of mercy, not of business; and they have traditionally shown little business sense. When a hospital's expenses go up it simply passes along the increase—to the government, to the insurance companies, and to the public. In the end the public pays in any case, either directly, or through taxes or higher insurance premiums. Yet many hospitals are in serious financial trouble.

Most hospitals are nonprofit institutions. Many nonprofit hospitals manage to pay their expenses only because they get direct subsidies. Some people think that such hospitals are so often in financial trouble precisely because they do not have to show a profit, since that is one reason why they have little incentive to economize. Some hospitals do have such an incentive because they are operated as profit-making institutions—the so-called "proprietary" (or investor-owned) hospitals. Studies have shown that an average hospital stay costs slightly less in a profit-making institution than in a nonprofit one. But investor-owned hospitals sometimes cut back on staff or close down unprofitable facilities that nonprofit hospitals tend to keep open.

Physician Extenders

Physicians have always been jealous of their powers, and in the past they tended to limit the role of nurses and anyone else who helped them. As medical care has become more and more expensive, that attitude has more and more been undermined. So-called "physician extenders" now do many of the more routine chores once done by physicians, so that they can spend more time on the most complex tasks. Physician extenders also provide skilled care. In both cases, the physician is ultimately responsible for their work.

Nurses. There are three broad categories of nurses, with subspecialties within each. Registered nurses (RNs) are prepared in teaching hospitals, community colleges, or 4-year colleges, and they take state licensing examinations. Practical nurses (LPNs), or licensed vocational nurses (LVNs), are also prepared in state-approved schools and they too must take licensing exams. Nurses aides may also receive some training, often provided by hospitals. In most states, however, they are not licensed.

Carmine Galasso

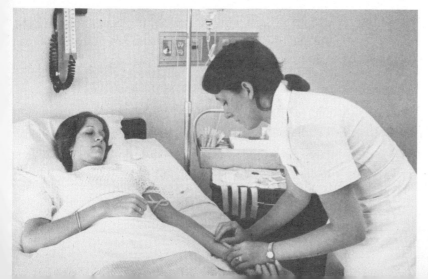

Nurse Midwives. A nurse midwife is an RN with additional training and practice in delivering babies. Some make deliveries at home and some work in the obstetric departments of hospitals (see Chapter 13).

Nurse Practitioners. Some nurse practitioners get only brief training; others have up to 2 years of it. Nurse practitioners examine and diagnose patients under a physician's supervision and they suggest treatments. They work in hospitals or in community health clinics.

Physicians' Assistants.   Physicians' assistants get academic training, generally in 2-year programs given by community colleges, universities, and medical schools. Some physicians' assistants qualify in specialty areas and work as surgeons' assistants, child health associates, and so on. Many physicians' assistants help diagnose patients; others operate sophisticated equipment in hospitals, clinics, and offices, or assist in surgery. Usually, they are not nurses.

A Mixed Report.   Some people once believed that physician extenders would be able to provide medical services at a lower cost than physicians could. But physicians do not, in general, reduce their bills even when much of the actual work in their offices is done by physician extenders. Physician extenders were also expected to bridge the "intimidation gap" between patients and physicians by making patients feel more at ease in a medical setting. But many physician extenders deal with patients pretty much as physicians do. These shortcomings do not mean that physician extenders have been useless—only that some overall goals have not yet been achieved.

The Government's Responsibility

Health care is to some extent a public responsibility and to some extent a private one. Providing for health care privately is not really a test of rugged individualism, because your ability to get private health insurance depends less on you than on your job or school: Many working people get health insurance as a fringe benefit of employment, but many others do not—those working for certain small businesses, for example, and part-time workers and the self-employed. Some of these people can afford to buy health insurance for themselves and their families, but about 24 million Americans cannot.

Socialized Medicine

In some countries, even some capitalist ones, health care has been made a government responsibility, like defense. In Britain, for example, the National Health Service (NHS) is a government department that owns the hospitals and employs many physicians and other health-care workers. Most services are free to patients. Alongside the NHS, there are some wholly private physicians who do not receive NHS fees and instead bill their patients.

The British system has its critics. Some people say that the NHS, like third-party payers in the United States, encourages waste, since people do not have to pay for the services they use. Certainly, the costs of the system have gone up rapidly. Moreover, nonemergency operations are very difficult to get, and in the recent past many British doctors emigrated to the United States, where they could earn more money.

National Health Insurance

Britain's National Health *System* in effect makes most doctors in that country government employees. National health *insurance* would also make health care a government responsibility, but it would do so without putting medical care under government control. You will remember that, right now, private health insurance is a bit of a lottery, something that some people get with their jobs and others do not. The government could make adequate health care less a matter of sheer luck by paying the insurance premiums of all Americans, regardless of their jobs.

Costs

Either a national health system or national health insurance—in fact, anything that made it easier for more Americans to get health care—would raise the cost of health care. It is for you as a citizen to decide what should be done. But you should bear in mind that if efforts to make health care easier to get are not combined with efforts to control its costs, the health-care system might well collapse.

Table 17–4.   Community Hospitals, Beds, and Services, according to Geographic Division

Geographic Division	Number of Hospitals	Number of Beds (1,000)	Beds per 1,000 Population	Occupancy Rate	Average Length of Stay in Days
United States	5,851	975.4	4.47	73.6	7.6
New England	259	51.0	4.16	77.6	8.1
Middle Atlantic	636	167.9	4.56	81.7	9.1
South Atlantic	809	149.6	4.33	73.7	7.4
East North Central	910	193.2	4.69	75.5	7.9
East South Central	484	68.0	4.86	74.2	7.0
West North Central	799	99.0	5.82	69.7	8.1
West South Central	853	100.8	4.57	68.0	6.5
Mountain	362	39.4	3.83	67.6	6.5
Pacific	739	106.5	3.57	66.5	6.4

[1] Ratios are based on 1978 preliminary estimates of the population.
[2] Percent of beds occupied.
Source: American Hospital Association, 1973–1979; U.S. Bureau of the Census, 1979.

In fact, the costs of health care will probably continue to rise, and rise dangerously, whatever may happen. In 1981 Americans spent about $280 billion dollars on health care; and it is estimated that in 1990 we might be laying out about $800 billion.

Choosing a Physician

Whatever you may think as a citizen about the proper extent of the government's responsibility for health care, as an individual you have to make up your mind about a much more concrete health-care problem: what physician to use. As a college student, you probably have access to the student health service and do not need to worry about choosing a physician. But you will have to make the choice eventually. Knowing where and when to begin the search is important. The best time to look is when you are well, so your judgment will be sound. This also helps the physician get a sense of what you are like normally. "Shopping" for a physician can be expensive, though, because you have to pay each time you visit one, even if you decide not to go back. So it is

---

Evaluating Your College Health Service

As a college student, you probably have access to a reasonably well-run health-care system: your college health service. If so, you are lucky.

Not all college and university health services are first-rate, of course; some provide very few services. In general, a top-quality college health-care service should offer at least 7 of these 12 kinds of services:

1. *Outpatient services,* or office visits with a physician or a nurse.
2. *In-patient services,* or bed care. When necessary, the health service should also be able to place students in a hospital.
3. *Mental health services,* including "crisis intervention" and short-term counseling.
4. *Athletic medicine,* medical supervision of sports and exercise programs.
5. *Dental services.*
6. *Rehabilitation services* for the handicapped. They should help the disabled to make full use of all of the college's facilities.

7. *Preventive medicine,* to encourage students to be vaccinated against contagious diseases and to help students with special medical problems, like diabetes or epilepsy, that require ongoing supervision.
8. *Health-education services,* to supply information on health-care matters and to encourage students to maintain good health habits.
9. *Environmental-health services,* to monitor such hazards as noise pollution, overcrowding, unsanitary conditions, and dangerous traffic patterns.
10. *Occupational-health services,* to make sure that the school provides safe, healthful working conditions for its employees.
11. *Health-emergency and physical-disaster plans,* to handle fires, epidemic illnesses, explosions, and so on.
12. *Research programs* to raise the quality of the health service.

a good idea to get a recommendation from a reliable source, such as another physician, the medical society or health department in your community, or a college health program.

When you make your first visit to the physician, think of it as a kind of detective job. You will want to find out about the physician's general attitude to medical care. Is the physician "conservative"—tending to rely on well-known procedures and practices—or more willing to try new cures? In your visit with the physician, you might refer to a news-making medical discovery. One physician might pooh-pooh the break-through; another might express cautious interest in it; a third might seem ready to grab a prescription pad or a scalpel at the mere mention of a new drug or surgical technique. You will have to decide which approach you are most comfortable with.

On other matters you can be more direct. You can ask what happens to patients on nights and weekends, and during the physician's vacation. Can routine lab tests be made right in the office, where they would be less expensive? The *way* the physician handles such questions is quite as important as the answers themselves; some physicians or their assistants will answer cheerfully and straightforwardly, others in a resentful and secretive manner.

Do not forget your own needs. Some patients are more comfortable with a physician of their own sex; some may prefer an older doctor or a young one. But do not be rigid: Some male physicians manage to create good rapport with women patients; an older physician has experience, while a younger one may be more flexible.

Communicating with a Physician

When you have found the right physician, you will want to get the most from every office visit. Here is some advice about how to do that:

- Speak clearly and to the point. Tell the physician what is really bothering you, no matter how embarrassing it is. Try to describe your symptoms (such as pain, itching, vomiting, fever, sleeplessness) as exactly as possible.

- The physician will probably want to know when your problem started; the more exactly you are able to pinpoint the time, the better.

- In order to prescribe drugs, the physician must know whether you have had undesirable side effects from drugs in the past. If you have, say so. Don't forget, too, that aspirins, birth control pills, and even vitamins taken in large quantities are all drugs.

- You may be asked about your personal and family background. If you have recently had a very upsetting experience, say so. Or if you have an emotional problem and the doctor does *not* ask about it you should speak up yourself. Don't forget that emotional problems affect physical health.

- If the physician prescribes medication or suggests treatment at home (exercise, for instance), make sure you understand what you are supposed to do. If you anticipate any problems, mention them while you are in the office.
- Follow instructions exactly. Get the drugs the physician prescribes and then take them *as prescribed.*

Even if you take drugs according to instructions, you may find that they do not work, or that they give you side effects. If you have *any* problems, call your physician at once. Do not try to deal with such problems yourself.

Finally, if any drugs are left over when you have recovered, throw them out. Never keep old drugs lying around; someone (including you) might take them by mistake at some time. And never assume that leftover drugs can be used again.

*Robert de Gast/Rapho/Photo
Researchers*

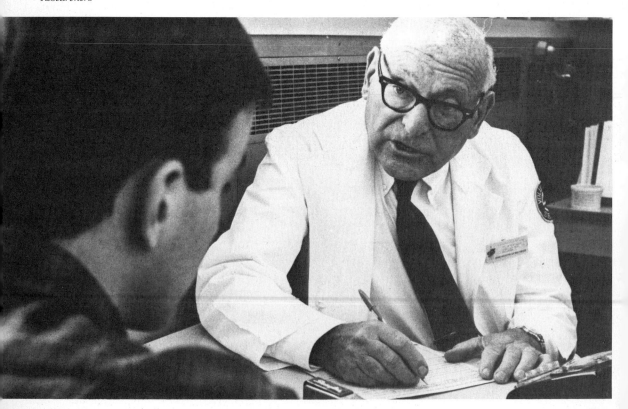

Choosing a Dentist

Many people regard the dentist's drill as an instrument of torture, and dentists as sadists. That is not really true, of course—in fact, much of the work at dental school is learning how *not* to hurt patients. Still, a visit to the dentist is usually no fun or worse. That makes it all the more important to choose your dentist carefully.

Many college students have dentists provided for them by their college health services. But since not all health services do so, you might have to go out and find a dentist before you have to find a doctor. Here are some guidelines to follow:

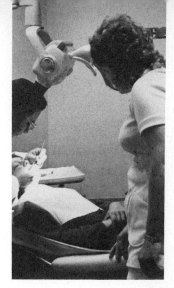

Jean Hollyman/Photo Researchers

- Even if your health service does not have a dentist, it can usually recommend one. For students, this is the best starting point.

- If for some reason that does not work, ask your doctor or call the local dental society.

- When you go for your first visit, the dentist should ask you to fill out a complete medical history, including allergies and adverse reactions to drugs. The dentist should take a set of x-rays.

- Either the dentist or the hygienist (the dentist's assistant) can *clean* your teeth, but the dentist should *examine* them.

- The dentist should *not* pull out teeth if they can be treated by other, less drastic means. The point of dental care is to *save* teeth.

- If complicated, expensive, and time-consuming dental work (on root canals, for example) must be done, the dentist should explain what is to be done; discuss other treatments, if any; arrange a convenient schedule of visits; and offer you several ways to pay your bill (at each visit, once a month, and so on).

- The dental work should be as painless as possible. The dentist should apply a topical pain killer to your gums before giving you shots of another pain killer and should wait until it has taken effect before beginning work. The dentist should have the kind of modern equipment, such as an air drill, that makes the work more efficient and less painful than it used to be.

- If you only need routine work, like a filling, the dentist should be able to do it in 1 or 2 visits.

- The dentist should encourage preventive dentistry by showing you how to take care of your teeth and gums yourself, every day.

If you go to a dentist who does not measure up, don't go back; just grit your teeth and start looking for another one.

SUMMARY

Many Americans believe that access to health care is a moral right that benefits the public as a whole. But health-care services are not, for the most part, provided through public funds. Since the 1960s health-care costs have skyrocketed, so they place a greater burden on society and its members.

The rapid increase in health-care costs stems from the rise of third-party payers (insurance companies and the government), from the high expense of health-care training and of high-technology medical equipment, from specialization among physicians, and from imperfections in the market for medical services.

Since 1900, and particularly since World War II, the technology of medical care has been greatly changed, and Americans have come to demand more and more health-care services. But people in many rural and inner-city areas, and members of minority groups, are not getting the health-care services they need, since physicians want to practice in cities (but not in slum neighborhoods) and in the suburbs.

Health care can be broken down into types, according to the way the patient gets it and to the place where it is given. Patients get primary care on their own initiative; but physicians refer them to secondary care, which is given by specialists. Tertiary care involves complex equipment and procedures in hospitals. Ambulatory care is for patients who can move about; patients in hospitals and other institutions get institutional care; and at-home care serves people who are laid up at home.

Health insurance helps people to pay for these expensive services, and everyone should have it. When you buy insurance, pay attention to what it does and does not cover. The federal government provides two kinds of insurance: Medicare, primarily for the elderly, and Medicaid, for the blind and disabled, aged, and poor, and for families that receive aid to dependent children. Proposals to establish a national health insurance system (which would help people buy private insurance) or a national health service (which would actually provide care) would raise the total cost of medical care. But they would also make those costs easier for people to bear.

Physicians and hospitals are responsible only for part of this country's health-care expenses. Another part is the cost of medicines, over-the-counter medicines, nostrums, and quackery. Let us take a look at these products and those who sell them —since we are all enticed by them every day.

Selected Readings

Brown, Andrew J. *Community Health: An Introduction for the Health Professional.* Mineapolis: Burgess, 1981. An excellent introductory text about the health-care system and its origins.

Cornacchia, Harold J. and Barrett, Steven. *Consumer Health: A Guide to Intelligent Decisions,* 2nd ed. St. Louis: Mosby, 1980. The title pretty much describes the book.

Raffel, Marshall W. *The U.S. Health System: Origins and Functions.* A relatively advanced text, for those interested in an in-depth appraisal of this country's health system.

Shipley, Roger R., and Plomsky, Carolyn G. *Consumer Health: Protecting Your Health and Money.* New York: Harper & Row, 1980. Chapters 5–7 provide a users' guide to the health-care system.

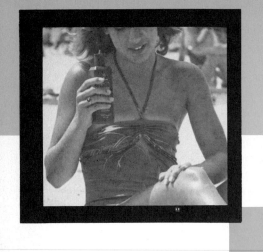

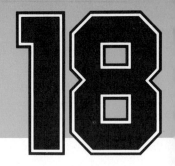

Health-care Products

chapter objectives

When you have finished reading this chapter you should be able to:

1. Appraise advertisements
2. Evaluate health professionals and health products
3. Explain why patients are vulnerable to quackery
4. Recognize the most important agencies that control quackery
5. File a consumer complaint

Television, magazines, billboards, and newspapers bombard us with ads that hawk drugs and cosmetics. Some of the most talented people in the United States create these ads, and they do so for very large sums of money. Using all the resources of art and science they promise you love, beauty, strength, relief from constipation—happiness, in a word.

Drugs can surely help people to live healthier, longer, and more productive lives. But all drugs are potentially dangerous and so are many cosmetics. Most people think that the government takes all the risk out of drugs and cosmetics by suppressing the really harmful ones. And they trust their doctors to prescribe only safe and effective drugs. They think, in short, that they do not have to use their own judgment when choosing and using drugs. They are dead wrong.

The Drug Industry

American companies make thousands upon thousands of health-care products: products for coughs, pain, and dry skin; for insomnia, constipation, and colds; for acne, body odor, and "tired" eyes. In fact, each organ, system, and limb of the body is served by dozens of products.

The Bettmann Archive

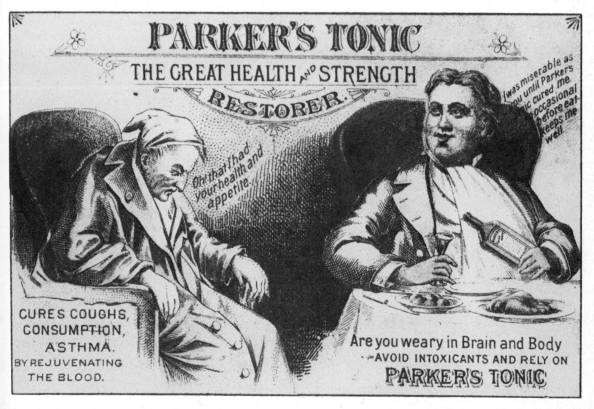

The choices are confusing. Let us take aspirin, for example. It is, to begin with, sold in many dosages (see Chapter 4) and under many brand names. You can buy it in the form of pills to chew on and pills to swallow, and in time-release capsules. The prices are as varied as the brands and forms. And aspirin is also combined with other drugs—in pain relievers, stimulants, antacids, and antihistamines.

The Cost of Health-care Products

Each year consumers spend billions on health-care products—in 1979 more than $2 billion. The health-care business is among the most profitable in this country.

Drug manufacturers make money by creating new products and selling them for a profit. Even if these new products are no better than products already on the market, they can make money. What really sells most health-care products is advertising and the sales force.

Brand Names and Generics

Most drugs have more than one name. First is the chemical name of the drug, the name that simply describes the drug's chemical content. Some companies sell drugs under these chemical names, and the drugs they sell are called *generics*. Usually, generics are cheaper than *brand-name* drugs. A brand name is simply a label that a manufacturer attaches to a drug and then advertises heavily, so you will remember it. For example, Allopurinol is a drug widely used to treat a disease called gout. Thrifty people buy it under that generic name. Several companies, however, produce exactly the same drug but sell it under the names Lopurin and Zyloprin. These brand-name products are usually about 60 percent more expensive than identical generic products.

Prescription and Over-the-Counter (OTC) Drugs

Prescription drugs are medicines that can be purchased only with the consent of a physician or dentist. They must be bought in a pharmacy (or drug store); and the pharmacist, a health professional who specializes in preparing and dispensing drugs, must place the doctor's instructions on the container. These instructions indicate the dosage of the drug and how often it should be taken.

An *over-the-counter (OTC)* drug can be bought by anyone, without a physician's consent or supervision. OTC drugs generally are less strong than prescription drugs and have fewer side effects; they usually are less harmful when misused.

Physicians bear most of the responsibility for the drugs they prescribe. But it is the consumer who selects OTC drugs. So it is the consumer who should be educated to make the right choices and ask the right questions.

And *you* are the consumer.

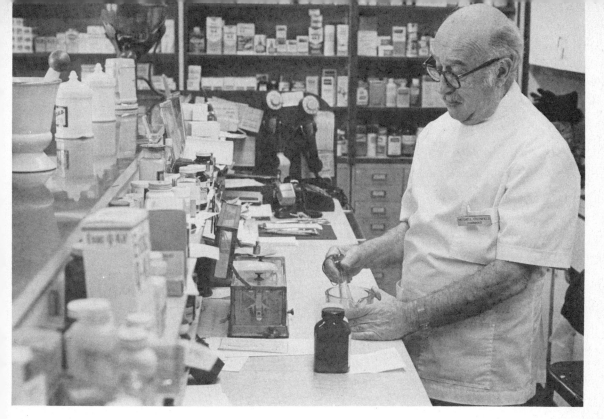

A pharmacist at work.

Ray Ellis/Rapho/Photo Researchers

Using Drugs

Side Effects

Although OTC medicines usually have fewer serious side effects than prescription drugs, *all drugs have side effects.* Manufacturers frequently claim that a drug is "safe." Some drugs are more safe than others, but each person reacts differently to drugs. Drugs that are safe for most of us cause problems for some people; one person's treatment may be another's poison.

An educated consumer should never take *any* drug without knowing its side effects. Ask physicians and pharmacists about strange medicines. Read labels. Do not assume anything about the quality, safety, or effectiveness of OTC drugs.

There are three kinds of side effects:

- *Dose-related:* Such side effects are predictable; they would affect everyone who took a certain amount of a drug. For example, if you take enough sleeping pills, you will become unconscious.
- *Allergic reactions:* Allergies are specific to individuals. Only people who are allergic (see Chapter 10) to certain dosages of a drug develop allergies to that drug.

- *Rare and unpredictable:* These reactions are specific to individuals but have unknown causes.

Certain kinds of people have more problems with drugs than other people do. Children are particularly sensitive, so their reactions to drugs should be watched with care. People with certain diseases—for example, diseases of the heart, kidney, or liver—cannot tolerate a number of drugs. And drugs taken by pregnant women circulate in their blood and enter the bodies of their unborn children, sometimes with fearsome effects. Nursing mothers even transfer drugs through their milk.

Drug Interaction

People sometimes take more than one drug at a time. Certain drugs, when combined, cancel out each other's effects (antagonism). Other combinations of drugs have an effect equal to the sum of the effects of each drug taken by itself (potentiation). But some combinations have an effect greater than that sum (synergy). That is why you should always tell physicians about all the drugs you are taking. Remember to ask physicians if the drugs they prescribe can be taken with common OTC products, like aspirin and antacids, and (if you are using them) with birth control pills or alcohol.

Some drugs should not be taken with certain foods. Caffeine and citrus fruits, for example, interfere with antibiotics; and tetracycline is less effective if you eat calcium-rich foods, like milk, after taking it. Some drugs, moreover, can create deficiencies of certain vitamins and minerals, so it is important to eat a well-balanced diet when taking drugs over a long period.

How to Take Medicine

Everybody knows the old rule, "Take two aspirin, plenty of liquids, and rest in bed." Sometimes that is all you have to do. Sometimes you have to follow more complicated rules. Here are a few:

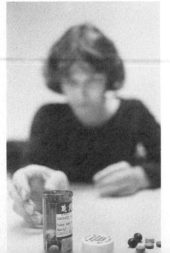

- *Set goals:* Know what the drug is supposed to do for you, and how quickly. If the drug does not seem to be working, tell your physician.
- *Avoid dependency:* Sometimes drug dependency (see Chapter 4) is more or less unavoidable, as when certain medicines are used over a long period of time to treat chronic illnesses—certain pain relievers in cases of arthritis, for example. Ordinarily, you should avoid using OTC drugs—including preparations for insomnia, constipation, and fatigue—that create dependency.
- *Take medicines as directed:* Follow the directions about how often to take medicines, and how much to take. Gobbling up more than you need will not make you more healthy.

- *Finish the prescription:* When physicians tell you to take a drug for a certain length of time, they have their reasons. Many drugs, for example, have a "cumulative" effect—they work by gathering strength as doses pile up in the body.

Drug Advertisements

When used correctly, many OTC drugs are safe and effective. But most people do not take a drug—at least at first—because it is safe and effective. They take it because the ad where they learned about it was effective. Sometimes these ads are more clever than the newspapers, magazines, and TV shows in which they appear.

Appraising Advertisements

Advertisers are trying to manipulate you. Ads are designed to make you feel insecure, to make you think that you have a problem and that a certain product is the solution. Be skeptical of all ads, especially of those using these techniques:

- *Pseudoscientific terminology:* One ad claimed that a certain product would improve the purchaser's love life by using "disguised hypnosis" to eliminate disorders in the "subconscious mind." You hesitate to doubt medical jargon like this because it has a ring of authority to it.
- *Testimonials:* Remember that no one recommends a product in an advertisement except for pay. He who pays the piper chooses the tune.
- *Sex appeal:* We have all seen ads in which a man puts on a brand of after-shave lotion and then walks through the streets, followed by beautiful strangers who seem to be panting for sex with him. Put on one of these brands and then walk through the streets yourself.

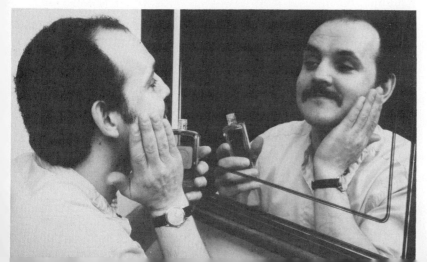

Can the difference between one brand of after-shave lotion and another make anyone more attractive to anyone else?

Ken Karp

Does the same thing happen to you? People *do* find good grooming attractive, but the difference between one brand of after-shave lotion and another is not going to have *any impact at all* on your love life—and neither will perfume.

- *Claims of "evidence":* References to laboratory studies and surveys are usually misleading, because most often they do not tell the whole truth, or they mix truth with falsehoods. Some ads claim that products were tested "by an independent laboratory." For all you know, the laboratory was in somebody's closet or desk drawer.

- *"Doctor's" Approval:* Once many people hear an official title they suspend judgment. "Doctor's approval" might mean one physician or 1,000. And what kind of "doctors" are they, anyway—witch doctors? Remember that the word "physician" has a legal meaning, but "doctor" does not; we can all call ourselves "doctors."

The Art of the Half-truth

Drug companies must comply with certain laws. They must place labels on all products. The labels must state the purpose of a product, give directions for its use, and warn of certain dangers. But these laws are few, and they force drug companies to tell the truth, but *not* the whole truth. Side effects, for example, tend to be minimized in ads.

The Truth, but Not the Whole Truth

The truths that ads contain are those that benefit the advertiser. What is *not* said is sometimes more important than what *is* said. And *how* the message is put is often more important than the *content* of the message.

People are manipulated by advertisements, among other reasons, because they cannot tell the difference between what an ad says and what it implies. An ad might say, for example, that a certain product "*may* end your itch." Taken quite literally that is no doubt true; after all, doing nothing at all *may* also end it. But most people assume the ad promises that the product "*will* end your itch."

Another favorite technique is to claim that a product is superior to "other products" on the market; since these products are not named the claim is too vague even to be false. Claims that cannot be false also cannot be true.

Guidelines for Buying OTC Drugs

OTC drugs should be used as a last—not as a first—resort. Before using them try adjusting your diet, getting more exercise and sleep, or dealing with your emotional life. Any serious or prolonged medical problem should be treated by a physician. Some minor problems are best treated by ignoring them, since drugs may either mask symptoms

MooMoo Milk tastes great. Keep your family healthy. Buy MooMoo Milk.

According to the above "commercial," does MooMoo Milk keep your family healthy? If you answered yes, you're probably in the majority, but you're wrong.

This is just one way advertisers make implied claims about their products that may not be true. The commercial doesn't say directly that MooMoo Milk keeps your family healthy, but psycholinguistic studies show that most people would get that impression. Recent research by Richard Harris of Kansas State University confirms that people don't discriminate between what is directly stated and what is implied. He gives other examples of ways in which consumers are misled by linguistic manipulation:

- The use of hedge words that weaken the statement, such as "Knock-out capsules *may* relieve tension."
- Using comparison adjectives that give no comparison, such as "Chore gives you whiter wash." The statement is undeniably true because it could be completed with any phrase, such as, "than washing with coal dust."
- Inadequate or incomplete reporting of survey or test results.
- Using a negative question, which implies an affirmative answer: "Isn't quality the most important thing to consider in buying aspirin?" The answer might very well be no, but the assumption is yes.

- The use of expressions such as "hospital-tested" or "doctor-tested" that give little information but lend an air of scientific respectability.

Harris tested people's responses to these misleading techniques. One hundred eighty students listened to tapes of 20 mock commercials of the type frequently heard on radio and television. They heard one of two versions of each commercial containing either implied claims, or only directly asserted claims. They then were asked to decide, based on what they heard in the commercials, whether certain statements about the commercials were true, false, or impossible to judge. Half the students in both groups were given an example of an implied claim and were specifically warned not to interpret such claims as asserted ones.

The students correctly rated an average of eight out of 10 of the asserted statements as true. But the students also judged seven of the implied claims as true. Even students who had been warned about implied claims rated more than half of them as true. Harris notes that the Federal Trade Commission, which regulates advertising on radio and television, has not defined a clear legal status for implied claims. What constitutes deceptive advertising is complex, and though the intent to deceive is clearly prohibited, it is difficult to substantiate.

Source: Sherida Bush Harris is at the department of psychology at Kansas State University, Anderson Hall, Manhattan, Kansas 66506.

(thus making you think you are well when you are not) or interfere with the process of natural healing. Cold medicines, for example, often do both (see Chapter 11).

When you do use an OTC drug use one that is effective. As we have seen, ads are a bad source of information; get your advice from a physician or a pharmacist, or from such books as the annual *Physician's Desk Reference* (available in most libraries) and the *FDA Consumer*, a periodical that often reviews health-care products. Shop around and compare products. Choose the drugs with the fewest side effects, and do not hesitate to buy the generic version.

Finally, certain home remedies are as effective as any drug you can buy without a prescription. For example, gargling with warm water mixed with a little salt is very helpful for a sore throat. A teaspoon of baking soda in water can relieve an acid stomach, and drinking lots of water does wonders for constipation. A long soak in a hot tub can relieve a lot of muscle aches and tension.

Specific OTC Products

OTC products are designed to relieve the common ailments created by the American way of life. Americans eat too much animal fat, drink too much alcohol, smoke too many cigarettes, get too little exercise, and abuse their bodies in many other ways; and the drug industry humors us by producing medicines that are supposed to make us healthy but do not force us to give up these and other unhealthy habits. Let us look at some of the most popular of OTC preparations.

The Common Cold

By far the most common of all communicable diseases (see Chapter 11) is the all-too-common cold. As we saw in Chapter 11, the common cold is incurable, and all efforts to cure it with commercial products (including those described below) may disrupt the body's natural healing processes. But people try to cure their colds anyway, and drug companies are happy to help them. Antihistamine pills and oral nasal decongestants may help to dry nasal passages and ease the misery of a cold, but they will not do anything to cure it or shorten its duration. Nose drops, too, relieve congestion. They should be used only as a last resort and only for a short time, since after a while they increase the congestion they are meant to relieve. All these medicines usually contain more ingredients than they need, and they sometimes cause fatigue, excessive dryness, or dizziness. They may also permit people who are sick to carry on with their daily routines and prevent them from getting the rest that would help them get over their illnesses.

Aspirin is sometimes useful for controlling the aches and pains of the common cold, but it may block the body's efforts to resist infection (see Chapter 11).

Cough Medicines

Remedies for coughs often contain useless ingredients like sugar, artificial color, and alcohol. An effective ingredient, often recommended by physicians, is *Dextromethorephan*. Other remedies may ease a dry throat and taste good, but they do little to relieve other symptoms.

Pain

Aspirin.   One of the safest, cheapest, and most effective of all pain relievers is none other than aspirin. In fact, it is one of the most effective of all drugs, and it can cause serious side effects, such as stomach disorders and internal bleeding. People who are sensitive to aspirin can take acetaminophen, which is sold under a number of brand names.

Premenstrual Tension.   Pain relievers have no effect upon premenstrual tension. Diuretics may help eliminate the water build-up associated with it, but they are dangerous and not very effective. It is wiser to deal with premenstrual tension by cutting down your intake of salt.

Menstrual Pain.   Aspirin is usually all you need to control mild menstrual pain. Other pain-relieving OTC drugs contain chemicals that may not be helpful or lead to unpleasant side effects. Severe cramps (dysmenorrhea) cannot be helped by any OTC drug. Severe pain is caused by hormones called "prostaglandins." New prescription drugs called "antiprostaglandins" (sold under several brand names) now offer much relief.

Stomach Problems

Diarrhea.   The most useful OTC drugs for controlling diarrhea contain kaolin and pectin. Certain prescription drugs containing codeine or other opium derivatives (see Chapter 4) control diarrhea even better, but they are addictive. Most attacks of diarrhea last only a few days; if you have one that lasts longer, see a physician. Diarrhea in children or older people should always be brought to a physician's notice.

Constipation.   Constipation usually cures itself without drugs. If, after 3 days, it does not, try a high-bran cereal, prunes or prune juice, or a few extra glasses of water. If *that* does not do the job after another 8 hours, you might want to try a mild laxative, especially if the constipation is caused by a change in your daily routine. OTC drugs containing dioctyl sodium sulfosuccinate are effective "stool softeners." Useful "bulk producing" laxatives contain psyllium or carboxymethylcellulose.

Indigestion.   Advertisements for indigestion are sometimes hilariously silly, but indigestion itself is painful enough. You can usually relieve stomach aches and burning sensations caused by overeating or by eating spicy or high-fat foods by using an OTC drug with aluminum hydroxide, magnesium hydroxide, or magnesium trisilicate. Better yet, eat more carefully. Prolonged, severe, or recurrent indigestion is a sign of a more serious problem; and using too much of these drugs can upset the excretory system.

Itching

Mild itching caused by dry skin can be controlled with an OTC hand or body lotion. More difficult cases may be helped by OTC cortisone products. Lotions to control itching from bites, plants like poison ivy, or drug reactions should contain zinc oxide or calamine. If the itching gets worse after you apply the lotion stop using it. See a physician for internal itching of the vagina or the rectum. You can relieve the pain from a bee bite by applying a paste of meat tenderizer and water. The itching from mosquito bites and poison ivy can be reduced by *brief* applications of hot water at 120 to 130 degrees Fahrenheit.

Sunburn.   Every so often, magazines and newspapers proclaim the dangers of too much exposure to sunlight, but sun worshipers ignore these warnings. An OTC spray or lotion with at least 20 percent benzocaine can reduce the pain of sunburn, and so can aspirin and a cool bath.

It makes more sense to prevent sunburn than to treat it. The most effective sunscreen lotions contain para-aminobenzoic acid, commonly known as PABA. It comes in a wide variety of strengths, each for a different kind of skin, and should be used according to directions.

It makes more sense to prevent sunburn, by using sunscreen lotions, than to treat sunburn.

Ken Karp

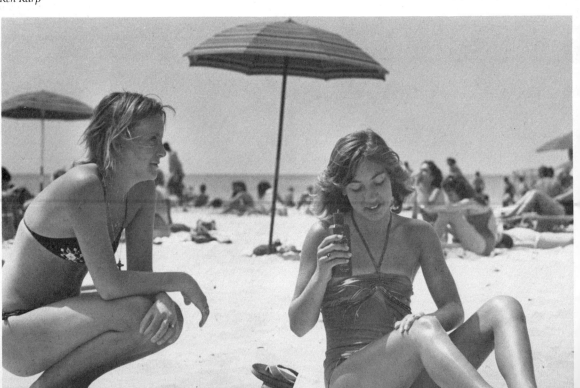

"Feminine Hygiene"

Tampons and Sanitary Pads.   Pads fit over the vulva and collect the menstrual discharge (see Chapter 13) as it passes out of the vagina. Tampons are inserted into the vaginal canal itself and absorb the flow before it leaves the body. Women with intact hymens (see Chapter 13) may have difficulty using tampons because the opening in the hymen (through which the tampon must be inserted) can be very narrow.

Tampons have recently come under scrutiny, since they have been connected with a rare (but sometimes fatal and widely publicized) disease called toxic shock syndrome (TSS). This is not a reason to stop using tampons, but it is a reason to be careful: Change tampons at least every 6 to 8 hours, use a sanitary pad for some part of each 24-hour day during menstruation, and avoid so-called superabsorbent tampons (which seem to be associated with TSS).

Choose any one of the 60 or so kinds of sanitary pads and tampons that seems most comfortable to you, but avoid scented or deodorant tampons or pads because they can irritate and cause allergies.

Genital Deodorants.   At a time of many unneeded things, genital deodorants for women are among the most unneeded. They are without medical or hygienic benefits but can cause irritations, burns, infections, itching, swelling, and lumps. They can also prolong or mask serious problems. Forget about them.

Acne

Acne is caused by overactivity of the sebacious glands, which produce an oily substance designed to lubricate the hair follicles. If the glands secrete too much oil, bacteria gather in it, and the body reacts with the inflammation response (see Chapter 11). Boil-like lesions break out and may cause pain, scars, and emotional problems. Acne can neither be prevented nor cured, but it can be controlled. Washing your face with soap and water several times each day might do the trick. If it does not, a number of OTC preparations may help control mild cases, but severe ones require medical attention.

There is no single ingredient that can help control all cases of acne—each person's skin is different and reacts to lotions in a different way. Some acne treatments may even compound the problem. Among the more-or-less effective ingredients are benzoyl peroxide, salicylic acid, resorcinol, and sulfur. Antibiotic preparations do not appear to have any effect.

Since acne is not a dietary disease it does not respond to dietary treatment. But cutting sweets, nuts, chocolate, and fried foods from your diet may reduce the inflammation.

Allergy

Stuffy noses, post-nasal drip, itchy eyes, and scratchy throats are not always caused by viruses; often the culprit is plant pollen blowing in the wind and causing allergies (see chapter 10). Allergies are not easily distinguished from certain viral infections (see Chapter 11), since they share many symptoms. The problem may be an allergy if it occurs in spring or fall, when plant pollens are present in the air, or if your symptoms last longer than two weeks. To find out exactly what, if anything, you may be allergic to, you have to see an allergist. If the allergy is short-lasting, OTC preparations with Chlortrimeton are the most useful ones to control the disorder. Allergies that do not respond well to this treatment require medical attention.

Cosmetics

We have seen that drug companies try to cash in on our hope that using drugs will make us healthy even if our life styles are not healthy. They also try to profit from the delusion that we can enjoy sexual and emotional intimacy with others merely by using cosmetics—without acting in ways that will promote intimacy. Even more than drugs, cosmetics expose the public to the blandishments of advertising, for a drug's manufacturer at least has to prove to the government that the drug is not dangerous, but the manufacturers of cosmetics do not really have to prove anything to anybody. Except the customer. Yet cosmetics, like drugs, can be dangerous if misused—they can cause skin problems, headaches, nasal congestion, and itching; and some of them contain carcinogens (see Chapter 10).

The sheer variety of cosmetics overwhelms. The brand names are as numerous as the color shades. Lost amid all the products and claims, the consumer finds it hard to choose. Let us take a look at a few categories of cosmetics and at the principles that should guide you when you make your choices.

Jim Anderson/Woodfin Camp & Associates

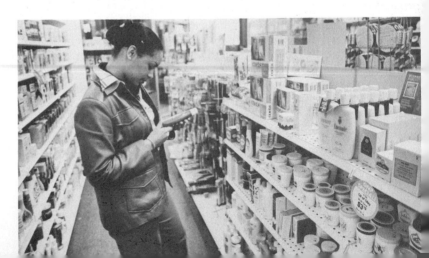

Mouthwashes

Breath sprays, drops, and washes have only a temporary effect; they do nothing for chronic bad breath (halitosis). Proper brushing and flossing of teeth is probably the best way to avoid bad breath; brushing the tongue is sometimes helpful too. Keep in mind that mouthwashes are not harmless; most contain alcohol, which can irritate and dry the mouth.

Deodorants and Antiperspirants

Antiperspirants are really drugs because they alter the function of the body by blocking perspiration. Deodorants are cosmetics because they diminish or mask body odor, which they do not prevent. But some deodorants also contain a chemical to inhibit odor-causing bacteria. The most effective antiperspirants contain aluminum chloride or aluminum chlorhydroxide. Aerosol deodorants are less safe than stick and roll-on products since the spray is inhaled and may hurt the lungs or irritate the eyes.

Eye Makeup

Eye makeup, mascara, for example, is safe when you first buy it. But after a time, mascara can become contaminated with microorganisms and infect the eyelid or even, if the cornea is scratched, cause blindness. As a rule, mascara should be discarded after 4 to 6 months' use; water-based mascaras should be thrown out even sooner.

If your lid does become infected, or if you scratch your eye with mascara, consult a physician and bring the eye makeup along for testing. Do not use mascara, eye liner, or eye shadow if you already have an infection.

Hair-care Products

Shampoos.   Shampoos are concoctions of detergents, wetting agents, water softeners, perfumes, and artificial colors; and some also have proteins, lemon, eggs, beer, and herbs. When you wash the dirt and oils out of your hair, you wash out all the ingredients, too, so all these extras seem to give little, if any, benefit.

Most people do not have to use a dandruff shampoo; it is usually enough to shampoo several times a week or, if need be, daily. If that does not do the job, get a shampoo with zinc pyrithione in it.

Hair sprays.   Hair sprays (used by men and women to keep their hair in place) mostly do not damage it, but they may harm the eyes, lungs, and clothes. Reduce these problems by spraying away from your nose, mouth, and eyes; by not inhaling while you spray; and by leaving the room immediately after you spray.

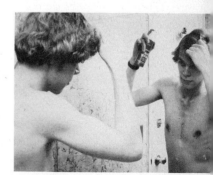

Hairsprays are used by men as well as by women.

Martin M. Rotker / Taurus Photos

Quacks and Quackery

Society teaches its members to respect authority, the authority of parents, teachers, and physicians, for example. At the same time, many people cannot tell a real authority from a "quack," someone who pretends to be an authority but who is not. This confusion and the respect usually granted to authority ensure that quacks are very numerous. And to make matters more confusing, even real and well-meaning authorities sometimes base their views on incomplete information and are sometimes proved wrong. Quacks, however, usually do not base their opinions on information at all; they want their products to *sell*, not to *work*. Often quacks persist, even when they know that their products and methods are harmful.

The Birth of Quackery

Fear is the breeding ground of quacks. People who are frightened and sick need comfort and relief. Quacks cater to these needs by promising easy cures. Quacks often acquire great reputations by claiming credit for curing people who have recovered through the body's natural healing processes. They manipulate our distrust of standard methods of treatment. They are sometimes easier for sick people to find than are legitimate practitioners. Quacks prey upon a population with an almost religious faith in the power of technology—a faith largely created by such real medical miracles as pacemakers, laser surgery, and kidney machines. Finally, some people fall into the hands of quacks simply because they know nothing about legitimate treatments.

How to Spot a Quack

Do not expect a modern-day quack to be an old-fashioned huckster, someone who talks loudly and rapidly, who looks like a circus clown. Some quacks are attractive, charming, soft spoken, and intelligent; some dress in laboratory coats and carry stethoscopes. Judge the qualifications of anyone claiming to be a health practitioner by using these rules:

- Make sure that anyone who treats you has a license from an accredited school. Get in touch with the local medical, dental, or osteopathic society for lists of their members.
- Ignore people who promise miracle cures for complex problems. Something that sounds too good to be true probably is.
- Be wary of testimonials from strangers. Accept only scientifically documented information. Consult your local or state board of health, or the office of the state attorney general, about anything that makes you doubtful, or look things up in a library.
- Distrust anyone who tries to stop you from going to a physician.

- Be wary of gadgets that are said to make it easy to reach difficult goals (losing weight, for example).

- Avoid "secret remedy" treatments with medications that are mysterious or that "cannot be explained." Avoid treatments "invented so recently" that no one has heard of them yet and treatments that are kept secret to "prevent them from falling into the hands of the big drug companies."

- Be skeptical of health practitioners who tell you that there is a conspiracy against them or that other doctors are jealous of them.

- Don't patronize practitioners who use meaningless titles, like "naturopath."

- Don't believe practitioners who blame their failure to cure you on your own lack of faith.

- Ignore anyone who insists on treating you outside of the United States to avoid government regulations.

- Distrust practitioners who demand large payments before they will treat you.

- Be skeptical of medical treatments sold through the mails. The Postal Service does not license mail-order advertisers, so a box number on the address of a product does not legitimize it. Don't assume that ads for mail-order products (or other products) in magazines, books, and newspapers have to be truthful. Ads in periodicals are screened only by the publishers themselves, and they are rarely investigated.

- Use your brains. One so-called cancer treatment requires patients to drink every hour juice made from vegetables and liver, and to submit to frequent coffee enemas. If something makes you laugh, it may well be absurd.

Nostrums

The quack's element is human weakness in all its forms, and each kind of weakness has bred its own kind of quack. Let us consider some nostrums, devices that are supposed to cure health problems but that do not.

Breast Developers.   Are your breasts big enough? Many women think not. The size of the breasts depends on heredity, hormones, and body weight. Exercise can affect the apparent size of the breasts, but in reality it can only enlarge the pectoral muscles behind them; the breasts themselves have no muscles. Lotions and creams cannot change the size or shape of the breasts and neither can vacuum caps.

Penis Enlargers.   Many men worry about the size of their penises even more than women worry about the size of their breasts. And like

Sole Searching

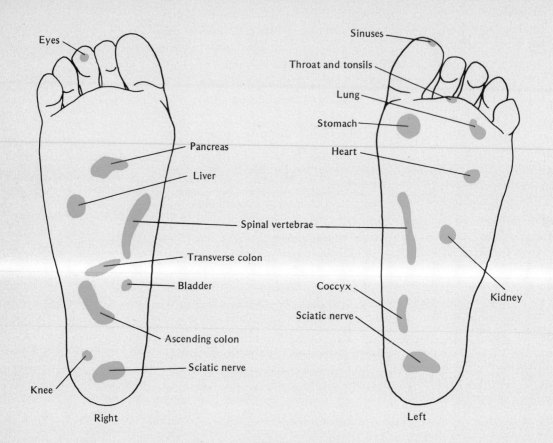

Eyes

Pancreas

Liver

Spinal vertebrae

Transverse colon

Bladder

Ascending colon

Sciatic nerve

Knee

Right

Sinuses

Throat and tonsils

Lung

Stomach

Heart

Coccyx

Sciatic nerve

Kidney

Left

Is it possible that the cure for bodily ills lies somewhere in the soles of the feet? Believe it or not, that's what practitioners of foot reflexology claim. According to this ancient Chinese practice, the nerve endings in your whole body are located in your feet. Corns, calluses, bunions and other lumps can clog these nerves and block energy flow. By massaging the spot on your sole that corresponds to the ailing part of your body (see above), you can release this energy and relieve pain. (Although this theory may sound incredible, the massage feels great anyway!) Using your thumbs, fingertips or a hard eraser, poke and prod your sole until you find the sore spot—then massage for 30 seconds. Another option: Use a carved wooden foot roller for an invigorating massage—it will stretch and relax your muscles.

Courtesy *Mademoiselle*, March 1981, p. 208. Copyright © 1981 by The Condé Nast Publications, Inc.

the breasts, the penis has no muscles, so it cannot be enlarged by vacuum pumps, pills, gadgets, or exercises.

Wrinkle Removers.   Dry skin may appear to be more wrinkled than moist skin, so any kind of lotion makes skin look smoother. But lotions to remove wrinkles can only tighten the skin slightly, and briefly. Pills or special diets have no proven effect at all.

Diet Nostrums.   Losing weight honestly—but effectively—is difficult (see Chapter 9). Millions of people are looking for a "magic wand"— pills, protein supplements, slenderizing equipment, reducing devices, anything at all—to help them reduce painlessly, without cutting down on food and without effort. Diet pills that contain amphetamines (see Chapter 4) can raise blood pressure, increase the risk of heart attack, and make people nervous and irritable. And in the long run, they do not promote weight loss.

Megavitamins.   Vitamins are no doubt important for your health and well-being (see Chapter 8). But "more" is not "better."

Health Foods.   Despite what many people think, "health foods" (see Chapter 8) are not superior in nutrition to other kinds of food. Nor can you be sure that any product actually is "organic."

Arthritis Aids.   Copper bracelets, "immune milk," sea water, yeast diets, and special drinks do nothing to help arthritis (see Chapter 10). Other "cures" that do not work are radioactive materials, colored lights, metal disks, and "uranium tunnels."

Acupuncture.   In the early 1970s, when contacts between the United States and mainland China were reopened, Americans became aware of acupuncture, a technique of traditional Chinese medicine in which sharp needles are inserted in various parts of the body to relieve symptoms of illness and pain. Acupuncture may in fact be effective for migraine, for psoriasis and other skin conditions, for depression, and for anxiety. But its usefulness has been exaggerated, and many acupuncture clinics have been taken over by quacks.

Dentistry.   "Denturists" are quack dentists (see Chapter 17). To get business, they usually charge less than real dentists. Although denturists are unlicensed, many display phony credentials. They often claim— falsely—to prescribe dentures legally and repair them. Denturists often give phony nutritional advice, too.

SELF-ASSESSMENT DEVICE 18–1: QUICK QUACK QUIZ

To assess your knowledge and understanding of health quackery, please answer the following "Quick Quack Quiz".

Circle the best answer: True or False

TRUE FALSE 1. In former years "quacks" were frontier medicine men who dispensed numerous elixirs designed to cure the ills that had plagued mankind since the beginning of time.

TRUE FALSE 2. Today quackers is still found in various forms.

TRUE FALSE 3. Quackery and faddism can be dangerous to health because they tend to prevent people from following sound health practices and receiving adequate health protection.

TRUE FALSE 4. Because of updated federal laws the U. S. consumer need no longer be concerned about false and misleading health information and products appearing on the market.

TRUE FALSE 5. Over-the-counter drugs are safe, when used according to the directions, for minor conditions and for temporary relief of symptoms.

TRUE FALSE 6. All those persons listed in the yellow pages as "Marriage Counselors" are qualified or their names would not be allowed to appear in the phone book under that title.

TRUE FALSE 7. A fairly large percentage of people in this country suffer from iron deficiency anemia ("tired blood").

TRUE FALSE 8. Properly synthesized and manufactured vitamins have the same value in respect to health maintenance as do "natural" vitamins.

TRUE FALSE 9. Malnutrition in this country is rampant because our food is grown on depleted soil.

TRUE FALSE 10. It is normal for a person in good health to experience occasional fatigue and lack of pep.

TRUE FALSE 11. Everyone should take vitamin pills just to be sure they are getting an adequate supply of vitamins.

TRUE FALSE 12. Yogurt has much the same nutritional value as milk.

TRUE FALSE 13. The body stores all the excess vitamins and minerals it receives for later use.

TRUE FALSE 14. There is no known preparation that by itself will effectively control weight.

TRUE FALSE 15. Losing and then regaining weight repeatedly produces unnecessary stress on body functioning and may be harmful to your health.

TRUE FALSE 16. The vibrating machines often found in health clubs have been scientifically proven effective in reducing weight.

TRUE FALSE 17. There are drugs, by prescription only, which have been shown effective in depressing appetite and thereby helpful in promoting weight loss.

TRUE FALSE 18. Sauna baths and rubber garments that cause the wearer to sweat have been proven to be effective in weight and fat reducing programs.

TRUE FALSE 19. No exercise, preparation, or mechanical device will develop the breasts.

TRUE FALSE 20. Electrolysis, the only way for permanent and safe hair removal, can cause permanent disfigurement if misused.

Source: Lanese, M. M. The Quick Quack Quiz. *The Physical Educator*, December 1973, pp. 217–218. Found in *Health, Quackery and the Consumer*, W. B. Saunders, Philadelphia, Publishers.

Sex Clinics How good a lover are you? A lot of people think they are not good enough, and worries of this sort cause some men to have problems sustaining erections and some women to fail consistently to reach orgasm. That is where the sex therapist comes in. Now, sex therapy is not all quackery by any means; much progress has been made in this field, and there are good private and university clinics that can indeed treat sexual problems. But at present, sex therapists are not li-

TRUE FALSE 21. Medical devices for diagnosing or treating human illness must be effective and safe in order to be marketed.

TRUE FALSE 22. In deciding whether to use unproven methods in attempting a cancer cure, the best source is the cancer patient who has already tried the method.

TRUE FALSE 23. There are now hormonal creams on the market that can prevent the wrinkles of aging.

TRUE FALSE 24. Acupuncture now is allowed in a few states on an experimental basis under the supervision of licensed doctors.

TRUE FALSE 25. Hypnotism can be an acceptable method of treating mental and emotional disorders if used by one of the few hundred physicians and psychiatrists in the U. S. fully qualified to practice it.

TRUE FALSE 26. Health cultists such as chiropractors have an inflexible theory concerning a single cause of all human illness.

TRUE FALSE 27. Self-diagnosis and self-treatment can endanger health.

TRUE FALSE 28. Early symptoms of stomach cancer may resemble those of stomach ulcer.

TRUE FALSE 29. Copper bracelets are effective in curing rheumatism.

TRUE FALSE 30. A good score on this quiz is your assurance that you are immune to the many forms of health quackery prevalent in the U. S. today.

26–30 correct . . . . Ralph Nader Buyer
21–25 correct . . . . Red Ribbon Consumer
11–20 correct . . . . Better Beware Buyer
0–10 correct . . . . Quack's Delight

1. True	11. False	21. False
2. True	12. True	22. False
3. True	13. False	23. False
4. False	14. True	24. True
5. True	15. True	25. True
6. False	16. False	26. True
7. False	17. True	27. True
8. True	18. False	28. True
9. False	19. True	29. False
10. True	20. True	30. False

censed, so it is hard to judge whether or not a clinic is legitimate. Quacks have stepped in and set up phony sex clinics, some of them little more than houses of prostitution, all over the country.

Aphrodisiacs. Bogus drugs that are supposed to improve sex drive—but do not—are called aphrodisiacs. The most common ingredient in these nostrums is the famous "Spanish fly," originally made from insects ground into powder and now from red pepper, which can irritate the urethra (see Chapter 13). Ginseng root is also used as an aphrodisiac.

Controlling Quackery

Controlling quackery is difficult. The American Medical Association (AMA) and the American Dental Association (ADA) attempt to police the actions of physicians and dentists, respectively. But for the most part, these organizations protect rather than control their members. Malpractice suits have weeded out some medical and dental frauds, but hardly enough to make a difference. Besides, most quacks are not physicians or dentists.

Since no organization can really control the great army of frauds, spotting and controlling fraud is more or less up to you, the consumer. It is up to you to ask the obvious questions before you buy a product or a service; and if you are gypped by a quack it's up to you to file a complaint and give evidence. But victims of fraud do not like to admit that they are gullible, so often they do nothing.

Efforts to control medical fraud might be more effective if more help were given by the publishers of newspapers and magazines. Right now, publishers do not have to check out the claims made in the ads they carry, and usually they *do not* check them out. That removes a chance to kill medical fraud close to its sources.

How to File a Consumer Complaint

Consumer complaints are sometimes ineffective because they have not been drawn up well. By following these rules, you can help make your efforts more successful:

- Report the complaint promptly.
- State the problem clearly.
- Describe the product or service completely. Include the product's code number, for example.
- Report your complaints about a product to its manufacturer and distributor, and to the store where it was purchased. Notify your local health department about problems with drugs, cosmetics, or foods.
- Save the product, but don't use more of it.
- If you receive ads through the mail for a probable fraud, take them back to the local post office.
- Make copies of letters, receipts, bills, and invoices. Write down the names of the people you speak to. Make it clear to them that you intend to take your complaint further if you are not satisfied with their responses.

If a reasonable amount of time has passed and you do not get satisfaction, follow these steps:

- Send copies of your complaint to the office of your state attorney general, to the local better business bureau, to the state and national office of consumer affairs, and to independent consumer groups.

- Get in touch with the Federal Trade Commission if your complaint is about unfair or deceptive ads or business practices. Write to newspapers and magazines, and radio and television stations, asking them not to run the ad.

- Notify the company or person you are complaining against of your actions.

- As a last resort, sue. Many states have small claims courts that handle cases involving up to $1,000 without lawyers.

SUMMARY

All drugs and even cosmetics are potentially dangerous. OTC drugs are less dangerous than prescription drugs. But before using any OTC drug you should try natural methods of healing, like eating more intelligently and getting more sleep and exercise. When you do use OTC drugs, follow the directions.

Think about the advertisements for health products before you act on them. Do not be manipulated by advertising. And be wary of so-called medical practitioners who offer you "easy" and "certain" cures for difficult and uncertain problems. Use your brains—ask yourself if the claims made for products and practitioners make sense. If these claims seem too good to be true they probably are not true.

Take responsibility for getting rid of quacks. When you are a victim of medical fraud, file a complaint and pursue it.

Suggested Readings

Cornacchia, Harold J., and Barrett, Stephen. *Consumer Health: A Guide to Intelligent Decisions.* St. Louis: Mosby, 1980. This book is designed to help people make decisions that protect their health and pocketbooks.

Health Insurance Institute. *Source Book of Health Insurance Data.* Washington, D.C.: Health Insurance Institute, 1979/80. This publication is an excellent statistical reference to the private health insurance system in the United States. Information is included about costs, staff, and geographic location of health services.

Schaller, Warren E., et al. *Health, Quackery, and the Consumer.* Philadelphia: Saunders, 1976. This book is concerned with the health care delivery system in the United States and its effects on the consumer. It also explains quackery and how to avoid deception.

Shipley, Roger R., and Plonsky, Carolyn G. *Consumer Health.* New York: Harper & Row, 1980. This book is a valuable source for consumer-related problems. It explains how to use health products and services effectively.

Subcommittee on Health and the Environment, Committee on Interstate & Foreign Commerce, U.S. House of Representatives. *A Discursive Dictionary of Health Care.* Washington, D.C.: U.S. Government Printing Office, 1976. This resource includes definitions of terms used in the health-care system. It provides useful information about health-care products.

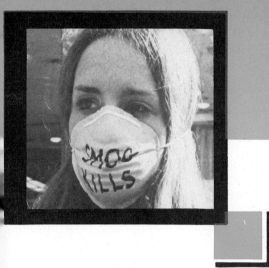

The Environment

chapter objectives

When you have finished reading this chapter you should be able to:

1. Recognize that the earth has a limited potential to sustain life
2. Identify the forces that contribute to environmental deterioration
3. Describe different kinds and sources of pollution
4. Discuss the social aspects of environmental problems
5. Explain how environmental quality could be improved

The Effect is . . .

Each small action, each shovel of dirt, each ounce of pesticide, each car exhaust, each jet plane, each backyard incinerator, each cow in the feedlot, each yard of asphalt or concrete covering the water-absorbing earth, each beer can in the barrow pit, each mile of interstate, each acre of block-filled land, each building on a flood plain, each pound of garbage, each acre of overgrazed land, each factory or refinery, and yes, each rocket shot into space has little effect. But cumulatively the effect is staggering and catastrophic.

Source: Wilson F. Clark, *Energy for Survival: The Alternative to Extinction* (New York: Doubleday, 1975).

Primitive peoples live in harmony with nature because they have to—it is far more powerful than they are, and everything they possess comes directly from it. But human beings longed from the first to be independent of nature, to challenge and to conquer it. Many of humanity's greatest achievements stem from this longing. These achievements have permitted larger and larger populations to make more and more demands on the earth and its resources. But our ability to make these demands is much greater than our ability to satisfy them. Many people have come to think that the ideal of conquering nature is unrealistic, and perhaps wrong. A new ideal—living with nature—has been born.

Despite the birth of this new ideal, human behavior goes on pretty much as before. Each year, the factories of the world create millions upon millions of products. And each year they create an enormous number of *by*-products. Some of these by-products are released into the environment through the air or the water, both of which they pollute. Very little has been done to repair the damage already inflicted on the environment, and little more has been done to prevent future damage.

Environmental Pollution

Air Pollution

All kinds of air pollution—the haze that often hovers over cities, especially in wintertime—come from the burning of fossil fuels: oil, coal, and gas. Various kinds of fuels, with many kinds of impurities, burned in various processes, produce many kinds of pollutants.

Air Pollutants.   Carbon monoxide, from the burning of gasoline in automobiles, is among the most important of these air pollutants. People who get caught in traffic jams often come down with carbon monoxide poisoning, whose symptoms include headache, nausea, abdominal pains, and (in extreme cases) temporary black-outs and loss of vision.

The hydrocarbons (compounds containing hydrogen and carbon) also left from burning gasoline are also significant air pollutants. Gasoline vapors mix with the nitrogen oxide in the air, and under the influence of strong light they form peroxides and ozonides. These react with one another and form a number of chemicals, which we see as the "blue haze," or photochemical smog, typical of many big cities. This smog is irritating to the respiratory tract and, like other hydrocarbons, may be carcinogenic (see Chapter 10).

Sulfur dioxide, a by-product from the smelting of ore that is high in sulfides, is another air pollutant. When mixed with water vapor, it forms caustic gases that irritate the eyes, nasal passages, and lungs, sometimes causing severe distress.

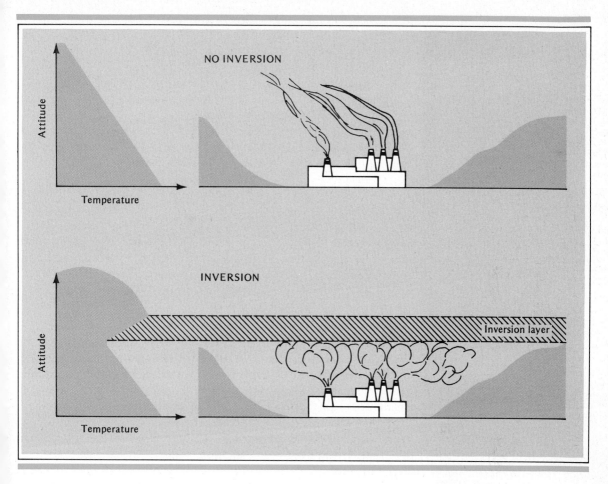

Figure 19-1. Normally, the higher the altitude the cooler the temperature (above). Temperature inversion occurs when air near the ground is held down by a layer of warmer air that prevents pollutants from rising (below).

Geographical and Weather Conditions. The presence of pollutants in the air does not itself cause air pollution. For most of the time, these pollutants rise high into the atmosphere and do not make people sick.

Inversion Layers. But in some areas wind patterns and the terrain (usually mountainous) create conditions that prevent the pollutants from escaping. The layer of cool air immediately on top of the ground is covered by a layer of warmer air—a so-called *temperature inversion.* This warmer air layer prevents the pollutants in the cooler air beneath it from rising. In some cities, smog is sometimes so bad that people with respiratory diseases have to stay indoors, and even healthy people have to cut back on outdoor activities. The famous smogs of Los Angeles are caused mainly by temperature inversions.

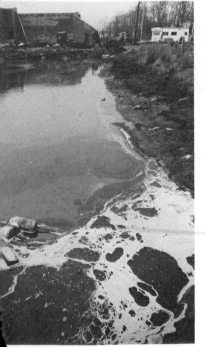

Water pollution.

Gordon S. Smith/Photo Researchers

Acid Rain. When coal is burned in steel factories and power plants, the sulfur within it is released into the air as smoke—garden-variety air pollution, in other words. This mixes with water vapor in the air, and the polluted water vapor condenses in clouds and falls to the earth's surface as rain. This rain has a high content of sulfuric acid and is therefore called *acid rain.*

Acid rain has killed all the fish in some lakes of the Adirondack Mountains in New York State, and it has killed off all the greenery in a 100-square mile area around Sudbury, Ontario. A copper plant in Sudbury happens to be an important source of the acid-rain problem, but the Adirondacks contribute very little to it. And that is one of the most sinister aspects of acid rain, which sometimes falls thousands of miles from its source.

Water Pollution

The Water Cycle. The total amount of water on our planet has not changed since it was formed. What does change, and change each moment, is the distribution of that water between three zones—the atmosphere (in the form of clouds), the earth's surface (including rivers, lakes, and oceans), and the part of the earth below its surface. Water constantly circulates from zone to zone in what is called the *water cycle.*

At any given time, most of the world's water is held on the earth's surface—in the oceans, rivers, and lakes. The sun, as it beats down upon the earth, causes this water to evaporate into the atmosphere, where the water forms into clouds. These clouds grow larger and larger until finally they condense. Rain then falls on the earth's surface, replenishing the water supply of the oceans, rivers, and lakes. The rain also seeps below the surface, into the water table, one of the main sources of human drinking water. The water in the water table is called ground water.

What is important about this water cycle, from our point of view, is that pollution in surface water, pollution in the atmosphere, and pollution on land eventually get into the ground water through the rain. Few things are as important for humankind as our supply of water. So it should be a matter of great concern that the quality of our water is getting worse and that we are using up our clean water much too quickly, disturbing the balance among the zones.

Industry and Water Pollution.   Chemicals, some of them dangerous, are used in every industrial process. And every industrial process creates by-products. Some of these chemicals can be reused, and some of the by-products are valuable. More often than not, however, they are worthless junk. In the past, useless chemicals and by-products were simply flushed into lakes and rivers, left to rot in fields, or buried.

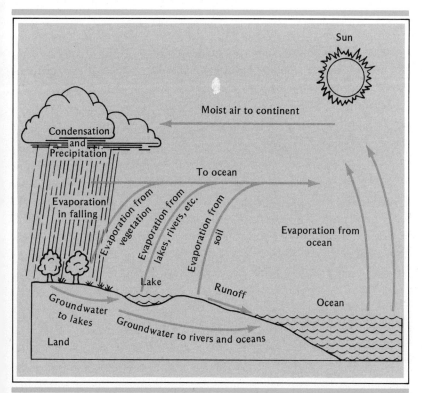

Figure 19-2.   The Water Cycle. The sun causes water on the earth's surface to evaporate into the atmosphere, where clouds are formed. The clouds condense, and rain falls to the earth, replenishing the water supply.

Chemicals and by-products flushed into lakes and rivers enter the water cycle directly and proceed to threaten or pollute all sources of water. Buried or stored chemicals and by-products enter the water cycle more slowly: First they seep into the ground, then into the ground water, and then into the water we drink. Since the 1970s the disposal of chemicals has been regulated more carefully. But these regulations are very hard to enforce.

Eutrophication.   Among the chemicals that seep into our sources of water are the fertilizers farmers use to get higher crop yields. When fertilizers enter lakes and streams, they encourage the growth of small plants called algae. By day these plants produce life-giving oxygen, but by night they produce carbon dioxide, which replaces oxygen. When the algae die, they sink to the bottom of the lake and rot, which uses up some of the lake's remaining oxygen. The lack of oxygen causes many of the fish that live at the lake's bottom to die. And if bacteria get into the lake through sewage and garbage, they use up more of its oxygen supply, and this kills the fish in the upper parts of the lake. In short, all the lake's fish are killed by the chemical enrichment of its waters, or *eutrophication,* and the lake becomes a slimy mess.

Toxic Wastes

Some industrial chemicals and by-products are, in themselves, fairly harmless. But some of them are toxic. The Environmental Protection Agency (EPA), a federal agency responsible for regulating environmental quality, estimates that each year American industries produce 770 billion pounds of wastes, 10 percent of them toxic.

Toxic wastes are dangerous whether or not they enter the water cycle. Some of them are poisonous and cause such problems as birth defects and cancer, both in humans and in wildlife. Some are corrosive; they can eat away storage containers and human skin. Some are reac-

How not to do it: a garbage dump.

Michael Hanulak/Photo Researchers

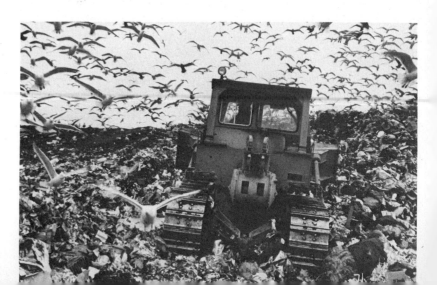

The Story of a Calamity

During the 1940s and early 1950s, the Hooker Chemical Company dumped chemical wastes from a factory in Niagara Falls, New York, into an abandoned waterway called Love Canal. Hooker acted quite legally, and in the actual dumping the company followed all the procedures it was required to follow. In 1953 Hooker sold the site to the local board of education for $1. The board then built a school on the landfill and sold adjoining lots to developers, who built houses on them. Particularly on warm days, the people who moved into those houses could smell chemical odors, but city officials told them not to worry.

The smell did not go away; it got worse. And the people in Love Canal suffered to an unusual degree from such problems as miscarriages, birth defects, and cancer. Finally, a young mother whose third child was mentally retarded got in touch with a local reporter. He found that the family's backyard was a chemical swamp, and the publicity from his articles led to further investigations. A state report later said that 5 out of 24 (nearly 21 percent) of the children born at Love Canal between 1958 and 1974 had birth defects.

The state closed the school in April 1978. In August President Jimmy Carter declared an emergency at Love Canal, and 237 families who lived in the first two rings of houses surrounding the old canal were evacuated by the state. Then the government money ran out. Others want to leave the area but cannot afford to; their houses, of course, are worthless.

Three other chemical dump sites were created in the same area, all of them larger than Love Canal and potentially more dangerous. It is pointless to try to fix the blame for this tragedy; the issue of toxic wastes is too complex. The important point is that there are hundreds of chemical dumps in the United States, and therefore hundreds of potential Love Canals.

---

tive, or unstable; occasionally they explode. Finally, some toxic wastes are ignitable—they can catch fire or give off poisonous gases or fumes.

Dumping. The heart of the problem of toxic wastes is the difficulty of getting rid of them. In the past—and perhaps, despite EPA regulations, in the present—hazardous wastes were dumped into landfills, ponds, fields, and lagoons. Often, they were not labeled, and the dump sites were just above supplies of drinking water. Some of the companies that specialized in disposing of wastes did not know their business, and these companies endangered the public. Of course, not all disposal companies were greedy, and not all of them were ignorant. But most of them did not—and still do not—have enough money to handle incoming wastes properly. (That means testing the barrels in which the wastes come and reinforcing the dangerous ones.) Fire is more than just a possibility at toxic-waste disposal sites; as one expert said, "It's not an 'if,' it's a 'when'."

Solid Wastes

Most of the kinds of pollution we have discussed so far are created by industry. Even industrial pollution is ultimately everyone's fault and everyone's concern, because industry produces goods for consumers, so it is ultimately consumer demand that creates the problem. (This is not to deny that industry plays an important role, too.) But the problem of *solid wastes* is for the most part created directly by consumers—by you. Solid wastes are the trash discarded by homes and businesses—everything from beer bottles to old screen doors. Several hundred million tons of it are churned out each year.

Solid wastes are by-products, and (as with other by-products) the problem is getting rid of them. Now, the trash of homes and businesses includes a lot of things that could be recycled (used again)—iron, steel, aluminum, and glass, for example—but only about 6 percent actually is. For recycling is a problem: Plants are expensive to build and operate, and our tax and transport systems favor new over recycled materials. Besides, the market for these materials is often poor.

Much solid waste that is not recycled is dumped into landfills and covered over by earth, whether it is first burned or not. But the number of landfill sites is small and falling. Some solid wastes are burned and then dumped in the ocean. Some are simply heaped up in empty lots, where they accumulate and become a health problem.

Pesticides

In 1962 a well-known writer named Rachel Carson (1907-1964) published a book called *Silent Spring* about the problem of *pesticides*, chemicals used by farmers to kill insects. Carson showed that pesticides harm human beings, birds, and fish, as well as insects; and she made

Spraying pesticides.

Joe Munroe/Photo Researchers

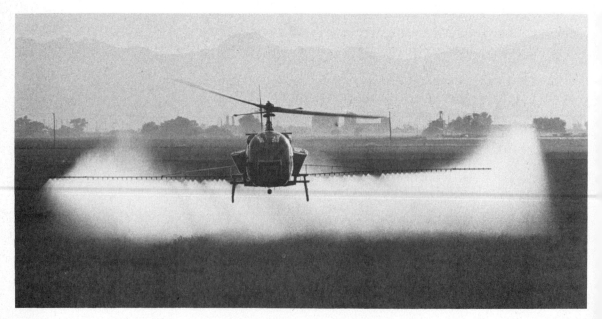

her point so convincingly and movingly that her book helped launch the environmental movement (see below).

In 1962 the most widely used pesticide was dichloro-diphenyl-trichloroethane—DDT—and although DDT was banned on January 1, 1973, it still gets into our bodies in many ways—mainly through eating animals that have eaten plants growing in formerly sprayed areas.

Pesticides are sprayed directly on many foods that we eat. Foods sprayed with pesticides are also eaten by animals that are eaten by us. Pesticides have entered the water cycle through ground water. Many Americans have a good deal of DDT in their bodies; for example, most mother's milk in this country would have too much DDT in it to be sold through interstate commerce.

It is hard to evaluate the long-term effects of pesticides on human health, since they have not been around very long and the body can rid itself of some—but not of others. High doses of DDT do kill birds and fish, and they also do accumulate in animal fat. This increases the risk of cancer, especially cancer of the liver, in humans who eat the meat (and fat) of such animals.

Heavy Metals

In April 1956 a 5-year-old girl entered a hospital in Minimata, Japan, a fishing village. Her brain was severely damaged, she was delirious, and she could neither talk nor walk. The girl was a victim of poisoning by mercury, one of the heavy metals. Mercury had been dumped into

Table 19-1. Poisons and Some of Their Effects

Poisons	Uses	Toxic Effects
Amides, Amines, & Imides	Plastics	Cancer and birth defects
Arsenic	Pharmaceutical products, such as boric acid	Skin and lung cancer
Benzene	A solvent in chemical processes	Leukemia
Cadmium	Electroplating; cadmium-silver oxide batteries; some other manufacturing processes	Kidney damage
Chromium	Paint pigment; electroplating processes	If swallowed: hemorrhages of the gastrointestinal tracts; inhaled through lungs: cancer of the respiratory tract
Copper	Many industrial uses	Irritation of the gastrointestinal tract
Esters & Ethers	Pesticides and herbicides	Destruction of brain nerves
Lead	Lead-acid batteries and pigments	Brain and bone damage
Manganese	Aluminum and steel; electroplating	Sleeplessness, leg cramps, spastic reflexes
Mercury	Chlorine, caustic soda, and other chemicals; metallurgical processes	Brain damage, birth defects; harms the central nervous system
Selenium	Electronic equipment, steel, pigments, ceramics, and glass	Eye, heart, and lung damage
Trichloroethylene (TCE)	A solvent	Gastrointestinal and nervous disorders

the local waters by a factory, and it had built up in fish—the staple of the local diet—and thus entered the bodies of the people of Minimata Bay.

The heavy metals—such as mercury, arsenic, cadmium, chromium, copper, lead, nickel, and zinc—get into human food in many ways. Lead, for example, is discharged into the air from automobiles and from lead smelting plants. It mixes with water vapor, falls to the earth's surface in the rain, and is absorbed by leafy vegetables; then it enters the bodies of the people who eat those vegetables. Mercury gets into our food through the ocean, which it enters through industrial pollutants. In the ocean, small plants absorb the mercury as they take in food from the water. When the plants are eaten by small fish they, too, are contaminated. The big fish eat the little fish; mercury therefore builds up in the bigger fish. The larger a fish may be, the more mercury it gets with every meal since the mercury continues to accumulate. At the top of the food chain, the bodies of the biggest meat-eating fish have concentrations of mercury that are much higher than those of the waters where these fish live, and sometimes they are unfit for human consumption.

When the heavy metals do get into our food they usually accumulate gradually and slowly affect the nervous system, which after a time starts to suffer from symptoms like those of Minimata disease.

Radiation

Back in the 1950s, the American public had a love affair with the atom. For military security the government relied, or claimed to rely, on the "maximum deterrence" of the H-bomb. And many people expected that atomic energy would some day provide most of the country's electrical energy, too. By the late 1970s, there were 73 atomic plants generating electricity in the United States. Many people still view atomic energy as the most realistic source of electricity for the near future, since we do not need to rely on foreigners for atomic energy. But many people are now scared of atomic energy, and since it is also expensive its future is doubtful.

One problem with atomic energy is the possibility that a reactor's nuclear core might melt down, releasing radiation into the air. This has come pretty close to happening, although it never actually has. But another important trait connected with atomic energy recurs all the time. When atomic energy is produced, radioactive by-products are produced along with it. Amazingly enough, no one has ever figured out what to do with these radioactive materials; the nuclear power industry has been allowed to expand for more than 25 years without coming up with a long-lasting solution. And a long-lasting solution is absolutely necessary, because some of this stuff will remain radioactive—and therefore dangerous—for *thousands of years*.

Meltdown!

It's been said that life imitates art. In 1979 a movie called *The China Syndrome* dramatized a fictional crisis in which the core of a nuclear reactor almost melted down and burned into the earth, releasing radiation. This catastrophe, which has never yet occurred, is called the "China Syndrome" because if a reactor in the United States were ever to melt down, some say it might burn straight through the planet, to China, on the other side of the earth.

In March 1979, shortly after the movie was released, an accident that might have led to the China Syndrome—but did not—took place at the Three Mile Island nuclear power plant, in Pennsylvania. A panel appointed by then-President Carter found that at least 30 tons of fuel in the reactor core had reached a temperature of no less than 4,000 degrees Fahrenheit. The meltdown point is about 5,200 degrees Fahrenheit. According to the commission, a bit of the fuel may actually have gotten that hot.

Right now, the nuclear power companies store their wastes in about 70 deep pools throughout the country. It is difficult to make these pools absolutely leakproof, so radioactive material is seeping out and entering the ground water and thus entering our water supplies. Earthquakes might eventually fracture the pools and release all of the dangerous wastes they contain. The fear of radioactive pollution of water is quite reasonable: Some years ago, 200,000 gallons of radioactive material stored at Hanford, Washington, leaked into the Columbia River.

Operational Problems.   Although the storage of wastes is the main problem with nuclear energy, actually operating the plants has created a few nightmares. Equipment failures are frequent, especially in the valves and pipes that regulate the reactors' cooling systems. The staffs of most nuclear power stations are not required to have much training. The Nuclear Regulatory Commission, the federal agency that is supposed to regulate the plants, is understaffed and cannot really do its job. Finally, utility companies, which own and operate the plants, sometimes cut corners on safety.

Three Mile Island Nuclear Plant.

Paul Concklin/Monkmeyer

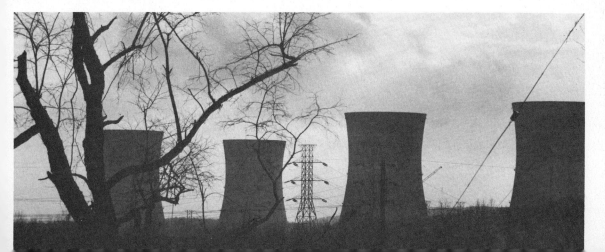

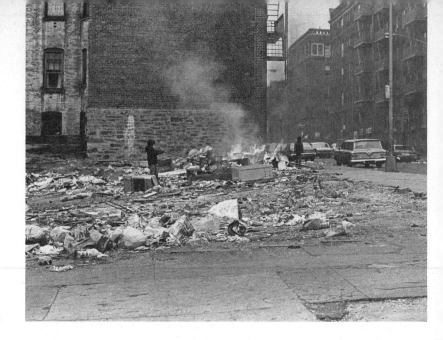

An urban slum.

A. W. Ambler/Photo Researchers

The Urban Environment

When people think of the environment they think of rural lakes and remote mountains. Yet most Americans do not live in the countryside. Don't the 70 percent of the American people who live in metropolitan areas have an environment? They do, but it is an urban environment.

This urban environment is in many ways really two quite separate and unequal environments: that of the rich and the middle class, on the one hand, and that of the poor, on the other. The problems of the urban environment show up most dramatically in the neighborhoods of the poor—the slums.

The Social Environment

Slums are ugly. The older buildings are dirty, overcrowded, and badly maintained. The new buildings, many of them in government-built housing projects, are also dirty, overcrowded, and badly maintained, and in addition they are dull to look at. Graffiti and garbage proliferate everywhere. Sometimes the housing stock in a slum becomes so bad that large areas are literally abandoned and fall to the arsonist's torch. This makes overcrowding elsewhere in the slum even worse. Crowding helps to raise crime rates and death rates.

Pests

You do not often think of cities as animal reserves, but cities (especially slums) provide homes for many species of animals. The most important of these is the species to which we ourselves belong—*homo sapiens*. Cities are also home to the animals that live off human beings, while contributing to human diseases. The three most important kinds of animal pests are rats, mice, and insects. These infest most parts of most cities; but the problem is worse in the slums because pests live off the city's garbage, and there is more exposed or untreated garbage in the slums.

Rats are a particular nuisance, for they are reservoirs of many infectious diseases (see Chapter 11), which they pass on to us by biting people and by contaminating our food and water supplies with their feces and urine. They also carry on their bodies a flea that is the reservoir of the bacterium that causes plague. Many cities have more rats than people. Rats get into houses and apartment buildings through open and unscreened doors and windows, through ventilators, under shallow or cracked house foundations, and through holes around electrical inlets and pipes. Even if you do not actually see them, you know that they are there if you see gnawing around doors, windows, utility lines, and packaged foods.

Noise Pollution

Noise is a more democratic problem than rats: It is probably no worse in poor neighborhoods than in rich ones. Sound is measured in decibels. At 0 decibels a noise becomes audible to a normal person. Ordinary breathing is 10 decibels, and whispering is 30. Heavy automobile traffic registers at 100 decibels, and the takeoff of a jet at 150. Some jets are even noisier; the Concorde, a supersonic transport plane (SST) made by the French and British, makes such a racket that it is permitted to land at only two airports in the United States. The noise from other jets becomes also, from time to time, a political issue.

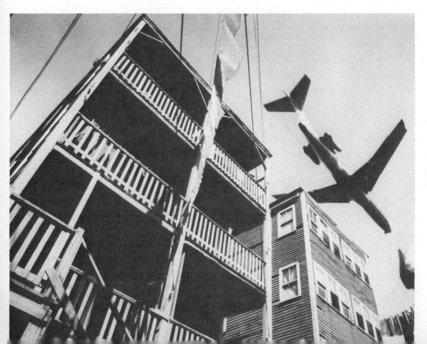

Noisy airplanes fly over rich and poor neighborhoods alike.
Michael Philip Manheim/Photo Researchers

Noise Pollution Scale

Sound	Intensity in Decibels	Sound	Intensity in Decibels
Human whisper	30	Printing press	97
Normal conversation	60	Farm tractor	98
City traffic	80	Punch press	105
Garbage disposal unit	80	Boiler shop	105
Vacuum cleaner	85	Textile looms	106
Garbage truck	85	Motorcycle	110
Food blender	93	Riveting gun	110
Subway train	95	Rock band (amplified)	114
Jackhammer	95	Drop hammer	130
Power lawnmower	96	Jet airplane	135 to 150

Noise may help produce such stress-related diseases (see Chapter 2) as hypertension and peptic ulcers. It also causes deafness. Still, noise pollution is easier to control than other kinds. Garbage collection, for example, causes a good deal of noise that might easily be reduced by requiring people to switch from metal garbage cans to rubber or plastic ones. Protective devices to screen out sounds are also widely available.

Social Action for the Environment

Conservationism and Environmentalism

The environmental movement is simply a new form of the conservation movement, which is over 70 years old. Back in 1908, Gifford Pinchot (then the head of the Forest Service) said that this country's natural resources should be used for the greatest good of the greatest number, for the longest period of time. That is still the movement's goal.

Environmental consciousness—the recognition that the earth and its resources are threatened—was shared by a very few people until 1962, when Rachel Carson's *Silent Spring* made more people aware of the harm done by pesticides. As this awareness spread, the threat to the environment became an issue of public debate and, finally, a political issue. The first fruits of that debate, the National Environmental Policy Act, came into effect on January 1, 1970, at the start of what many people call the "environmental decade." The act is still the cornerstone of federal legislation on the subject.

This and other laws really did reduce the level of water and air pollution; the amount of carbon monoxide in the air, for example, has been going down in the United States by about 7 percent a year since the

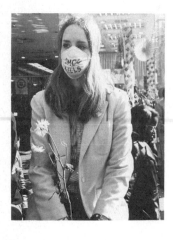

Earth Day, April 22, 1970, was a milestone for the environmental movement.

Winston Vargus/Photo Researchers

early 1970s; and there are fish again in such places as New York's once-dead Hudson River. But preserving the environment is not cheap; it costs money, and the expense is passed on by industry to consumers. Since these additional expenses may reduce a product's sales, industry by and large opposes environmental regulation. Besides, most of us care more about ourselves than about anything else.

Even people who are sympathetic to environmentalism do not always agree on how to serve the cause. For example, environmentalists think that oil should be conserved. But some of them think that it should be conserved by raising its price; others think it should be conserved by rationing.

Future of the Spaceship Earth: Population and Other Problems

The problem of the environment is worldwide, but as yet there are no worldwide solutions. One nation can easily undo what another nation does, and some problems that affect the world as a whole seem to be utterly beyond control. The most important of these is over-population.

Too Many People

The planet earth now holds about 4 billion people. By the year 2000 it will hold 8 billion. Even now, about half of the world's people are *always* hungry, and many others are often so. Since between now and the year 2000 the world's population may grow more rapidly than its food supply, by 2000 it is possible that even more people will be starving.

Table 19–2. Population Projections, by Region: 1978 to 2000

Region	1978	1985	1990	2000
World, total	4,258.7	4,829.8	5,275.3	6,198.6
More developed	1,115.9	1,168.9	1,205.8	1,272.3
Less developed	3,142.7	3,660.9	4,069.5	4,926.4
Africa	442.5	544.5	630.4	828.1
Latin America	349.4	420.6	478.4	608.1
Northern America	242.2	258.5	270.5	289.5
East Asia	1,107.9	1,203.6	1,274.5	1,405.9
South Asia	1,352.8	1,606.1	1,802.6	2,205.3
Europe (excl. Soviet Union)	480.2	492.4	501.2	520.2
Soviet Union	261.6	279.6	291.6	311.8
Oceania	22.1	24.4	26.2	29.6

(In millions. Source of data presents 3 series of projections. Figures shown here are for *medium series*)
Source: U.S. Bureau of the Census, *Statistical Abstract of the United States, 1980* (101st ed.), table 1574, p. 900.

How many human beings could this planet of ours support? Some people speculate that if the world's food resources were developed and used with all possible efficiency, about 30 billion people might be kept alive in a state of chronic near-starvation. At the moment, the world's population is growing by about 2 percent each year; and at that rate, it will take 100 years to reach this limit. If population were to grow more rapidly—and this is not impossible—the maximum might be reached in 60 or so years.

And in 60 years many of you will still be alive.

Too Few Resources

Population becomes overpopulation when there is not enough of the most important of all resources: food. But food is not the only resource that is in short supply. By the year 2000 the industrial countries may face critical shortages of such raw materials as mercury, tin, helium, and petroleum. America's coal reserves will probably last much longer. But water, the essence of life, is already scarce in some parts of the United States, and the shortage will spread to other parts of the country.

Too Few Solutions

The problems of population and resources are essentially global in scope. But there are no truly global political institutions to deal with

Figure 19–3. World Population, 1975 and 1979, with Projections to 2000.

Source: U.S. Bureau of the Census, *Statistical Abstract of the United States, 1980* (101st ed.), table 1571, p. 896.

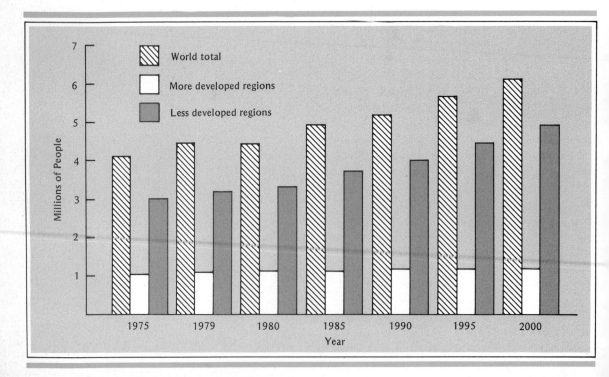

Goals

In the long run, the mind and conscience of humanity can achieve great things. But we may not have much time. If the human race is going to survive, we shall have to reduce the rate of population growth and give up the idea that consuming material things is good in itself. Below are a few goals that could help us do that. If they seem utopian—we're in a lot of trouble.

Among the goals that might help us survive—and survive as human beings—are the following:

- Getting all societies to accept the two-child family norm as quickly as possible.
- Seeking a more equitable distribution of the world's resources between rich and poor countries.
- Striving through science to increase food production, while reducing consumption of vital resources, such as oil.
- Emphasizing activities, like education and music, that do not use up raw materials.
- Setting up research and planning centers to deal with natural resources and to anticipate future needs.
- Passing laws to limit the weight and horsepower of trucks and automobiles.

This isn't a complete list of worthwhile goals. Try to think of others.

them, and it is not clear how to reconcile the conflicting interests of different countries. Nor is it clear what the rich countries owe to the poor ones, or what the present owes to the future. One expert has suggested, for example, that a billion people could live on the food eaten by only 220 million Americans. Yet since virtually all this food is produced in the United States, it might be argued that it is simply ours, and that we have no obligation to share it with others. Even if we share it, how should we do so? Some people say we should only help countries that are politically sympathetic to us. Others think we should only help countries that have a real chance for survival and should abandon those that do not, much as hopelessly wounded soldiers on a battlefield are often left to die so that medical aid can be used to save those who are less seriously wounded.

Two things *are* clear: The problems of the poor nations will certainly affect the rich ones; we ourselves, for example, already feel the effects of starvation abroad in the form of very high rates of illegal immigration. And whatever the present may owe to the future, the future is not far away.

SUMMARY

Human beings, particularly in the Western countries, once regarded the earth as a limitless storehouse of resources. Humanity's job, in that view, was to conquer those resources and dominate the earth. More and more people now realize that humanity must learn to live in harmony with nature, not in a contest against it.

But others have yet to outgrow older attitudes, whose consequences affect us in the form of pollution. Water and air pollution were the first kinds to be recognized and (in the United States) dealt with effectively. As a result, the levels of water and air pollution have been reduced here, although the environmental problems caused by sludge, solid wastes, heavy metals, toxic wastes, and radiation still await effective action. In great measure, these problems are due to our failure to find safe and permanent ways of getting rid of these substances.

Cities—where most Americans live—have their own environmental problems. Some of them, like solid wastes, and rats and other pests, affect slums more than the other parts of cities. But other problems, noise, for example, affect all parts about equally.

The environmental movement, which emerged in the 1960s and grew in the 1970s, is a more broadly based and better-publicized form of the older conservation movement. Both seek to preserve the environment for the greatest good of the greatest number. The movement has helped to enact laws to protect the environment. But this protection costs money and curtails profits and so is opposed by much of industry.

Despite these disputes, the United States is moving to solve some of its environmental problems. In the world as a whole the story is different. Many countries are indifferent to these problems; others fail to deal with them effectively. And the world's population may be growing more rapidly than its resources. The problems of the future—problems that will affect both rich and poor countries—are not far away.

Suggested Readings

Berry, James Wesley. *Chemical Villains: A Biology of Pollution.* St. Louis: Mosby, 1974. A reference for the in-depth study of the biological aspects of environmental pollution.

Eckholm, Erick P. *The Picture of Health: Environmental Sources of Disease.* New York: Norton, 1977. A study of the effects of the environment on the health of humans.

Ehrlich, Anne, and Ehrlich, Frank. *Human Ecology: Problem and Solutions.* San Francisco, Freeman, 1973. A good source for the way humans relate to their environment—it cites some of the problems and some of the solutions.

Freeman, A. Myrick. *The Benefits of Environmental Improvement: Theory and Practice.* Baltimore: Johns Hopkins University Press, 1979. A practical look into the benefits gained from various improvements in the environment.

Hafen, Brent Q. *Man, Health and Environment.* Minneapolis: Burgess, 1972. This book relates the effects of the environment on humans and human health.

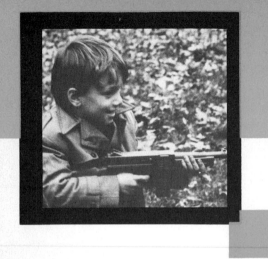

20

Violence

chapter objectives

When you have finished reading this chapter you should be able to:

1. Recognize the scope of violence in the United States
2. Explain the different theories of violent behavior
3. Discuss the impact of violence on society
4. Explain the role of family violence
5. Distinguish between individual violence and social violence

Through religion, through schooling, through the mass media, and in hundreds of other ways, society teaches its members that violence is bad. Yet acts of violence are common. Murder, for example, is the second leading cause of death among people aged 15 to 24, right ahead of suicide, itself a form of violence. Young adults are more likely to die from violence than from cancer and more likely to be disabled by violence than by heart disease; violence, in fact, helps to cause heart disease.

Something, somewhere is going terribly wrong. But what?

The Roots of Violence

The Impaired Self-image

Self-esteem—feeling good about yourself—is the basis of mental health (see Chapter 1). People fail to develop self-esteem when they fail to achieve such important life goals as financial and professional success. These failures breed feelings of self-hatred, uselessness, inferiority, and anger, feelings that isolate people from society and make them think that its rules, which do not benefit them, somehow do not apply to them either. These are the people who overcome society's restraints

Figure 20–1. Half of all murders are committed with handguns.

Source: U.S. Department of Justice, FBI Uniform Crime Reports, *Crime in the United States 1979.* Release date September 24, 1980, p. 12.

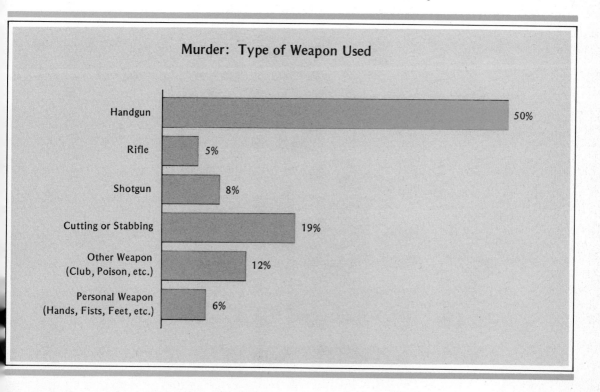

Murder: Type of Weapon Used

Weapon	Percentage
Handgun	50%
Rifle	5%
Shotgun	8%
Cutting or Stabbing	19%
Other Weapon (Club, Poison, etc.)	12%
Personal Weapon (Hands, Fists, Feet, etc.)	6%

Definition

Murder and nonnegligent manslaughter, as defined in the Uniform Crime Reporting Program, is the willful (nonnegligent) killing of one human being by another.

The classification of this offense, as in all other Crime Index offenses, is based solely on police investigation as opposed to the determination of a court, medical examiner, coroner, jury, or other judicial body. Not included in the count for this offense classification are deaths caused by negligence, suicide, or accident; justifiable homicides, which are the killings of felons by law enforcement officers in the line of duty or by private citizens; and attempts to murder or assaults to murder, which are scored as aggravated assaults.

Trend

Year	Number of Offenses	Rate per 100,000 Inhabitants
1978	19,555	9.0
1979	21,456	9.7
Percent change	+9.7	+7.8

Source: U.S. Department of Justice, FBI Uniform Crime Reports, *Crime in the United States 1979*. Release date September 24, 1980, pp. 6–7.

on violence, for violence gives such people a sense of power, self-worth, purpose, and achievement.

Social Frustration. Americans tend to assume that anyone, however poor, can become anything—a millionaire, a movie star, a lawyer, what have you. We all want to become rich, famous, and successful; and we

Learning violence: 1.

Bonnie Freer/Photo Researchers

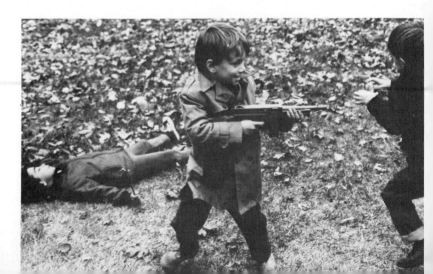

all compare ourselves with people who have actually done so. This pressure for success is one of the great sources of stress in our society, for people who do not measure up to their hopes do not develop self-esteem.

The pressure, and the feelings of failure that, often go along with it, are sometimes so strong that, according to Robert K. Merton (1910–   ), a famous American sociologist, they sometimes cause people to behave violently. Most people at first seek success in ways that are approved by society—getting good grades, for example. But some people cannot do these things, and others find that virtue does not pay. The pressure to succeed still bears down upon them, so they turn to other ways of achieving success, especially to violent ones.

Violence as a Learned Response

Behaviorist theories of violence attempt to explain how we *learn* to act aggressively, not the *drives* that produce aggressive acts. The behaviorists say that human beings at birth have no disposition to violence and, in fact, do not even know how to behave violently. This knowledge has to be learned, either through observation or direct experience. Most violent people first observed violence or became victims of it in their own families (see below). Some people learn habits of aggression by taking part in organized violence, as soldiers, for example, and sometimes they have much trouble returning to civilian life because they cannot forget the violence that was drilled into them. Others learn habits of violence because they are born into (or become part of) the "subculture of violence," groups that consciously reject society's rules, including its rules about violence.

Reinforcement.   People do not always imitate the behavior they see, and they do not always repeat a particular kind of behavior after they have done it once. They need a reason to learn any kind of behavior and such reasons are called "reinforcement" (see Chapter 1). Reinforcements for violence might include money or prestige. And when people see violence rewarded they are the more ready to behave violently themselves ("vicarious" reinforcement); the sight of punishment for violence makes them more cautious.

Kinds of Violence

Domestic Violence

About 50 million Americans a year (out of 226 million in 1980) suffer from violence inflicted by close relatives. Of these 50 million, 6.5 million are children. But they are avenged by the 8 million or so children (18 percent of the total) who each year injure their parents. And in 16 per-

Learning violence: 2.

Jason Laure/Woodfin Camp & Associates

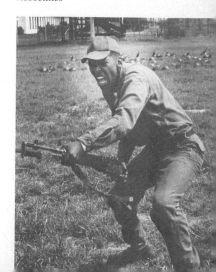

Aggravated Assault

Definition

Aggravated assault is an unlawful attack by one person upon another for the purpose of inflicting severe or aggravated bodily injury. This type of assault is usually accompanied by the use of a weapon or by means likely to produce death or great bodily harm. Attempts are included since it is not necessary that an injury result when a gun, knife, or other weapon is used which could and probably would result in serious personal injury if the crime were successfully completed.

Trend

Year	Number of offenses	Rate per 100,000 Inhabitants
1978	558,102	255.9
1979	614,213	279.1
Percent change	+10.1	+9.1

Source: U.S. Department of Justice, FBI Uniform Crime Reports, *Crime in the United States 1979.* Release date September 24, 1980, p. 19.

cent of American marriages, husbands or wives have physically abused their spouses.

These violent families are the breeding ground of violence in general, for in them children first come by feelings of self-hatred and learn to behave violently.

Child Abuse.   Children who are abused by their parents live in all parts of the United States and come from every social class. And their parents are not, as a group, any more prone to severe mental illness than other people.

What then makes a child abuser?

Child abusers almost always report that, as children, they themselves were victims of abuse. They often say that they got little warmth or support from their parents. As adults they often lack self-esteem and rarely feel happy. They distrust other people and usually do not seek out adults for support or help. Their goal in life is merely to escape punishment, criticism, and ridicule.

Child abusers do not perceive their own children as real people. They think that children exist to please their parents—indeed, that children belong to their parents. Child abusers, in fact, are childish. Unconsciously, they want to become children themselves, and they want their

How to Spot Child Abuse

These signs may indicate that children are being abused by their parents:

- Repeated bruises, burns, and cuts, and no good explanation for them.
- Very shy or very aggressive behavior.
- Frequent wandering or lack of supervision.
- Isolation of the family.
- Parental indifference to a child's needs.

own children to become the loving parents they never had. When child abusers have to cope with the stresses of living in the real world, such as unemployment or divorce, they turn to their children for help and support. But children are too young to understand such problems fully, and the abuser responds with resentment, anger, and violence to the child's inability to help. Most child abusers are not aggressive outside the home; on the contrary, they are shy and submissive people who deposit their anger within the family.

Child abusers are partly responsible for the epidemic of violence in American society, for it is they who pass on the idea that violence is an acceptable way of solving problems. Children who are physically punished by their parents learn that violence is a legitimate means of discipline. But some of them do not learn that violence is legitimate only within very narrow limits. Later in life, they often turn to violence themselves, and quite commonly they grow up to be child abusers.

Abuse of Spouses.   In the 1970s the women's movement made the abuse of women by their husbands a national issue. But spouse abuse itself is as old as marriage, and it is hard to say if it is more common now or less so, though it certainly is common: Each year husbands severely injure about 1.8 million or so women. Abuse of husbands, too, is quite common, though it would be hard to say how common. One study claims that the number of abused husbands and wives is about equal. Women, however, are more likely to tolerate abuse (mainly because they have difficulty supporting themselves) and are more likely to be injured seriously. But women often resort to what one expert calls "protective reaction violence": Wives who anticipate attacks by their husbands often attack first, and forcefully.

Spouse abuse and child abuse have common roots. Spouse abusers, like child abusers, treat their families as means to their own childish ends by using their families to relieve frustrations. In many families, the husband abuses the wife, the wife abuses the older children, and the older children abuse the younger ones.

Preventing Domestic Violence.   Families infected by domestic violence are usually so isolated from other people that they cannot ask for help. Breaking through this isolation is often the most important—and difficult—part of helping them, and that is why programs for counseling these families are necessary. Self-help groups like Parents Anonymous give support to parents who have abused (or fear abusing) their children. About 500 local programs have been set up to help battered wives, and a number of counseling programs for their husbands exist, too. The police have been reluctant to arrest husbands who abuse their wives, but they are feeling more and more pressure to do so.

Where to Find Help

Child Abuse

- Parents Anonymous (800 421-0353; 800 352-0386 in California): A national organization of self-help groups for parents who either abuse or fear they will abuse their children.
- National Center on Child Abuse and Neglect (Department of Health and Human Services, Box 1182, Washington, D.C. 20013): Write for information on child abuse or for the location of your area's resource center.

Spouse Abuse

- Office on Domestic Violence (Department of Health and Human Services, Box 1182, Washington, D.C. 20013; 202 472-4205): Information and materials on spouse abuse.
- National Coalition Against Domestic Violence (1728 N Street N.W., Washington, D.C. 20036; 202 347-7015): An organization of women's shelters and domestic-violence programs across the country.

Street Crime

Levels of murder, assault, robbery, and rape began to move up in the late 1960s. In 1970 there were 365 violent crimes, mostly street crimes, for each 100,000 Americans. By 1979 the number had risen to 535 per 100,000. These statistics are controversial and probably should not be taken at face value. But it is certain that there is an awful lot of street crime in the United States—more than in other industrial countries. In the cities, the level of crime may have stopped rising in the late 1970s, though it did not go down. But in the suburbs and in rural areas it continues to rise, and to rise dramatically.

Why should this situation have come about in this nation, a nation that has always prided itself on its law and order? Can the causes be traced back to our rugged-pioneer tradition, to our you-can-have-what-

High Noon (the Hollywood Western): Good against Evil on Main Street.

Museum of Modern Art

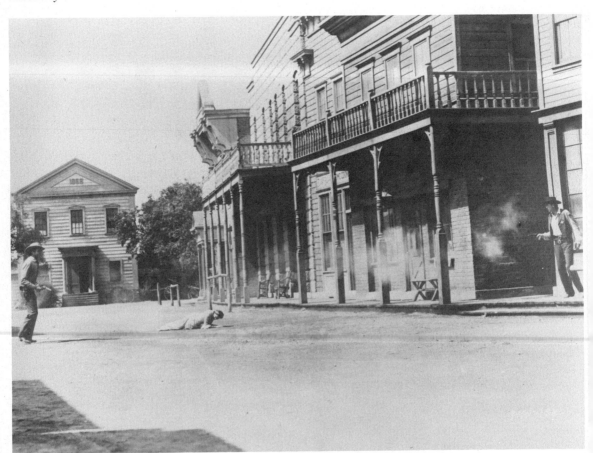

ever-you-want-if-you-want-it-enough philosophy, to our alleged loss of religion?

Why?   The causes of American street crime are debated with vigor. Police officials blame a loss of respect for law and moral values, a lack

Figure 20–2.   Crime Clock for the United States. *Source:* U.S. Department of Justice, FBI Uniform Crime Reports, *Crime in the United States 1979.* Release date September 24, 1980, p. 5.

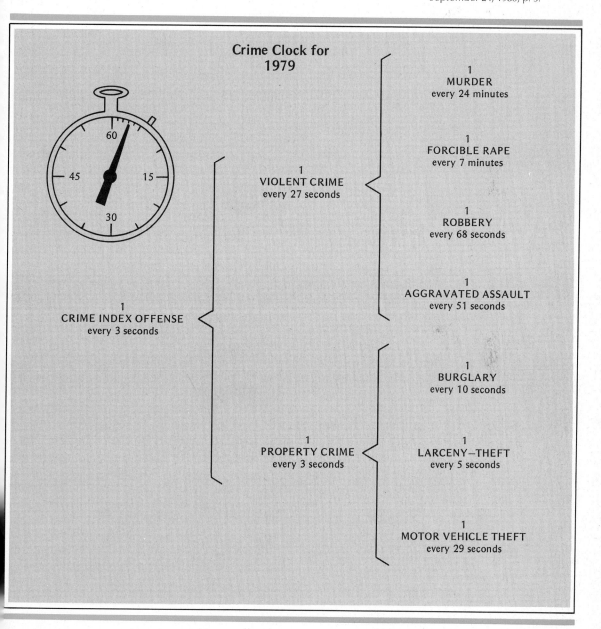

Crime Clock for 1979

1 CRIME INDEX OFFENSE every 3 seconds

1 VIOLENT CRIME every 27 seconds

1 MURDER every 24 minutes

1 FORCIBLE RAPE every 7 minutes

1 ROBBERY every 68 seconds

1 AGGRAVATED ASSAULT every 51 seconds

1 PROPERTY CRIME every 3 seconds

1 BURGLARY every 10 seconds

1 LARCENY–THEFT every 5 seconds

1 MOTOR VEHICLE THEFT every 29 seconds

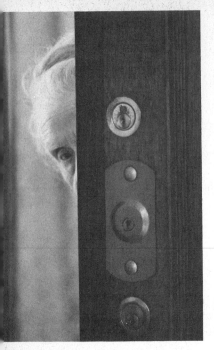

Jan Lukas/Rapho/Photo
Researchers

of self-discipline, and drugs. Some studies suggest that 50 percent of street crimes are committed by drug abusers who need money to support their habits, and misuse of alcohol also plays a major part. Some people argue that poverty is the ultimate cause both of drug misuse and street crime. Others point out that street crimes are mostly committed by young adults, and young adults are now a larger part of our population than they were at most times in the past (see Chapter 16). It is young adults—especially those belonging to minority groups—who have the highest levels of unemployment and, therefore, of poverty.

Helping the Victims. Until recently, law enforcement officials tried to find and punish criminals and largely ignored the victims of crime. Yet these victims need help, and a few hospitals and mental-health clinics now provide support groups and outpatient counseling for them.

Whether or not victims of crime get help, it is normal for them to go through a phase similar to grief and mourning (see Chapter 16) after the death of a relative or friend, and this phase should not be cut short. Some people find it very difficult to recover from a crime and need quite a long time to do so.

Rape

Rape is a crime of passion but not of sexual passion, for rapists are weak men who try to assert themselves by dominating and humiliating people, usually women. Insecurity and contempt are the passions behind rape, not lust. Rapists are not particular about the women they attack; on the contrary almost any woman—of any age, size, or appearance—will do. The rape of a man by a man is usually inspired by the same motives that cause men to rape women.

Many rapes are physically brutal, and many tear apart their victims' emotional lives. Sex—even legal, "normal" sex—still creates much guilt, doubt, and fear. Rape creates even more of these feelings. The victims' inability to protect themselves makes them feel shame and self-hatred. They wonder if they will ever feel safe in their bodies again. They do not know if they will be viewed as victims of a horrible crime or as temptresses partly responsible for it. The trial, if it comes to that, may be as much their trial as the rapists', for the defendants' lawyers can accuse the victims of lying (there are rarely witnesses) or of being promiscuous. In the latter case, their sex lives may be examined in detail.

Preventing rape means making compromises. Women must be cautious about where, how, and when they move about, and if they must err, let it be on the side of caution. When a woman is confronted by a rapist and cannot escape, she should try to talk him out of his design. Sad to say, if the rapist is armed, most police officials think it is wiser to submit.

Forcible Rape

Definition

Forcible rape is defined as the carnal knowledge of a female forcibly and against her will. Assaults or attempts to commit rape by force or threat of force are included in the statistics shown here; however, statutory rape (without force) and other sex offenses are not included in this category.

Trend

Year	Number of Offenses	Rate per 100,000 Inhabitants
1978	67,131	30.8
1979	75,989	34.5
Percent change	+13.2	+12.0

Source: U.S. Department of Justice, FBI Uniform Crime Reports, *Crime in the United States 1979*. Release date September 24, 1980, pp. 13–14.

Violence in the Schools

Each year about 9,000 teachers and students in the United States are assaulted sexually. Some 70,000 teachers are injured so seriously that they have to get medical treatment. The yearly damage to school property runs to $600 million. The worst of it is that many teachers cannot teach and many students cannot learn, because their schools are filled with fear.

Why? The reasons for this state of affairs are similar to those which produce violence in general. Many school children are plagued by poor self-esteem—in part because they do poorly in school. Through school violence, they attempt to lash out at their troubles: It gives them revenge, a sense of purpose, and a feeling of power and achievement.

Some people blame school violence—and many other problems as well—on what they call "permissiveness." They think that parents and schools have given students too much freedom at too early an age, and that courts are too easy on youthful criminals. Young people, they argue, do not want freedom so much as a clear sense of limits. When young people are given freedom without such limits, they abuse it, or so this argument runs.

Finally, many people think that television, radio, the newspapers, and the magazines promote violence in the schools by publicizing it so very much.

The Cost of Violence

We pay for violence in many ways. First, two-thirds of all violent crimes cause physical injury. When someone is murdered or seriously injured, the victim's family may lose its source of income; the community may lose a productive worker; and the local, state, and federal governments may lose tax dollars. The victim may have high medical bills and, if not capable of working, may be forced to live on welfare or disability payments; and the government—that is, the taxpayers—must pick up the tab. Even so, government compensation to victims of crime rarely pays back more than a small part of any victim's loss.

The cost of crime.

Richard Hutchings/Photo Researchers

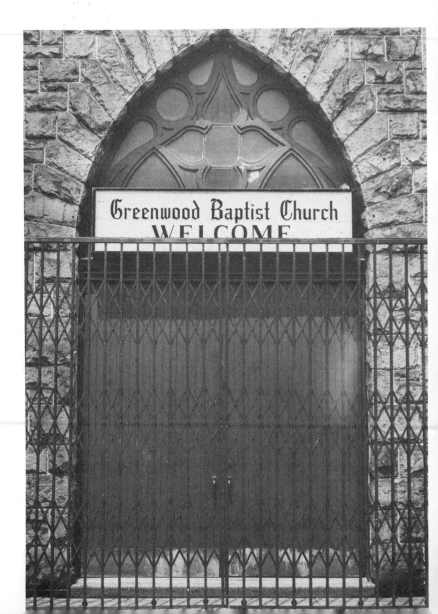

"I Want Your Money . . ."

It may be broad daylight or late at night. It may be in your own home or in some strange neighborhood. But the chances are substantial that at some point in your life, you will be the victim of violent crime. It helps if you have already thought out some basic strategies.

Any robber with a weapon has you at an insurmountable disadvantage. Do not try to be a hero. Even people with decades of training in the martial arts will not resist an opponent with a knife or a gun. In this situation, a safe escape, not holding on to your wallet, counts as an unqualified victory. A can of repellent like Mace will be of little use. By the time you get it out, a robber could shoot or stab you several times.

Police officials also advise against trying to negotiate to keep some of your things. The longer you delay a mugger, the more nervous he will be that someone will observe the crime and call the police. In reaching for your wallet, move slowly and calmly, explaining what you are doing. Otherwise, you may startle the mugger into attacking.

Source: *Time*, January 23, 1981, p. 21.

Violence against property is expensive, too. Arson, the deliberate setting of fires, destroys an enormous amount of property each year. Vandalism costs an immense amount of money; merely replacing the broken windows of American public schools takes between $4 million and $5 million annually. In New York City, vandalism raises the costs of building construction by about 30 percent.

Violence also has hidden, indirect costs. When people fear crime, they start to live differently, at least if they can afford to. They take taxis instead of buses. They put locks and burglar alarms in their houses, and they buy weapons. Businesses hire guards and put up gates and grillwork over their windows, and they pass the costs along to us. In one way or another, everyone pays for the high cost of violence.

Finally, one part of the cost, the emotional cost, is paid by the victims alone. During the crime, they fall under an enemy's power and lose control over their fates and bodies. Some people never overcome the fear and terror of this moment and are uncomfortable in public places or in their own homes for the rest of their lives. Even when the victims are not in physical danger, as when a home is burgled, they experience what experts call a "violation of self," for most people regard their homes as a part and parcel of themselves.

Collective Violence

So far we have only examined the kinds of violence that individuals commit against other individuals. All modern societies forbid this kind of violence and punish it. But society tolerates, and even exalts, another kind of violence: the violence of one society against another—war.

Why are these two kinds of violence treated so differently? The reason is that every society has both a positive and a negative aspect. Belonging to a society in the positive sense means sharing its customs and beliefs, its moments of triumph, and its moments of shame. Belonging to it in the negative sense means *not* belonging to another society. Societies are mutually exclusive; you can be an American and a member

Table 20–1.   Casualties in World War II

Country	Men in War	Battle Deaths	Wounded
Australia	1,000,000	26,976	180,864
Austria	800,000	280,000	350,117
Belgium	625,000	8,460	55,513[1]
Brazil[2]	40,334	943	4,222
Bulgaria	339,760	6,671	21,878
Canada	1,041,080	32,412	53,145
China[3]	17,250,521	1,324,516	1,762,006
Czechoslovakia	—	6,683[4]	8,017
Denmark	—	4,339	—
Finland	500,000	79,047	50,000
France	—	201,568	400,000
Germany	20,000,000	3,250,000[4]	7,250,000
Greece	—	17,024	47,290
Hungary	—	147,435	89,313
India	2,393,891	32,121	64,354
Italy	3,100,000	149,496[4]	66,716
Japan	9,700,000	1,270,000	140,000
Netherlands	280,000	6,500	2,860
New Zealand	194,000	11,625[4]	17,000
Norway	75,000	2,000	—
Poland	—	664,000	530,000
Romania	650,000[5]	350,000[6]	—
South Africa	410,056	2,473	—
U.S.S.R.	—	6,115,000[4]	14,012,000
United Kingdom	5,896,000	357,116[4]	369,267
United States	16,112,566	291,557	670,846
Yugoslavia	3,741,000	305,000	425,000
TOTAL	84,149,208	14,942,962	26,570,408

[1]Civilians only.   [2]Army and navy figures.   [3]Figures cover period July 7, 1937–September 2, 1945, and concern only Chinese regular troops. They do not include casualties suffered by guerrillas and local military corps.   [4]Deaths from all causes.   [5]Against Soviet Russia: 385,847 against Nazi Germany.
[6]Against Soviet Russia: 169,822 against Nazi Germany.
Source: U.S. Bureau of the Census.

of the Boy Scouts, for example, but not an American and a European. Often this sense of not belonging to other societies degenerates into a feeling of hostility against them. Members of different societies find it easy to accept clichés and rumors about each other: They forget that societies, like people, have a right to differ, and that these differences are precious. Yet members of different societies often hate each other for their very similarities: Each society denounces "them" for doing the same things it finds heroic in "us." These sad and dangerous attitudes kill the moral sense. They delude us into thinking that people in other societies are not fully human. They lead to violence, to war, to genocide, and to misery in every other form.

Nuremberg, Germany, September 1945—a few months after the end of World War II. *UPI*

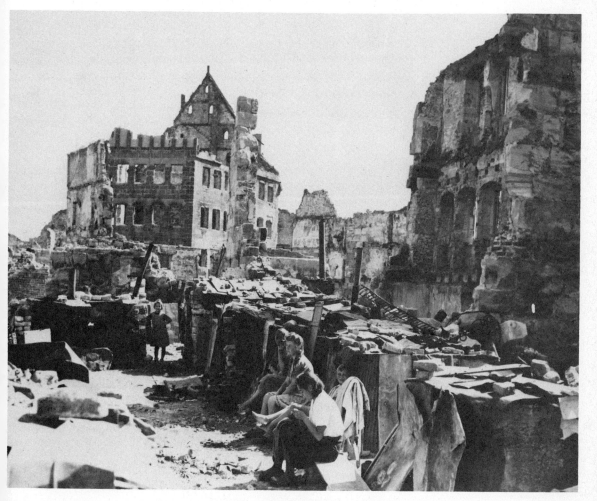

SUMMARY

Violence in American society affects almost everyone, but it affects young people in particular because they are most often the victims and the criminals. In some schools, violence became so widespread in the 1970s that it got in the way of teaching and learning.

Violence, according to some experts, has its roots in feelings of inferiority, feelings that sometimes make people attempt to gain self-respect in any way they can—violence, for example. Behaviorists maintain that habits of violence are learned, as everything else is learned, through observation, imitation, and reinforcement.

Feelings of inferiority are often generated within the primary family group, parents and children, and it is here that violence is learned. Child abusers teach their children that violence is an acceptable way of coping with problems. Like spouse abusers, they try to use their children to bolster their own fragile self-esteem. The children of child abusers often become child abusers themselves. These families are the breeding ground of violence.

The level of violent crime rose in the United States throughout the 1970s. Crime's total cost—physical, economic, and emotional—rose, too. The emotional cost of rape is particularly high, but in the 1970s an effort was made to help the victims of rape and also those of other crimes.

People who commit violent crimes are mostly, in society's eyes, failures. Yet their failures in part are society's failures. For it is society that has failed to create real opportunities for all its members, on the one hand, but that still subjects all of them to relentless pressures to succeed, on the other. The reality is so different from the ideal that many people lose self-esteem and cannot cope with the stresses of failure. Sometimes the result is individual sickness: drug taking or mental illness. And sometimes the result is violence, a social sickness. These problems will continue to plague us until everyone in our society has a real chance to develop self-esteem and everyone accepts a personal responsibility to make the most of that chance.

Suggested Readings

Cole, Michelle. *The Tyranny of the Meek Violent Sheep.* New York: New York Times Books, 1980. This book defines the passive and the psychic violence that affects our daily lives.

Hartup, Willard W., and De Wit, Jan. *Origins of Aggression.* The Hague: Mouton, 1978. This book includes a variety of articles on aggression and its development.

Hornstein, Harvey A. *Cruelty and Kindness.* Englewood Cliffs, N.J.: Prentice-Hall, 1976. A book on the human potential toward violence and aggression—a new look at aggression and altruism.

Newman, Braeme. *Understanding Violence.* New York: Harper & Row, 1979. This book delves into the diverse aspects of violence.

Scherer, Klaus R., et al. *Human Aggression and Conflict.* Englewood Cliffs, N.J.: Prentice-Hall, 1975. An investigation of conflict and aggression from the point of view of psychology and sociology. Causes and motivational aspects are explored.

Newsweek. "Plague of Violent Crime," March 23, 1981, p. 50.

Science. "Identifying the Dangerous Individual," April 17, 1981, p. 310.

Society. "Crime and Unemployment," July/August 1980, p. 2.

U.S. News & World Report. "Toll of Violence: 1.3 Million," April 13, 1981, p. 70.

Appendix:
First Aid and
Safety

objectives

When you have finished reading this appendix you should be able to:

1. Make up a first-aid kit
2. Help out in an emergency
3. Keep a safe home
4. Know where to get help when sudden illness strikes

Would you know what to do if you had an automobile accident and everyone in your car but you were injured? Or if someone in your house or dorm were to swallow a poison? Or if a friend were to overdose on a drug? Remember: It will be too late to learn after an accident. "Be prepared"—the Boy Scouts' motto—is more than a slogan; it can save lives—your own, perhaps.

How can you prepare yourself? First, become familiar with the first aid and safety tips discussed below. Second, find out if an emergency medical service (EMS) exists in your community. EMS means more than just an ambulance; it includes first aid, hospital services, and rehabilitation, and a communications system that ties them all together. Find out how to call the nearest EMS; you can start by checking the phone book for a special emergency number. Third, take a course in cardiopulmonary resuscitation (CPR, see below) from the American National Red Cross or the American Heart Association. Finally, in any emergency, no matter what sort, keep calm and do your best. That is all anyone can ask of you.

First Aid.   What is first aid? It means immediate care given to victims of injuries or sudden illnesses. Putting on a bandage is first aid, and so too is attempting to stop serious bleeding. Sometimes first aid is enough, but often it is only the first step in treatment. People with serious injuries or illnesses must be taken to hospitals or to physicians.

Table A–1.   Suggested First-Aid Kit Contents

First-Aid Item	Use
Activated charcoal	To bind and/or absorb poison
Adhesive bandages (Band-Aids)—different sizes; plastic-coated to avoid sticking	Open wounds
Adhesive tape—1- and 2-inch rolls—1 roll of each size	To hold dressings and bandages in place
Alcohol (70%)—1-pint bottle	For poison ivy; to sterilize; to cool body (except infants)
Alcohol wipes—towelettes—12	To clean hands
Aspirin—5 gr.—and Tylenol	Depress pain
Baking soda—small container	In case of delayed medical attention for third-degree burns and/or shock
Bandage—3 x 1-inch roller	Finger bandages
Bandage—3 x 2-inch rollers	To hold dressings in place
Bulb aspirator	Suck blood and other secretions from back of throat
Calamine lotion—bottle, 4 to 6 ounces	Poison ivy, poison sumac, poison oak, and soothe minor bites and stings
Constriction band made of rubber tubing	Bites and stings
Cotton applicators—1 package	To make swabs
Cotton (sterile) half-ounce package	Swabs
Dimes and nickels	For pay-telephone calls
Elastic wraps (Ace bandages) 2- and 3-inch width, 1 can	To hold dressings
Emergency telephone numbers: doctor, fire and police departments, hospital, poison control center	To reach those who can assist

Table A–1.   Suggested First-Aid Kit Contents (continued)

First-Aid Item	Use
Epsom salts	For a laxative in case of poisoning
First-aid book	As a guide on what and what not to do
Flashlight and extra batteries	To examine throat; for vision in darkness, signaling
Hot-water bottle	Relief of pain
Ice bag (plastic)	To reduce swelling; for burns; for relief of pain; the bag itself without ice can cover third-degree burns
Kerlix gauze rolls—two	To cover wounds
Kwik Kold, 5″ x 10″—two	For instant cold pack
Matches	To sterilize needles, scissors, dressings
Measuring cup and spoons	For measuring
Medicine dropper	To rinse eyes
Needles	To remove splinters
Oil of cloves	To place on cotton for toothache
Paper and pencil	To record information and send messages
Paper drinking cups	To give drinks; to cover eye injuries
Penlight	For contraction of eyes; to examine nose and throat
Plastic bag—(Ziploc)—1 gal. size	Carry water, waterproofing, airtight dressing
Rescue ("space") blanket	Body temperature control, signaling, water repellent protection
Safety pins—12, various sizes	To tie bandages
Salt (table)—dilute with water before administering	For delayed treatment of shock and burns; for treatment for heat cramps
Scissors—1 pair	Cutting
Sharp knife or razor blade	Cutting
Snakebite kit	Treatment of snakebite
Soap (mild)	Cleaning wounds
Splints—2 or 3, different lengths	Splinting broken arms and legs
Sterile dressings (gauze)—2 x 2, 4 x 4, 6 x 6 inches	To cover wounds
Sterile eye pads—3 or 4	To cover injured eyes
Sterile gauze (also called roller gauze)—rolls in widths up to 3 inches, 1 each	To cover wounds
Sterile soap—liquid, 4 to 6 ounces	Cleaning
Sugar cubes—small container	Insulin shock
Syrup of ipecac—one ounce	To induce vomiting in poison cases
Tackle box	To store and transport supplies listed
Thermometer—1 oral, 1 rectal	To determine body temperature
Tongue blades	To splint broken fingers
Towel	Drying
Triangular bandages—at least 4, with material for making more	Bandages, tourniquet, sling, splint stabilization
Tweezers—1 pair	To remove small splinters
Wire ladder splints—1	For splinting fractures

Not Recommended:
See Consumers Union, *The Medicine Show*, New York: Pantheon Books.
   Mercurochrome, Merthiolate, iodine
   Ammonia—aromatic spirit, inhalant ampules
   Boric acid
   Over-the-counter burn ointments

Source: Alton L. Thygerson, *Study Guide for First-Aid Practices*, Englewood Cliffs, N. J.: Prentice-Hall, 1978. By permission.

Before we consider specific first aid treatments, let us call to mind a few general rules. The first is always to handle injured people gently, and not to move them unless you have to, because movement often causes further injury. If they are conscious, speak to them gently and kindly and let them know that help is on the way. Second, do not get in touch with emergency services (the police, for instance) until you have made the victim's condition more stable. Third, when you do call for help, give clear information about the number of victims, their location, and the extent of their injuries. Make sure that you are understood.

A Glossary of Specific First Aid Problems and Treatments

Bleeding

Place a clean bandage or cloth over the bleeding wound and press down on the bandage with your hand. (If you do not have a cloth or bandage, use your hand or an object.) When the bandage gets soaked with blood, put another bandage over it, but do not take off the first one. Should the bleeding be in the arm or leg, keep the wounded area raised.

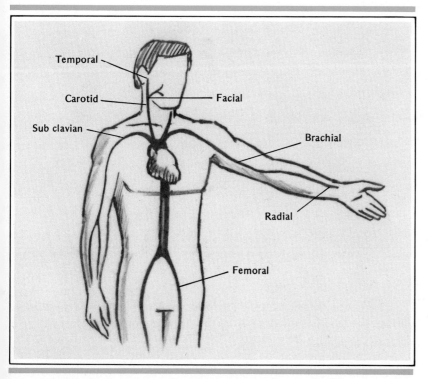

Figure A-1.   The pressure points.

Pressure Points.   If profuse bleeding does not stop after a few minutes, put pressure on the pressure point nearest the wound. The major pressure points are the temporal, carotid, facial, subclavian, brachial, radial, and femoral. Remember to keep pressing on the wound itself, even as you work on the pressure points; you can do this by placing a bandage or cloth over the wound and tying it tightly.

Tourniquet.   As a last resort—to be used only in cases of extensive bleeding—you can apply a "tourniquet" by wrapping a cloth on the limb above the wound and twisting the cloth very tightly. Tourniquets that are made too tight can cut off all blood supply to the area and so may cause victims to lose part or all of a limb. They should be used only in extreme cases, when the victim might otherwise die. The tourniquet should not be concealed, and the victim should be watched carefully.

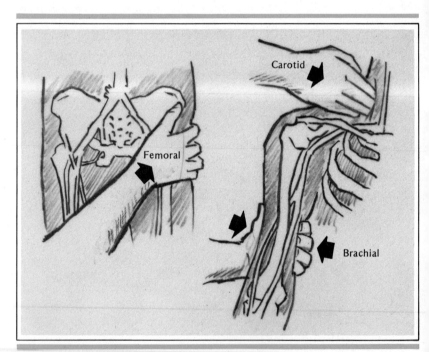

Figure A–2. Applying pressure to a pressure point.

Breathing Problems

Anyone who stops breathing for more than 4 to 6 minutes may suffer permanent brain damage or may die. Emergency aid for people who have stopped breathing—artificial respiration—consists of blowing air into the victims' mouths so that the rescuers supply oxygen to the victims until they begin to breathe or until medical help comes.

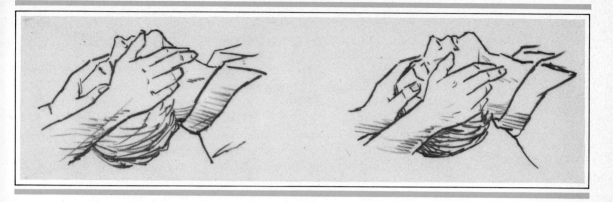

Figure A–3. Finding the neck pulse.

Give artificial respiration to anyone whose breathing has stopped but whose pulse is still beating; if the pulse is beating, blood is still circulating. (To check the pulse, put your first two fingers—not your thumb—on the side of the victim's neck, a little below the chin. Do not rely on the wrist pulse.) If the pulse is not beating, give cardiopulmonary resuscitation (CPR). (See entry for CPR below under Heart Attacks.)

Treatment.   Give artificial respiration as follows:

1. Put one hand under the back of the victim's neck, and keep the victim's head tilted back.
2. Press your other hand down on the victim's forehead, then pinch the victim's nose with the thumb and index finger, so air will not get out and keep the nose pinched closed during the following operations.

Figure A–4. Artificial respiration.

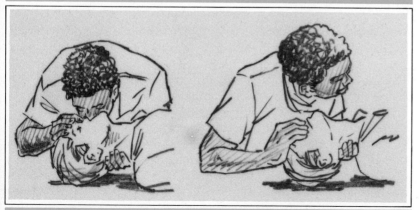

3. Take a deep breath, and make a tight seal with your mouth around the mouth of the victim.

4. Blow four quick, full breaths into the victim's mouth to give the victim's lungs a quick supply of oxygen.

5. Inhale and blow again, forcefully but easily. Make sure the victim's chest is moving up and down. If it is not, inhale and blow still more forcefully. A moving chest means that air is going into the lungs.

6. If the victim still cannot take in air without your help, tilt the victim's head far back, so that the jaw sticks up and out.

7. Take your mouth away from the victim's for a few seconds to let the victim breathe out. But keep the victim's nose closed.

8. Take another deep breath, make the tight seal (step 3), and blow into the victim's mouth again.

9. Let the victim breathe out.

10. Continue breathing and stopping, 10 or 12 times a minute, until the victim starts to breathe or until emergency help arrives.

Broken Bones

Never move a victim with a broken (fractured) bone unless you have immobilized the bone—that is, kept it from moving so that sharp bone edges cannot cut vital tissue.

Treatment.   Immobilize a broken bone by tying a "splint" to the area of the broken bone to prevent movement. The splint does not have to be stiff; you can use newspapers, rolled-up blankets, or the like. (If the splint *is* stiff, wrap soft cloth around it, if possible, where it touches the skin.) Make the splint long enough to include the joints above and below the broken bone. Tie it to the area of the broken bone with bandages, a cloth, or clothing. Do not tie it too tightly; you will know that it is too tight if the victim's fingers or toes either swell or turn blue.

Burns

Burns are caused by fires and also by hot liquids, electricity, certain chemicals (like lye), and radiation. First-degree burns are the least serious kind, second-degree burns cause blisters, and third-degree burns leave raw and charred flesh. People with some second-degree and all third-degree burns should be taken to hospitals or physicians.

Treatment: First-degree Burns.   First-degree burns may be caused by too much exposure to the sun (sunburn) or by brief contact with hot objects (like clothes irons), hot liquids, or steam. The skin may turn red, and there may be swelling or pain. Put cold water—never ice water—on the burn. Gently wash dirty skin with soap and water. If you like, put a clean, dry bandage on the burn.

Treatment: Second-degree Burns.   Second-degree burns are caused by very bad sunburn, longer contact with hot liquids or steam, flash burns from kerosene or gasoline, and direct contact with flames. Skin is red, spotty, or wet looking, and blistered. These burns are very painful. Put cold water—never ice water—on the burn until the pain goes away. Wash the burn gently with soap and water, then blot (don't rub) with a clean towel or cloth. Do not break the blisters. Put a clean, dry bandage on the burn or, to keep oozing flesh from sticking to clothing or bedding, use a plastic wrap. Keep burned hands and feet raised; keep burned fingers and toes separated from each other. Those with facial burns should sit up. Victims of such second-degree burns should go to the hospital or to physicians.

Treatment: Third-degree Burns.   Longer contact with hot liquids, steam, or flames, and contact with electricity or chemicals like lye, causes third-degree burns. Layers of the skin are lost, or they are white or charred-looking; and hair pulls out easily on the skin. But there is little pain because nerves have been destroyed. Cover burns with a clean cloth, a bandage, or a plastic wrap, like Saran Wrap. Treat the victim for shock (see below). Give artificial respiration if the victim cannot breathe or cardiopulmonary resuscitation (see below) if you cannot feel the neck pulse and are trained in CPR. Keep burned hands and feet up; keep burned fingers and toes separated from each other. People with facial burns should sit up, and they should be watched to see if they develop breathing problems.

Do *not* put cold water on the burn—it may cause or worsen shock. Do not pull off burned clothing that sticks to the burn.

Chemical Burns.   If possible, get directions on first-aid treatment for the specific chemical involved. (Look on the container, if it is available.) Wash the chemical off the skin with large amounts of water. Treat victim for shock; if breathing has stopped, give artificial respiration; and give CPR if you have been trained in it and cannot feel the victim's neck pulse.

Choking on Food or Other Objects (the Abdominal Thrust)

Suppose you were having dinner with friends and someone suddenly choked on a piece of food. Your friend would not be able to breathe or talk and might turn blue in the face (for lack of oxygen). If your friend got no help, death would come in about 4 minutes.

If you know how to give this help—the abdominal thrust, sometimes called the Heimlich maneuver—you will be able to help remove the object (often, but not necessarily food) that your friend is choking on. In fact, if you should choke on something when you are *alone,* you can do the abdominal thrust on yourself.

By the way, choking on objects is not uncommon—it is the 6th leading cause of death by accidents. You can help prevent choking on food by eating slowly, by chewing your food carefully, by not swallowing big lumps of food, and by not getting excited or talking too much while you eat. Do not gulp your food, even when you are in a hurry.

Treatment.   When the victim is sitting or standing, you do the abdominal thrust as follows:

1.   Stand behind the victim and put your arms around the victim's waist.
2.   Put your fist against the victim's waist, just above the belly button and under the rib cage.

Figure A–5.   The abdominal thrust (sitting up). Note: the proper way to grasp and press is shown at bottom.

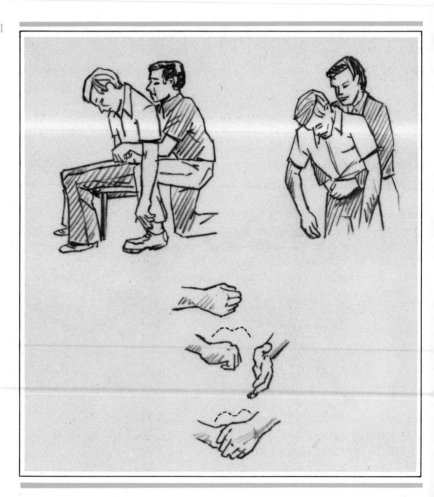

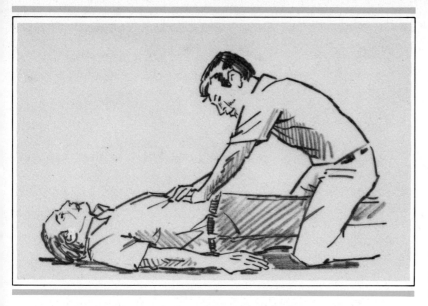

Figure A–6. The abdominal thrust (lying down).

3. Grasp your fist with your other hand, and press your hands into the victim's waist with a quick upward push. Press the abdomen, do not squeeze it.
4. Keep pressing until the swallowed object pops out of the victim's mouth.

   Should the victim be lying face up, the abdominal thrust is performed differently:

1. Kneel across the victim's hips.
2. Put your hands one on top of the other, at right angles. Put the heel of the bottom hand on the victim's waist, just above the navel and under the rib cage.
3. With a quick upward push, press your hands into the victim's waist. Press the abdomen; do not squeeze it.
4. Keep pressing until the swallowed object pops out of the victim's mouth.

Heart Attacks

   Each year 1 million people suffer heart attacks, and nearly two-thirds of them die—more than in any other kind of medical emergency. And half of the deaths take place before the victims get to a hospital.

   Heart attacks often occur when people are under physical, mental, or emotional strain. But not necessarily—heart attacks can strike at any time. The ability to recognize the symptoms of a heart attack is the beginning of first aid for one. These symptoms are as follows:

- Strong, steady pain in the center of the chest. Victims may feel "squeezed," "crushed," or even "stabbed." The pain may spread to the left shoulder, the left arm, the neck, or the stomach.
- Sweating, nausea, or difficulty in breathing.
- Shock.

Remember that heart-attack victims may deny, to themselves and others, that they are sick, so you have to pay careful attention to the signs of illness and then make up your own mind.

Treatment.   If you have received training in cardiopulmonary resuscitation (CPR), give it (see below). If not, there are still things you can do.

If you have not been trained in CPR. Get the victim into the most comfortable position—usually sitting with legs up and knees bent. Loosen clothing around the victim's neck and chest. Then:

1. Keep the victim warm.
2. If the victim cannot breathe, give artificial respiration.
3. Call emergency help—an ambulance, the local EMS, the police, the fire department. If possible, call the family physician.
4. If you are driving the victim to the hospital yourself, carry the victim to the car with care, and keep the victim sitting up during the trip. Drive quickly but carefully.

Cardiopulmonary Resuscitation (CPR). CPR is useful not only in cases of heart attack but also for shock, drug overdoses, drowning—whenever the heart stops beating and breathing ceases. *It is not a good idea to give CPR unless you have been taught how to do it* in a course given by the American National Red Cross or the American Heart Association. The guide below is meant to give you some idea of what CPR involves.

To receive CPR, the victim should be lying face up, on a firm surface, with feet propped up. The steps in CPR are as follows:

1. Kneel down next to the victim.
2. Use the middle and index fingers of whichever of your hands is the closer to the victim's feet to find the lower edge of the rib cage. Move your fingers along the rib cage to the notch where the ribs join the breastbone. Put one finger on the notch and then move the other finger next to that finger.

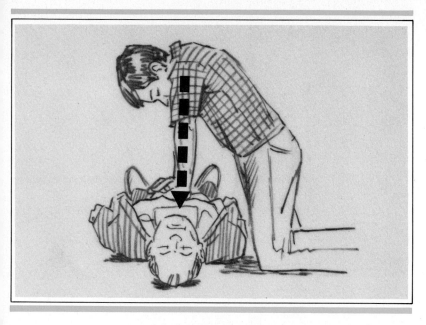

Figure A–7. CPR: Proper position for cardiac compression.

Figure A–8. CPR: One rescuer.

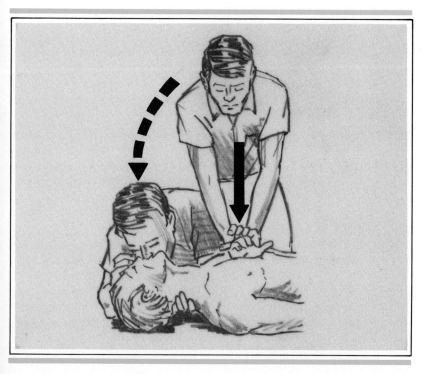

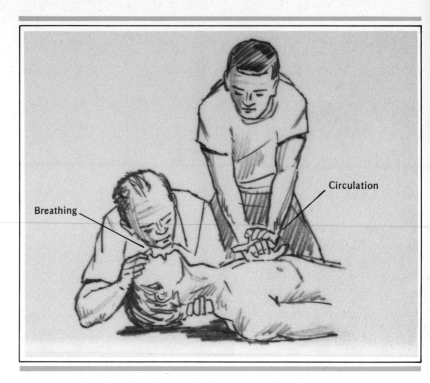

Figure A–9. CPR: Two rescuers

3. Put the heel of your other hand on the lower half of the breastbone, just next to the index finger that found the notch.
4. Put the first hand on top of the hand on the breastbone, so that the heels of the two hands are in the same position—along the breastbone. Keep your fingers off the victim's chest.
5. Move forward so that your shoulders come almost directly over the victim's chest.
6. Keep your arms straight (do not bend your elbows), then push hard enough to press the victim's breastbone down 1½ to 2 inches. Then relax.
7. Push down and relax 15 times, counting out for each push "1 and 2 and 3 and 4," and so on up to 15.
8. Then blow two quick breaths into the victim's mouth.
9. Continue the 15 intervals of pushing and relaxing, followed by the 2 breaths.

If there are two rescuers, one should push and relax, counting "one—one thousand, two—one thousand, three—one thousand, four—one thousand, five—one thousand." After "five—one thousand," the second rescuer should blow one breath into the victim's mouth. Then five more intervals of pushing and relaxing, and another breath into the mouth. Thereafter, the pushing and relaxing (60 times each minute) should go on while breath is blown into the victim's mouth. If this sounds complicated, you can at least understand why courses should be taken to learn the technique.

Overdose on Drugs

People who overdose on drugs may become sleepy, lose consciousness, or become anxious or depressed. Some drugs cause hallucinations (seeing or hearing imaginary scenes or voices); some cause death. People overdose both by accident and by design.

If you come across someone who has overdosed, do not start giving lectures; give first aid and (if necessary) get the victim to a physician or a hospital. After recovery, the victim might benefit from professional counseling.

Treatment.   Handle a case of drug overdose as follows:

1. If breathing has stopped (and this is the most common cause of death in drug overdoses) give artificial respiration. If the victim's pulse has stopped and you have been trained in CPR, give it.
2. Treat for shock (see entry below).
3. Keep victims awake by shaking them gently, walking them around the room, or talking. Or use wet towels on their faces and bodies.
4. If victims are conscious, try to make them vomit. But do not make unconscious or semiconscious victims vomit since they can choke on stomach contents coming up.
5. Lay semiconscious or unconscious victims on their sides.
6. If victims are hallucinating or extremely excited, try to calm them by talking gently and kindly. Keep them from hurting themselves. You may have to restrain them in some way.
7. If the victims are bleeding, stop the bleeding. If they have broken any bones, immobilize them.
8. If you can, find out which drug the victim took, how much of it, and when. As you ask these questions be tactful and friendly; your aim is to help the victim, not to be nosy or pass judgment.
9. Get the victim to the hospital or to a physician.

Shock

In medical jargon, "shock" has a special meaning: the failure of the circulatory system to supply enough blood to the body, whose functions are thus disrupted. Medical (or "traumatic") shock can, and often does, set in when the body is very badly injured, burned, or poisoned; heart attacks or stroke can cause shock, and so can very bad allergic reactions

Figure A–10.   Treatment for traumatic shock. To improve the circulation, people suspected of being in shock are positioned with feet elevated, as in a, and b. If the person is having breathing problems, the head and shoulders should be elevated, as in c. If the person is unconscious, turn the person to the side, as in d. And if bones may be broken, leave the person in the position found, as in e.

(see Chapter 10) and inability to breathe. An injury that might cause only mild shock in one person could cause severe shock in another. If not treated, severe shock can lead to death.

Shock is marked by cold, clammy skin; a fast but weak pulse that can be felt on the side of the neck, but not in the wrist; rapid but shallow breathing; restlessness and anxiety; vomiting, fainting, and dizziness; and extreme thirst. Victims do not necessarily suffer from all these symptoms, and sometimes they do not suffer from any of them. That is why you should always treat for shock *anyone* with serious injuries, for these almost always cause shock, with or without clear symptoms.

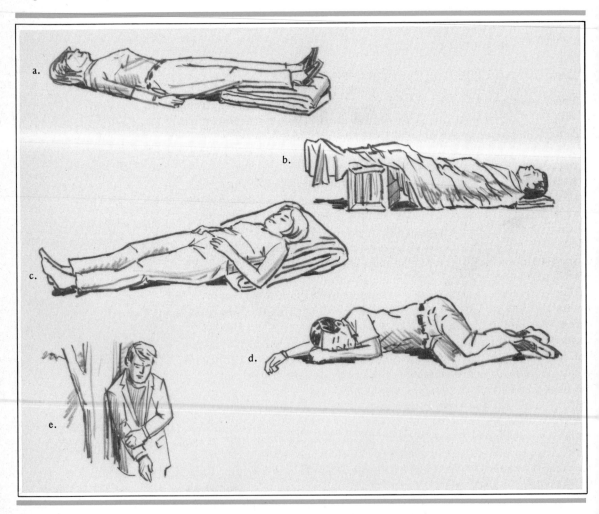

Treatment.   Follow these steps in treating shock:

1. Lay the victim face up, with the head lower than the feet. But if the victim is having trouble breathing or if the face is red, prop up the head and shoulders.
2. If you think the victim may have a head injury, keep the head level with, or slightly higher than, the feet.
3. Place unconscious victims on their sides.
4. Keep the victim warm.
5. If bones are broken, put a splint on the injured area before you move the victim.
6. Loosen the victim's clothing and shoes.
7. Call an ambulance, the police, or some other emergency service.
8. Reassure the victim that help is on the way and that you are doing all that can be done.

Safety in the Home

There is a place where 33 percent of all injuries—including 22 percent of all fatal injuries—occur. Among the injuries that commonly occur in this dangerous place are burns, electric shock, gunshot wounds, drowning, broken bones, chemical poisoning, and suffocation. This pit of dangers is the American home.

Just about all of these injuries could be prevented with a little care and common sense. Here is how.

In the Kitchen.   Use appliances carefully. Read the warning labels, and tack them up, if possible, in a place where you will always be able to see them. Never get an electrical plug wet, because you can get a severe shock if you plug it into a socket.

When you cook, do not let pot handles project beyond the stove—otherwise you or someone else will bump into and upset them. Always be sure to turn off electric-stove burners after using them; someone might accidentally touch a burner that seemed to be off but actually was very hot. To avoid grease fires, keep the stove and the oven clean. But if grease should catch fire, do not use water to put it out—instead, smother the fire with a pan lid or a plate. Keep a fire extinguisher in a handy place in the kitchen—and know how to use it.

Finally, never use kerosene, spot remover, or other flammable liquids on or near a stove.

In the Bathroom.   When you are soapy and wet, it is easy to fall in the shower or tub. Do something about that by making the tub or shower stall less slippery. One way is to buy and use stick-on pieces

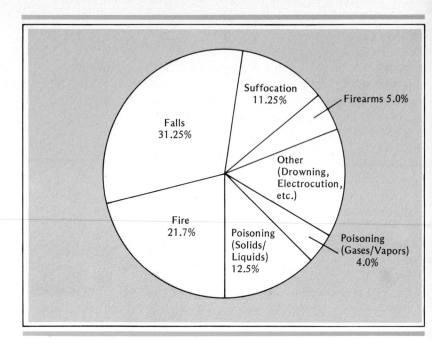

Falls
31.25%

Suffocation
11.25%

Firearms 5.0%

Other
(Drowning,
Electrocution,
etc.)

Fire
21.7%

Poisoning
(Solids/
Liquids)
12.5%

Poisoning
(Gases/Vapors)
4.0%

Figure A–11.   Causes of deaths in the home.

with rough surfaces. Or get a large rubber mat with suction cups on the bottom. Older people should consider having metal bars installed just over their tubs so that they have something to hold on to when getting in or out.

To prevent electric shocks, be careful not to let electrical appliances like radios or hair dryers fall into the water. Never use electrical appliances while you are in the tub or shower even if they are designed for that purpose.

For Every Room in the House.   Have strict rules for everyone, including children, about putting things away. Anything left lying around the house—toys, books, shoes, sports equipment—can be a tripper-upper. Keep stuff off the stairs. Families with pets should look out for their bones, rubber mice, and the like. Larger items, such as bikes, should be kept in places where nobody will fall over them.

Smokers should bear in mind that the habit can be a fire hazard. They should put out all cigarettes, pipes, and cigars completely, in an ashtray. *And no one should ever smoke in bed.*

Frayed wires on lamps and other electrical items should be repaired by trained electricians, or else the items should be replaced. Do not hide electrical cords under rugs.

Work out a plan of escape in case of fire, and make sure that everyone in your house knows the plan. Put "tot stickers" on the windows of rooms where children sleep so the fire company can find them quickly. Buy and install smoke alarms.

Children.   Never leave very young children alone in a house or in a separate part of the house, even for a few minutes. Keep soaps, detergents, medicines, flammable liquids, and other harmful chemicals away from children. Do not let them play with matches. Children like to explore, and they have to be *taught* the difference between what is dangerous and what is safe—something adults may take for granted. A child may think a piece of soap is a candy bar—until it is too late. Just in case, know the number of the local poison-control center.

People with swimming pools should be careful to keep unwatched children away from them.

Older People.   Older people frequently fall, and a broken bone may take much longer to heal in an older person than in a younger one. Keep track of the movements of older people and be ready to help them. If you know older people who are ill and housebound, call them regularly.

Table A–2.   Sudden Illness

Type	Cause(s)	Signs/Symptoms	First Aid
Head Area			
Earache (otitis media)	Bacterial infection	Severe ear pain (sometimes throbbing) Fever Rupture of eardrum releasing pus	Apply heat to ear Rest Nasal decongestant Pain reliever Use vaporizer, steamy shower Consult doctor
Toothache	Irritation or infection Lost fillings Broken tooth	Broken tooth Pain May or may not have swelling	Pain reliever, don't hold tablet in mouth Rinse mouth with salt water solution Consult dentist Insert cotton with oil of cloves in cavity Apply heat or cold compress
Headache	Tension and muscle spasms in neck, scalp, and jaw	Pain, fatigue	Pain reliever Massage or heat applied to back of upper neck Rest with eyes closed and head supported

Table A–2. Sudden Illness (continued)

Type	Cause(s)	Signs/Symptoms	First Aid
Head Area (continued)			
Sinusitis	Infected sinus	Pain in face under the eye(s) and opposite the bridge of the nose Headache Fever Runny nose	Alternating hot and cold compress to forehead and cheeks Apply decongestant nose drops to each nostril Increase humidity—use vaporizer Drink extra fluid Consult doctor
Respiratory			
Asthma	Form of allergic reaction Weather change or exertion can induce attack	Pants for breath Wheezing sound Coughs a lot and spits up white mucus Cyanotic lips and nails History of previous attacks	Reassure victim Rest in sitting-up position Extra fluids—warm liquids May have own medication Avoid smoke Get away from cause Vaporizer
Hyperventilation syndrome	Anxiety	Dizziness Blurring of vision Shortness of breath Fainting Pounding of heart Tingling of hands or around mouth	Reassurance Rest in quiet place Breathing into paper bag
Skin			
Boils	Hair follicle gets plugged Staphytococcus germ	Swelling the size of a pea to a walnut Area is red and tender Pus	Warm, moist soaks Do not squeeze
Contact dermatitis	Allergic reaction	Localized skin rash Itching Redness, swelling	Discover cause of the rash Wash red with usual soap and water If possible, leave rash exposed to air Relieve itching—keep area cool and wet, or try warm water, bathing in ½ cup of baking soda in warm bathtub

Table A–2.   Sudden Illness (continued)

Type	Cause(s)	Signs/Symptoms	First Aid
Skin (continued)			
Hives	Allergy	Itchy Pink or white slightly raised bumps	Discover cause Consult doctor
Musculoskeletal			
Backache	Inadequate exercise Awkward or heavy lifting Poor posture Mental stress Improper sleeping positions	Pain in the back Difficult to walk and/or move	Cold packs initially Rest on back with knees propped up Pain reliever Massage back Consult doctor
Neck pain	Muscle, ligament, bursal, or nerve inflammation	Stiff, painful neck	Heat from hot compresses or hot water bag Massage neck Pain reliever
Urinary Tract			
Painful, frequent urination	Bacterial or viral infection Excessive use of caffein-containing beverage	Pain or burning during urination Frequent, urgent urination Blood in urine	Drink a lot of fluids and fruit juices Avoid alcohol, coffee, and spicy foods Consult doctor
Urine retention	Prostate gland enlargement	Pain in lower abdomen Urgent desire to urinate, but can't	Sit in warm bath Avoid alcohol, coffee, and spicy foods Consult doctor
Gastrointestinal			
Abdominal pain	Appendicitis Food poisoning Dysentery Ulcer Gallbladder attack Many other causes	Cramping Stomach pain	Avoid solid foods—sips of water or other clear liquids, no ice chips Warm bath Rest quietly Do not give laxatives or enemas Do not give strong pain medication Do not apply heat to area Consult doctor

Table A–2.   Sudden Illness (continued)

Type	Cause(s)	Signs/Symptoms	First Aid
Gastrointestinal(continued)			
Constipation	Not taking time to go to bathroom Change in diet, work, activity Emotions	Passage of hard, dry stools	Avoid laxatives if possible—use stool softener or gentle laxative Drink extra water, juice Eat fruits, vegetables
Rectal pains, itching	Constipation Straining at the stool Heredity	Itching Pain	Soften stool—more fresh fruits and fiber or mild laxative Keep area clean Consult doctor
Diarrhea	Inflammation of the intestines	Discharge of watery stool, usually repeated several times a day	Avoid solid foods, spicy foods, fruit, alcohol, and coffee Sip clear liquids Suck ice cubes Later applesauce and other mild foods Bed rest Consult doctor if blood or signs of dehydration appear
Food poisoning	Bacteria	Stomach pain Cramping	Nothing to eat or drink until vomiting has stopped Sip water or eat ice chips Progress to mild foods Bed rest Consult doctor
Ulcers	Open sore on the inner wall of digestive tract or stomach	Burning pain, gas, vomiting, or belching Dark brown particles like coffee grounds in vomitus indicate bleeding ulcer Black, tarry stool indicates upper gastrointestinal bleeding	Antacids to neutralize gastric acid Avoid alcohol, coffee, tea, and carbonated drinks Eat more often Slow down and relax Consult doctor
Gallstone colic	Passage of a stone through bile duct from gallbladder to the small intestine	Pain just below right ribs Severe spasms	Bed rest No food or liquid Eat ice chips Consult doctor

Table A–2.   Sudden Illness (continued)

Type	Cause(s)	Signs/Symptoms	First Aid
Gastrointestinal (continued)			
Hernia	Heavy lifting Heredity	Bulge in abdomen May be painful	Place on back with hips higher than shoulders, draw knees up to relax abdominal muscles Do not push back Don't lift or perform strenuous exercise Consult doctor
Appendicitis	Inflammation of appendix	Pain around navel at first, later settling in the lower right side of abdomen; usually continuous and sharp; not always severe	Consult doctor, do not give a laxative; do not give anything by mouth except ice chips

Source: Alton L. Thygerson, *Study Guide for First-Aid Practices,* Englewood Cliffs, N. J.: Prentice-Hall, 1978. By permission.

Suggested Readings

Anderson, Gail V., Haycock, Christine E., and Zydlo, Stanley M. *The American Medical Association's Handbook of First Aid & Emergency Care.* New York: Random House, 1980. A resource that deals with mishaps and misfortunes and the emergency care that should be provided for them.

Hafen, Brent Q., and Peterson, Brenda. *First Aid for Health Emergencies.* St. Paul: West, 1977. This book tells how to survive health emergencies. It offers advice on prevention as well as lifesaving steps to aid victims if emergencies occur.

Glossary

abortion Removal of the products of conception from the uterus. *See also* Suction curettage; D and C; Hysterotomy; Induced labor

"acid" *See* LSD

acid rain Rainfall having a high content of sulfuric acid; caused by sulfur-laden industrial smoke mixing with water vapor in the air condensing into clouds, and falling to the earth's surface as rain.

active coping Coping that results when people assume they can control their own behavior and patterns of interaction—for example, problem solving, relaxation techniques, exercise, therapy. *See also* Reactive coping

active immunization The practice of injecting small amounts of a disease agent into a healthy person in order to stimulate the production of antibodies.

acupuncture A traditional Chinese medical technique in which sharp needles are shallowly inserted into various points of the body to relieve pains and symptoms of illness.

adaptation mechanism A fixed sequence of reactions between the mind and the body; consists of three stages: (1) reflex reactions to stimuli, (2) emotional responses, and (3) thought and planning.

addiction The compulsive need to take a habit-forming drug regularly in order to feel its physical effects or to avoid the discomfort of not taking it. *See also* Withdrawal symptoms

additives Substances added to processed foods in order to improve color, flavor, and nutritional value or to prolong shelf life.

aerobic exercises Exercises that strengthen the heart muscle, increase the amount of oxygen taken in by the lungs, and thus produce a training effect—for example, long-distance swimming, running, jogging, and bicycling. *See also* Training effect

alcoholic A person who has become physically addicted to alcohol, who can no longer control the use of it; an alcoholic often goes on periodic "drunks" and must continue to drink to avoid withdrawal symptoms.

allergy A disease of the immune system in which too many antibodies are released to fight a particular antigen; severe and persistent inflammation often results and blood pressure may drop dangerously.

alveoli Small, fine air sacs in the lungs, in which oxygen exchanges occur.

ambulatory (outpatient) care Medical care provided by clinics or physicians' offices to patients who are well enough to travel under their own power.

amino acids Organic substances composed of carbon, hydrogen, oxygen, and nitrogen that are linked together to form proteins. Eight are "essential"—the body requires them but cannot produce enough of them to meet its needs. *See also* Enzymes

458

amniotic sac   The bag of fluid that surrounds and protects a child in the uterus.

anaerobic exercises   Exercises such as sprinting that demand much extra oxygen but do not last long enough to produce a training effect. *See also* Training effect

analgesic drugs   Painkilling drugs, such as opiates and other narcotics.

anaplasia   Failure of body cells to function normally, especially cancerous cells.

androgen   A male sex hormone produced in the testes and adrenal cortex; causes male secondary sex characteristics.

androgynous personality   A sex role identity that allows people to follow their natural personalities and blend so-called traditional male and female traits.

"angel dust"   *See* PCP

angina pectoris   Strong pressure and squeezing pain in the chest as a result of too little oxygen reaching the heart.

anorexia nervosa   A psychological condition in which a person, usually a female between the ages of 10 and 20, is obsessed with losing weight and resorts to devious means and self-starvation to achieve it.

anorgasmia   Total inability to reach an orgasm.

anoxia   A lack of oxygen, causing body cells to die.

antagonism   A drug interaction in which two drugs taken together cancel each other's effects.

antibiotic   A substance, produced by a microorganism, that has the capacity to kill or inhibit the growth of another microorganism, such as a disease germ. Penicillin, Tetracycline, and Terramycin are common antibiotics.

antibodies   Chemicals, produced by the body cells, that combat, destroy, or neutralize the harmful effects of infectious agents; the production of antibodies creates immunities.

antigens   Chemicals, in infectious microorganisms, that injure the body's cells and stimulate the body to produce antibodies.

anxiety   Generalized feelings of uneasiness, apprehension, or fear, often without an apparent cause.

aorta   A large blood vessel, on the left side of the heart, that carries blood from the heart to arteries serving the rest of the body.

aphrodisiacs   Bogus drugs and other substances that are supposed to improve the sex drive.

apostat   The apetite control mechanism in the brain.

arthritis   A disease of the bones and joints resulting in painful stiffness and swelling; two common forms are rheumatoid arthritis and osteoarthritis.

assertiveness training   A form of therapy that helps people overcome their lack of self-confidence by identifying their rights and dispelling ideas that prevent assertiveness.

asthma   A kind of allergy that repeatedly obstructs the lung's air passages; often causes bronchitis.

atherosclerosis   Hardening of the arteries, caused by accumulations of fat within the arteries' walls.

at-home care   Medical care or treatment to patients who are too ill to leave home, provided by nurses, rehabilitation therapists, and other health-care professionals.

autonomic nervous system   The part of the nervous system that controls automatic body actions, such as heartbeat, breathing, and digestion. *See also* Voluntary nervous system.

bacteria   Microscopic one-celled plants of various shapes that live and reproduce outside of body cells; they cause many fatal diseases.

basal body temperature (BBT)   The lowest temperature of a healthy person during waking hours.

basal metabolic rate (BMR)   The minimum expenditure of energy needed to maintain the activities of cells and body functions, such as respiration and blood circulation.

B-complex vitamins   Water-soluble vitamins, such as thiamin, riboflavin, niacin, B_6, and B_{12}.

behaviorism   A branch of psychology holding that thought is a body function, that emotions are a product of hormones, and that all behavior is the product of conditioning. *See also* Conditioning

benign tumor   A slow accumulation of normal cells surrounded by a capsule or membrane.

Berne, Eric   American psychiatrist who has developed the concepts of time structuring and transactional analysis in his study of human interaction.

blood alcohol level (BAL)   A measure of the amount of alcohol in the bloodstream; a BAL of .02 means that there are .02 mg of alcohol for every 100 ml of blood in a drinker's body. A reading of .10 is a legal measure of drunkenness.

body type   *See* Endomorph; Ectomorph; Mesomorph

brain death   Death as a result of loss of oxygen to brain cells in the cortex, midbrain, and lower brain; leads to clinical death.

breech presentation   A birth in which the baby appears buttocks first.

bronchioles   The airways in the lungs.

caesarian section   The delivery of a baby by means of an incision in the mother's abdomen.

calisthenics   Isotonic exercises that stress a certain muscle group, such as push-ups, sit-ups, and leg-lifts.

calorie   A measure of the energy contained in a unit of food.

carbohydrates   Food substances that are the body's most important source of energy; may be simple or complex. Simple carbohydrates include the various sugars and are found in sugar-sweetened products, milk, and fruit; complex carbohydrates contain starch, glycogen, and cellulose and are found in whole grains, legumes, and vegetables.

carbon monoxide (CO)   A gas, found in cigarette smoke and automobile exhaust, that reduces the body's oxygen supply by preventing red blood cells from absorbing oxygen. Can cause poisoning marked by headache, nausea, abdominal pains, black-outs, and loss of vision.

carcinogens   Cancer-causing substances, such as some food additives and the tar in cigarette smoke.

carcinoma   A cancerous tumor growing from epithelial tissues.

cardiologist   A physician who specializes in treating heart disease.

cardiomyopathy   A chronic disorder of the heart muscle, usually involving an enlargement of the muscle itself and the obstruction of the valves.

cardiorespiratory fitness Fitness of the heart and lungs; best promoted by aerobic exercise.

cardiovascular diseases Diseases of the heart or blood vessels; the chief cause of death in the United States.

Carson, Rachel (1907–1964) Writer whose book *Silent Spring* (1962) discussed the extent and effects of pesticide pollution and thus helped launch the environmental movement.

cell pathology The process of cell destruction that often accompanies disease.

cellulose A complex carbohydrate found in plants; indigestible by humans.

cerebellum A part of the brain that directs physiological functions, such as muscle coordination and maintaining body equilibrium.

cerebral angiography A technique that determines brain death on the basis of whether blood is being circulated to the vital centers of the brain.

cerebrovascular accident *See* Stroke

cerebrum The part of the brain that directs thought and judgment.

cervical plug Mucous, in the mouth of the cervix, that prevents bacteria and the like from entering the uterus and infecting an unborn child.

chancre A sore or ulcer formed at the entry site of an infecting organism, as in syphilis.

chemotherapy Treatment with anticancer drugs; often produces unwanted side effects, such as nausea, weight loss, mood changes, and hair loss.

cholesterol A substance, found in animal cells, that is necessary for some physiological processes but may be a factor in atherosclerosis.

chromosome A structure, in the nucleus of a cell, that carries genes. Every human body cell carries 23 pairs of chromosomes, or 46 in all. Every human germ cell carries only 1 of a pair, or 23 in all.

chronic bronchitis A respiratory disease in which the airways of the lung become irritated and blocked with mucous; often found in cigarette smokers.

chronic obstructive lung disease (C.O.L.D.) A cluster of diseases, including asthma, emphysema, and chronic bronchitis.

chlamydia Microscopic organisms having features of both viruses and bacteria; cause Trachoma and certain sexually transmitted diseases.

circumcision A surgical procedure for removing the foreskin of the penis, usually right after birth.

cirrhosis A liver disease often found in alcoholics; caused by replacement of active cells by scar tissue; symptoms include abdominal tenderness, weight loss, and high blood pressure.

classical conditioning A type of learning in which subjects associate a neutral stimulus—one that does not elicit a response—with a stimulus that automatically does elicit a response.

climacteric The broad complex of physical and emotional symptoms, in males, that accompanies the onset of middle age.

clinical death Functional death—that is, when the body systems, such as the cardiovascular and respiratory systems, have stopped working; may be reversed by cardiopulmonary resuscitation. *See also* Brain death; Medical death

clinical depression A severe form of depression, characterized by stupor and lack of movement.

coitus interruptus A contraceptive method in which the man withdraws his penis from the vagina before he ejaculates.

collateral vessels A network of small blood vessels within the heart generated by physical exercise; in case of a heart attack, these vessels will continue to deliver blood within the heart.

colostomy Surgery that connects the colon to the outside of the body to permit the discharge of wastes.

coma An unconscious state caused by the death of cells in the midbrain.

common-law marriage A marriage entered into without legal formalities; in some states it becomes legal after 7 years of living together.

common-source epidemic A high level of a communicable disease; it occurs when a number of people have been exposed to the same agent at the same time—for example, food poisoning. *See also* Propagated epidemic

communicable disease A disease—for example, tuberculosis—that is caused by living creatures, microorganisms transmitted from host to host.

conception The fertilization of the ovum by the sperm cell.

conceptus The product of conception—of the union between the ovum and sperm—from the moment of union to the moment of birth; goes through several stages, from zygote to fetus.

conditioning A learning process in which a human or an animal is taught to react to a stimulus by making a certain response. *See also* Classical conditioning; operant conditioning

congenital defects Defects present from birth but not transmitted genetically; instead, they are caused by accidents in the womb. Examples include malformations of the heart, limbs, and mouth; some nervous system abnormalities; and deafness caused by maternal rubella.

conscious A level of awareness that encompasses whatever we are attending to at any given moment; it also includes perceptions, judgments, and memories. *See also* Preconscious; Unconscious

contraception Preventing conception by interfering with the process in which a sperm cell fertilizes an ovum, the production of ova, or the implantation of a fertilized egg.

cool-down A period of brisk walking or some stretching exercises, after vigorous exercise, in order to prepare the body for normal activity.

coping The mind's or body's attempt to make the adjustments that maintain homeostasis when dealing with an event or its effects. This attempt may be conscious or unconscious, short-term or long-term. *See also* Reactive coping; Active coping; Defense mechanisms

coronary thrombosis A heart attack in which a sudden clogging of blood vessels shuts off the blood supply to the heart and so great numbers of the heart's muscle cells die.

corpus luteum A follicle, in the ovary, that has burst, sent its ovum to the fallopian tube, and closed; it then produces progesterone.

cortisol A hormone that inhibits the production of antibodies.

Cowper's glands Pea-sized structures at the base of the penis; secrete pre-ejaculatory fluid into the urethra.

crowning During birth, the appearance of the baby's head as it emerges from the birth canal.

cryotherapy The application of extreme cold to body cells and tissues.

cunnilingus A form of oral sex in which the vulva and clitoris are licked.

d and c (dilation and curettage) A method of induced abortion, in which the walls of the uterus are scraped with a curette.

DDT (dichloro-diphenyl-trichloroethane) A pesticide that was sprayed to control insect pests, especially on food crops. Its accumulation in the fats of domesticated animals increases the risk of cancer in humans who eat such animals.

D sleep *See* REM sleep

death *See* Clinical death; Brain death; Medical death

defense mechanisms Short-term ways that humans use to cope with stressors attacking the weak points in personality make-up. *See also* Regression; Rationalization; Segregation; Projection; Repression

denturist Quack dentists who specialize in prescribing and repairing dentures.

depressants A group of drugs, including barbiturates and alcohol, that depresses the central nervous system. Depressants cause symptoms of drunkenness, build tolerance, and create addiction in users; withdrawal symptoms are severe.

depression Negative or hostile feelings toward oneself and others; characterized by exhaustion, boredom, and worry; caused by various forms of loss, such as loss of a parent, friend, stage of life, or self-esteem. *See also* Clinical depression; Manic depression

dermatologist A physician who specializes in treating skin disorders.

diabetes mellitus An inherited inability to produce insulin; as a result, glucose builds up in the blood, and unused fats break down into ketoacids, which then destroy brain tissue and can cause coma or even death.

diphtheria A highly contagious bacterial infection, usually in young children; marked by swelling and obstruction of the throat.

disease The whole pattern of responses made by an organism to the abnormal functioning of cells, whatever the cause. *See also* Communicable disease; Noncommunicable disease; Local illness; Systemic illness

distillation A process in which fermented alcohol is treated to produce pure alcohol; whiskey, vodka, and rum are made by this process. *See also* Fermentation

distress According to Hans Selye, a researcher, negative stressors arising from frustration of inner or outer needs; they weakens us and make us vulnerable to even more stressors. *See also* Stressors; Eustress

diuretic A drug that increases the flow of urine.

DNA (deoxyribonucle acid) Part of the gentic material that is found in the cell chromosomes; determines heredity and individual development.

Down's syndrome (mongolism) An inherited condition in humans, caused by an extra chromosome, characterized by distorted features and mental retardation.

dream analysis   A psychotherapeutic technique in which a patient's dreams are discussed to discover the unconscious urges or wishes they are held to conceal.

drug potency   The amount that must be taken to produce the desired effect; the smaller the amount needed, the more potent the drug.

drugs of abuse   Drugs—almost always mood-altering drugs—that are taken to help cope with stress and thus are taken too often.

Durkheim, Émile (1858–1917)   French sociologist who identified various forms of suicide and believed it to be caused by social forces.

Dysfunction   Menninger's term for mental imbalance that results from unsuccessful copying with stress; consists of five levels, ranging from the "jitters" to suicidal impulses.

dysmenorrhea   Painful menstruation.

dyspareunia   Painful sexual intercourse.

ectomorph   A person who tends to be slender.

ectopic pregnancy   Pregnancy resulting from implantation in a fallopian tube, instead of in the uterus.

ego   Freud's term for the force in the personality that screens information from the outside world and imposes reason and order on the id. *See also* Id; Superego

embryo   A developing human individual from the time of implantation to the 8th week after conception. *See also* Zygote; Fetus

emphysema   A respiratory disease in which the lung tissues lose their elasticity and small air sacs break; often found in cigarette smokers.

empty calories   Calories derived from substances, such as soda or alcohol, that have few nutrients or none.

encounter group   A group of from 6 to 20 people who focuses on improving interpersonal relationships by means of frank self-disclosure and confrontation.

endometrium   The membrane lining the uterus; either receives a fertilized egg or passes from the body during menstruation.

endomorph   A person who tends to be plump.

enzymes   Substances in the digestive tract that break down amino acids into smaller, less complex compounds. *See also* Proteins; Amino acids

epidemic   *See* Common source epidemic; Propagated epidemic

epidemiologist   A scientist who studies the occurrence of a disease as it spreads through large populations.

epididymus   A complex system of storage canals coiled at the back of the testes; acts as a maturation chamber for sperm cells.

epithelial tissue   Tissue that forms the skin, the glands, and the linings of the respiratory, gastrointestinal, urinary, and genital systems.

erectile inhibition (impotence)   Inability to get an erection; may be primary, in which case it is long-lasting and has physical causes, or secondary, which is temporary and usually has emotional causes.

Erikson, Erik (1902–   )   Neo-Freudian psychologist who created a theory of the ego's development through eight overlapping stages. Failure of the ego to overcome or resolve conflicts at one stage causes trouble in later ones.

estrogen A hormone, produced in the ovaries, that stimulates the development of secondary sex characteristics in females and helps make the endometrium ready to receive the fertilized egg.

etiology A branch of science dealing with the sources, causes, and origins of diseases or abnormal conditions.

eustress Hans Selye's term for stressors, such as success, rewards, or achievement, that result in growth, strength, and resistance to distress.

euthanasia The practice of painlessly putting to death persons suffering from incurable diseases or conditions.

eutrophication Chemical pollution, in lakes and streams, that encourages the growth of algae, which uses up the oxygen and thus kills off any animal life.

existential therapy A form of therapy that helps patients to find authenticity in their lives and to deal with their anxieties in a "godless," arbitrary universe.

fallopian tube Either of the pair of tubes that conduct the egg from the ovary to the uterus.

fats (lipids) Energy-rich fuels used by the body; found in animal products and vegetable oils. Fats help support and protect vital organs, insulate the body, and store certain vitamins. *See also* Saturated fats; Polyunsaturated fats

fat-soluble vitamins Vitamins such as A, D, E, and K, all of which, when digested, are stored in body fat; since they are not excreted in the urine, a new supply of them is not needed every day. *See also* Water-soluble vitamins

fellatio A form of oral sex in which the penis is licked and sucked.

fermentation A process in which sugars or starches are converted into alcohol by the action of yeasts, molds, or bacteria.

fertility awareness Contraception methods that attempt to pinpoint the time of ovulation, so that a woman may refrain from sexual intercourse when she is most fertile; includes the Rhythm Method; the Basal Body Temperature Method, and the Cervical Mucous Method.

fetal alcohol syndrome (FAS) A set of abnormal signs in infants born to mothers who have used alcohol heavily while pregnant. Signs include smaller-than-normal size at birth, particularly in the head; delayed mental development; and poor coordination.

fetishism Sexual excitement aroused by inanimate objects or by body parts not usually considered erotic.

fetus The developing human from the 8th week after conception until birth.

fiber A non-nutrient food component that, while indigestible, is important to digestion; dietary fiber helps prevent constipation and colon cancer.

flavor enhancers Artificial substances, such as MSG, that are added to food to change our perception of its flavor.

follicles Egg sacs located in the ovaries.

follicle-stimulating hormone (FSH) A hormone, secreted by the pituitary gland, that simulates the ovaries to grow and to produce estrogen.

fomites Objects that transmit disease indirectly, such as contaminated toys, clothing, bedding, and surgical instruments.

foster care   The temporary placement of children in private homes.

free association   A psychoanalytic technique in which the patient tries to uncover unconscious motives in dreams and behavior by telling the analyst whatever comes to mind.

Freud, Sigmund (1856–1939)   Viennese physician who founded psychoanalysis and developed a theory about the unconscious forces in the personality. *See also* Ego; Id; Superego; Unconscious

fructose   Fruit sugar.

fungi   Multicelled plants that travel by spores and exist both in microscopic forms, such as yeast, and in large colonies, such as mushrooms; cause such human infections as athlete's foot, ringworm, and candidiasis.

gastritis   Heartburn or upset stomach caused by an injury to, or the reaction of, the protective lining of the stomach and intestines.

general adaptation syndrome   Hans Selye's term for the three stages of response to stress: alarm, resistance, and exhaustion.

general practitioner (GP)   A physician who has a general or family practice. GPs deliver babies at home, make house calls, and treat a wide range of illness and injuries.

generic drugs   Drugs sold under their chemical names, not brand names.

genes   Biological building blocks of heredity; arranged on chromosomes. *See also* Chromosome; DNA

genetic disease   A disease that is transmitted from parent to child through the genes—for example, cystic fibrosis, hemophilia, and muscular dystrophy.

German measles   *See* Rubella; Measles

Gestalt therapy   A form of therapy that helps patients achieve wholeness by integrating, in their everyday lives, their thoughts, feelings, and actions.

Glasser, William   American psychologist who developed reality therapy, a method of psychotherapy that encourages patients to explore their present lives and accept personal responsibility for fulfilling their own needs. *See also* Reality therapy

glycogen   A variety of carbohydrate (a starch) that is stored in the body.

glucose   A sugar produced by the digestion of carbohydrates; is the first substance the body uses for energy.

gossypol   A male antifertility agent derived from the cottonseed plant.

grief   Sudden emotional suffering caused by the death, or the impending death, of another; considered to be a medical syndrome with physical and emotional symptoms, such as weeping, exhaustion, appetite loss, restlessness, and depression. *See also* Mourning

ground water   Water in the water table; below the earth's surface.

group practice   A medical practice in which two or more physicians share office space, nurses, and often patients.

gynecologist   A physician who specializes in treating the female reproductive system for disorders and for prevention

hallucinogens   *See* Psychedelic drugs

HCG (human chorionic gonadotrophin)   A hormone produced by placental tissue; its presence indicates pregnancy.

466

health maintenance organizations (HMOs)   Organizations that offer preventive medical services dispensed by groups of salaried physicians at little or no cost to members above a fixed monthly fee.

heart attack   *See* Coronary thrombosis; Myocardial infarction

heart murmur   A sound made by defective heart valves as they momentarily let blood flow back into the heart.

heavy metals   Metals such as mercury, arsenic, lead, nickel, and zinc; enter the human food chain from industrial pollution. Heavy metals slowly accumulate in the body and affect the nervous system.

herd immunity   An immunity that occurs when people live within populations that have high levels of immunity to certain diseases.

Heroin   An opium derivative, the most powerful narcotic, and the one most widely abused; originally developed as a treatment for morphine addiction. *See also* Opiates; Methadone

hermaphrodite   A person whose body is partly male and partly female due to hormone imbalances in fetal life.

heterosexuality   Sexual relationships between people of opposite sexs.

hierarchy of needs   Maslow's term for a series of needs that unfolds in a fixed sequence over the life span. Lower needs, such as those for food and security, must be met before the higher ones, such as those for esteem and self-actualization can be satisfied. *See also* Self-actualization

histamine   A substance released by injured body cells; alters the blood vessels near the site of injury to permit plasma, containing antibodies and white blood cells, to move into the area.

holistic health   Recognition of the physical, social, and psychological aspects of health and of their interrelatedness.

homeostasis   The narrow range of adjustments the body makes to keep working in a balanced way. If greater adjustments are required, the body is under stress. *See also* Stress; Coping; Defense mechanisms

homosexuality   Sexual relationships between people of the same sex.

hormones   Chemicals produced by the endocrine glands; profoundly affect all body functions. *See also* Androgen; Estrogen; Insulin; Progesterone; Testosterone.

hospice   A residence that serves the needs of the dying; provides special treatment such as painkillers and special diets; encourages friends and relatives to spend as much time as possible with the dying patient.

host   A living plant or animal that shelters a parasite.

hydrogen cyanide   A poisonous gas found in cigarette smoke; responsible for smoker's cough.

hymen   A membrane located at or across the vaginal opening; in young girls, protects the vagina from harmful microbes.

hyperplasia   The uncontrolled growth of cells, as in cancer.

hypertension   High blood pressure caused by clogged blood vessels, slowed blood flow, and a continuously pumping heart.

hysterectomy   Surgical removal of the uterus and, often, the ovaries and fallopian tubes.

hysterotomy   Surgical removal of a fetus.

id   Freud's term for the unconscious force that is the source of energy in the personality, especially the sexual and aggressive drives. *See also* Ego; Superego

illicit drug   A drug that is not used in a legal way, even if it is not an illegal drug.

immunity   The body's natural or acquired ability to produce antibodies to combat, destroy, or neutralize the effects of infectious agents.

immunication   *See* Active immunization; Passive immunication; Herd immunity

impotence   *See* erectile inhibition.

incidence   The number of new cases of an acute, short-term disease that develop during a specified period of time.

induced labor   A method of induced abortion in which salt water is injected through the abdomen into the uterus to bring about the onset of labor, in which the dead fetus and the placenta are then expelled.

infection   The entry into the body and the reproduction there of a disease-causing microorganism.

infectious disease   A communicable disease that is transmitted from person to person.

infectivity   The ability of microbes to lodge and multiply in a human host.

inflammation response   An allergic reaction in which blood flows to the site of a cell injury, and massive amounts of plasma escape from the blood vessels, producing swelling, redness, and high body temperature.

inherent insusceptibility   A physiological state that renders some people, with or without antibodies, immune to certain infections.

institutional care   Medical care provided by hospitals, rehabilitation facilities, and nursing homes.

insulin   A hormone, produced by the pancreas, that is used by the liver and by muscle cells to store and use glucose and fats. Inability to produce sufficient insulin results in diabetes.

interferon   A substance manufactured by body cells that keeps viruses from reproducing within cells.

internist   A physician who specializes in internal medicine—medicine of the body systems as a whole.

interpersonal sexuality   Mutual emotional and physical sexual relationships between people.

intimacy   An honest, open relationship that develops when people care about each other and share insights; occurs in friendships, marriage, work, or between people in times of great stress.

intrapersonal sexuality   The sex drive within each person as manifested in sexual fantasies and masturbation.

inversion   A reversal of the atmospheric temperature gradient in which a layer of warm air traps a layer of cooler air beneath and keeps it from rising; causes air pollution, smog, and related health problems in industrial areas.

investor-owned (proprietary) hospitals   Hospitals that are operated as profit-making institutions.

isometric exercises   Exercises in which one set of muscles is tensed against another without movement; require little oxygen beyond what is ordinarily consumed and produce little or no training effect.

isotonic exercises   Exercises, such as push-ups and sit-ups, that strengthen selected muscle groups through movement; require little extra oxygen and produce only a small training effect.

IUD (intrauterine device) A contraceptive device, such as a plastic or copper coil, sometimes containing hormones; placed in the uterus by a physician.

ketoacid A product of fats that are unused as a result of diabetes; destroys brain tissue and causes diabetic coma

labia majora Lips of skin, fatty tissue, and delicate membranes; protect the female genital area.

lactose Milk sugar.

laparotomy A surgical method for sterilizing women in which the fallopian tubes are cut and tied by a special device inserted through small incisions in each side of the abdomen; may be reversible.

leprosy A chronic contagious disease caused by a bacterial infection; marked by large nodules on the surface of the body, loss of sensation, paralysis, wasting of muscles, and body deformities.

leukemia A form of cancer in which the bone marrow produces large numbers of abnormal white blood cells.

leukocytes White blood cells.

limbic system The brain area that is the source of emotions.

lipids *See* Fats.

local illnesses Pathological changes in a single group of cells that make up one of the body's organs or systems—for example, lung cancer or appendicitis.

LSD (lysergic acid diethylamide) A psychedelic drug that causes hallucinations and weakens self-control. Flashback effects may occur days, weeks, or months later.

lumpectomy The removal of a cancerous tumor from the breast, but not the removal of the breast itself or adjacent tissues and muscles.

lutenizing hormone (LH) A hormone, secreted by the pituitary gland, that causes a follicle in the ovary to burst and send an ovum toward the fallopian tube nearest it.

lymphocyte A special kind of white blood cells, one that is part of the process of immunity.

lymphoma A form of cancer in which the spleen and lymph nodes produce abnormally large numbers of lympocytes.

macrobiotic diet A diet that excludes all foods of animal origin; usually includes brown rice, sesame seeds, and seaweed; can be dangerous to health.

major medical policy A health-insurance policy that pays hospital and physicians' fees over and above those paid by a subscriber's regular hospital and medical insurance.

malignant tumor A fast-growing accumulation of cancerous body cells that is surrounded by a capsule or membrane.

malnutrition Any deviation from a person's normal nutritional needs; refers to diets that contain too many, as well as too few, calories. *See also* Undernutrition

mammary glands Milk-producing glands located in the breasts.

mammogram An X-ray photograph of the breasts.

manic depression A form of mental illness characterized by wide swings of mood—from depression to elation.

marriage *See* Monogamous marriage; Serial monogamy; Trial marriage

Maslow, Abraham (1908–1970) American psychologist who believed that normal, healthy personalities grow by progressing through a hierarchy of needs. *See also* Self-actualization

mastectomy The partial or total removal of a breast, adjacent lymph-node tissue, and underlying chest muscles.

masochist A person who derives pleasure from being hurt by others.

masturbation Self-stimulation of the genitals.

measles A contagious viral disease marked by a cough and raised red circular spots on the face and body. *See also* Rubella

medicaid A government program that pays hospital, medical, and certain other expenses of the poor, blind, and disabled of all ages.

medical death Death as defined by an absence (after 12 hours) of spontaneous voluntary movement, brain-controlled reflexes, and electrical energy in the brain.

Medicare A government program that pays the hospital and medical expenses of people aged 65 and over who paid Social Security taxes.

medulla The part of the brain that directs the body's physiological functions, such as breathing.

Menninger, Karl (1893–   ) American psychiatrist; founded the Menninger Clinic in Topeka, Kansas, and developed theories of mental dysfunction and suicide, among others.

menopause The permanent end of the monthly menstrual cycle; occurs in middle age and may be accompanied by physical symptoms and intense emotional reactions.

menstrual cycle The 28- to 30-day cycle during which an ovum ripens, passes into the uterus, and together with the endometrium, passes from the body.

mental health The ability to adjust to one's society an cope with life's demands; based on a feeling of self-esteem and trust in others. Mentally healthy people plan ahead, set ambitious but attainable goals, and adopt realistic and optimistic attitudes toward life.

mesomorph A person who tends to be muscular and is neither markedly plump nor slender.

metabolism Chemical reactions, within body cells, that transform nutrients into energy. *See also* Basal Metabolic Rate

metastasis The breaking off of cancerous cells from their original areas of accumulation and their growth at other sites in the body.

methodone A synthetic narcotic used to wean addicts away from Heroin and other narcotics; in regulated dosages, does not produce a "high" but does allevaite withdrawal symptoms.

midwife A nurse or other childbirth assistant trained to deliver babies.

minerals Inorganic elements, such as calcium, phophorus, iron, and zinc, which serve nutritional functions similar to those of vitamins and are vital to many body functions.

Minimata disease A disease caused by mercury poisoning; marked by delirum, paralysis, and brain damage; first observed in Minimata, Japan, in 1956.

miscarriage A spontaneous abortion, usually caused by errors in fetal growth.

mongolism *See* Down's syndrome

monogamous marriage A marriage between one man and one woman.

monosodium glutamate (MSG) An artificial flavor enhancer commonly used in restaurants and processed foods.

morning sickness A sign of pregnancy; marked by nausea and revulsion against food; often abates after the first trimester.

mourning A prolonged bereavement over the death of another person; marked by an initial stage of numbness and followed by stages of despondency, depression, and guilt, and then by gradual re-entry into active social life. *See also* Grief

multiple sclerosis (MS) A disease in which the outer coating of the brain and nerve cells breaks down, disrupting messages from the nerves to the organs they control.

mumps A contagious viral disease marked by fever and swelling of the salivary and other glands.

myocardial infarction The sudden clogging of the vessels in the heart or leading to the heart; permanently destroys heart muscle.

narcotics A group of drugs, including the opiates and some synthetic drugs, that both excite and depress the nervous system; are highly addictive and produce severe withdrawal symptoms. *See also* Opiates; Synthetic narcotics; Methadone

neo-Freudian A psychologist who builds theory based on Freud's ideas but emphasizes social and cultural factors.

neoplasm Abnormal growth of body cells; may be benign or malignant.

neurosis A broad class of behavior patterns resulting from stressful events; marked by phobias, anxiety, or compulsive behavior and obsessive thoughts.

nicotine A stimulant drug found in cigarette smoke; constricts blood vessels and raises blood pressure.

nocturnal emission In men, an orgasm that takes place during sleep as a result of a sexual dream.

noncommunicable disease A disease that is not caused by the invasion into a body of living organisms.

non-nutrients Food components, such as fiber and other roughage, that pass undigested through the intestinal tract but still are important to digestion.

nostrum A device, medicine, or remedy that is supposed to cure a health problem, but does not.

nutrient A component of food used directly by the body—carbohydrates, fats, minerals, proteins, vitamins, and water.

obesity A disease marked by excessive body fat. Other symptoms include shortness of breath, fatigue, and body pains.

obsessive-compulsive syndrome Mental dysfunction characterized by persistent recurring thoughts (obsessions) and ritualistic behavior (compulsions), both of which are partly outside the victim's control.

occlusion A blockage of an artery, especially the coronary artery, preventing the flow of blood.

operant conditioning A type of learning in which a subject voluntarily elicits a response, which is then reinforced; widely used to help people stop smoking and to treat alcoholism. *See also* Reinforcement

ophthalmologist A physician who specializes in treating eye disorders.

opiates A subgroup of narcotic drugs that include opium and its derivatives: codeine, morphine, and Heroin. While widely abused, opiates are valuable in medicine for their painkilling properties.

organic foods Foods grown without chemical pesticides or chemical fertilizers.

outpatient care *See* Ambulatory care

overload The principle that in order to increase fitness you must increase the demands you make on your body.

over-the-counter (OTC) drugs Drugs that can be bought by anyone, without a prescription.

ovum The female egg cell, or sex cell, which unites with sperm to form the conceptus.

oxygen debt An effect of anaerobic exercises, those in which more oxygen is used up than the body can take in; produces dangerous accumulations of waste products in the muscles.

Pap test The microscopic examination of cells from the cervix or uterus to detect the early stages of cancer.

parasite An organism that lives in or on another living organism, obtaining from it part or all of its food.

Parkinson's disease A chronic nervous system disease that causes uncontrolled shaking and other motor difficulties.

particulates Minute particles of substances found in the air, especially in polluted and smoke-filled air, including nicotine and tar, a carcinogen.

passive immunication The practice of injecting antibodies directly into the body to confer immunity.

PCP (phencyclidine hydrochloride; "angel dust") Originally used as an anesthetic, this psychedelic drug is taken for its ability to produce vivid mental imagery; a killer.

peak experience Maslow's term for moments or periods of joy from fulfillment or feelings of oneness with the universe.

pediatrician A physician who specializes in treating children.

pertussis (whooping cough) An infectious inflammation of the air passages with a convulsive spasmodic cough sometimes followed by a crowing intake of breath; caused by a bacterium.

pesticides Chemicals used by farmers and gardeners to kill insects; especially widespread dusting of crops.

pharmacist A health professional who is licensed to prepare and dispense drugs for medicinal purposes.

phobia An intense, illogical fear of certain objects (animate or inanimate) or classes of objects.

photochemical smog A kind of air pollution caused by chemicals in gasoline exhaust under the influences of sunlight; irritating to the respiratory tract and may be carcinogenic.

physician extenders Various kinds of nurses, nurse midwives, nurse practitioners, and physicians' assistants, all of whom provide skilled medical care and do many routine chores once done by physicians.

pinworm An intestinal roundworm that causes intense rectal itching.

placenta A disk-shaped mass of tissue rich in blood vessels that

472

grows from the inner wall of the uterus to provide an exchange of materials between mother and fetus.

pleasure principle The tendency in the personality to wish to immediately satisfy sexual and aggressive drives.

polygenic disorders Disorders, such as diabetes and hypertension, that are caused by the interaction of many genes in combination with appropriate environmental factors.

polyunsaturated fats Fats found in many liquid vegetable oils, such as those made from corn, safflower seeds, and soybeans.

potentiation A drug interaction in which the effect of two or more drugs taken together equals the sum of the effects of each drug taken by itself.

preconscious Freud's term for thoughts and feelings that we are not aware of at any given time but that can become conscious without any difficulty at a suitable moment. *See also* Conscious; Unconscious

pre-ejaculatory fluid In men, a fluid that is secreted by the Cowper's glands that counters the acidity of the urethra and cleans it.

prescription drugs Medicines that can be purchased only with the consent of a physician or dentist; must be bought in a pharmacy, and the pharmacist must place the physician's dosage instructions on the container.

prevalence The number of people suffering from a chronic, long-term disease in a given population at a particular time.

primary care Medical help from a general practitioner or internist that patients seek out on their own; provided in physicians' offices or clinics. *See also* Secondary care; Tertiary care

progesterone A female hormone produced by a corpus luteum; causes the endometrium to grow engorged with blood and nutrients.

projection A defense mechanism in which a person attributes his or her own faults to another person.

proof The amount of alcohol in a product; a proof number equals twice the percentage of alcohol in a beverage (a bottle labeled 100 proof contains 50 percent alcohol).

propagated epidemic A high level of a communicable disease; results from the direct or indirect transmission of an agent from one host to another—for example, gonorrhea. *See also* Common source epidemic

prostaglandins Hormones that may cause severe pain, as in headaches and menstrual cramps.

proteins Organic compounds, composed of amino acids, used by the body to repair and build body tissues; available from animal meat, fish, poultry, milk, nuts, and various grains. *See also* Amino acids

prostate gland A gland surrounding the male urethra, just below the bladder; prostate secretions fortify and protect sperm by providing them with an alkaline coating.

protozoa Microscopic, one-celled animals that live and multiply in animal hosts; cause such infections as malaria and amoebic dysentery.

psoriasis A chronic skin disease marked by red patches covered by white scales.

psychedelic drugs A group of nonaddictive drugs, including LSD, peyote, and PCP, that cause distortions of perception and violent swings of mood. Effects may include tremors, rapid heartbeat, and sleeplessness.

psychoactive drugs Drugs that change the user's body chemistry and affect mood or perception.

psychoanalysis A now-traditional "talk therapy" in which patients attempt to use free association and dream analysis to find the unconscious motives that are held to underlie their problems.

psychosis A mental dysfunction in which a person can no longer control aggressive or regressive impulses and withdraws into a fantasy world; can be caused by functional, organic, or genetic factors. *See also* Manic depression; Schizophrenia

quarantine Limiting the free movement of infected people.

rabies An acute viral disease that attacks the nervous system of warm-blooded animals; is always fatal when untreated; transmitted by the saliva from the bite of an infected animal.

rationalization A defense mechanism in which a person wrongly blames circumstances for personal failures.

reactive coping A form of coping in which people feel themselves to be at the mercy of events or crises and either fight thoughtlessly or flee; these responses may lead to frustration, tension, fatigue, and stress-induced illnesses, or to acts of self-indulgence. *See also* Active coping

reality therapy (RT) William Glasser's method of psychotherapy, which seeks to lead people to stop denying the real world and instead to accept responsibility for fulfilling their needs for self-esteem and for giving and receiving love.

recommended dietary allowance (RDA) Nutritional guidelines, determined by the U.S. government, that estimate how much of a given nutrient is required to maintain good health.

regression A defense mechanism in which a person reverts to childish behavior.

reinforcement In conditioning, either rewarding desirable behavior, such as solving math problems, or punishing undesirable behavior, such as overeating or smoking.

REM (rapid eye movement) sleep The stage of sleep in which the eyes move rapidly from side to side and in which dreaming occurs.

renal disease specialist A physician who specializes in treating kidney diseases.

repression A defense mechanism in which a person completely erases conflicts from consciousness.

reservoir The place where agents of human diseases live—usually in the mucous membranes. Rodents, domestic animals, insects, plants, soil, manure, compost, and dust also act as reservoirs of disease.

resistance The sum of all the body's defenses against infection.

rickettsia Microscopic organisms related to viruses. Rickettsia live outside body cells but multiply within them; they are transmitted to humans by fleas and ticks and cause, among other diseases, Rocky Mountain spotted fever and typhus.

risk factor A physical condition or a practice that is statistically associated with a disease.

ritual Berne's term for a form of long-term coping that consists of shallow exchanges between people.

Rocky Mountain spotted fever A rickettsial disease marked by chills, fever, pains in muscles and joints, and a reddish purple skin eruption; transmitted by the bite of the Rocky Mountain wood tick.

role model   A person who serves as a model of behavior to others.

roughage   The indigestible portion, mostly cellulose, of plants.

rubella (German measles)   An acute contagious disease usually affecting children and young adults; marked by a red skin eruption, mild symptoms, and a short duration. May cause fetal deformities, such as cataracts.

sadist   A person who derives pleasure from hurting others.

sarcoma   A cancerous tumor growing from connective tissue, such as cartilage, bone, or muscle.

saturated fats   Fats that are found in animal products and some vegetable oils.

schistosoma   A parasitic worm that lives in the blood and lymph and spreads its eggs to many organs, where they cause painful irritations and inflammations.

schizophrenia   A mental dysfunction characterized by withdrawal into a fantasy world, belief that one's thoughts are controlled by others, inability to think, delusion, mood disturbances, odd movements, and violence. May be caused either by heredity or by life experiences, or both.

secondary care   Medical care involving a visit to a specialist or hospital. *See also* Primary care; Tertiary care

secondary sex characteristics   Traits that appear at puberty to distinguish one sex from the other. In males, they include deepening of the voice, growth of facial and body hair, and enlargement of the sex organs; in females, widening of the hips, growth of body hair, and development of the breasts and sex organs.

segregation   A defense mechanism in which thoughts are made into groupings that have no basis in logic.

self-actualization   Abraham Maslow's term for the highest state of human development. At this stage, people make full use of all their skills and talents.

self-esteem   The belief that we enjoy the respect of others and that we are worthy of respect; self-esteem increases our self-confidence and leads us to fulfill our artistic and creative needs.

Selye, Hans (1907–   )   A leading researcher in the field of stress, which he defined as the General Adaptation Syndrome (G.A.S.).

seminal vesicle   A gland in the male reproductive tract; temporarily stores semen before ejaculation.

seminiferous tubules   A complex system of canals, within the testes, that is the site of sperm production.

senility   Impairment of the thought processes in old age; caused by hardened blood vessels in the brain; marked by memory loss, disorientation, emotional disturbances, and intellectual decline.

sensor receptors   Structures in the nervous system found in the eyes, ears, nose, and skin that transmit messages to the brain about conditions in the environment.

serial monogamy   The practice of entering into a number of monogamous marriages. *See also* Monogamy

sex-role stereotypes   A culture's fixed beliefs about which jobs, rights, and privileges are appropriate to each sex.

sexual fantasy A sexually stimulating daydream.

shock therapy A physical therapy in which a mild electric current is briefly passed through the brain, often producing convulsions and temporary coma; used for severely withdrawn, depressed, or excited mental patients.

small pox A very contagious and dangerous viral disease marked by high fever, successive stages of skin eruptions, and scar formation. Mainly eradicated by the 1970s through world-wide vaccination programs.

smegma A thick secretion that accumulates under the foreskin of the penis; implicated in cancer of the penis and (in women) of the cervix.

socialization The way in which a person is brought up and taught to be a part of society.

solid wastes 1. Trash discarded by householders and businesses, much of it recyclable; is usually dumped into landfills and covered over with earth. 2. Excrement eliminated through the large intestine and the rectum.

solo practice A medical practice consisting of one physician in one office.

specialists Physicians who treat only one part of system of the body, or only one group of people, such as children or women.

sperm viability The ability of a sperm cell to swim quickly toward the ovum and fertilize it.

STDs (sexually transmitted diseases) A group of diseases—gonorrhea, syphilis, herpes, and nongonococcal urethritis are the most common—that are spread by sexual contact. Most are spread by bacterial infections.

sterilization A long-term method of contraception that involves cutting or tying the fallopian tubes in women or the vasa deferentia in men. *See also* Vasectomy; Tubal ligation; Hysterectomy

stimulants A group of drugs—for example, nicotine, cocaine, and amphetamines—that excite the central nervous system. Long-term effects include feelings of restlessness and irritability, weight loss, paranoia, and a tendency to violence.

stress According to Selye, "the nonspecific response of the body to any demand made upon it." Stress can be caused both by pleasant and unpleasant events. *See also* General Adaptation Syndrome; Eustress; Distress

stressors Sources of stress arising from inner causes, such as lack of self-esteem, or from outer causes, such as a contagious disease, rush-hour traffic, or social pressures. May lead to a breakdown of the body and thus to disease.

stroke (cerebrovascular accident) A disruption of the brain's blood supply; results in the death of brain cells.

subconscious *See* Preconscious

sucrose Table sugar.

superego Freud's term for the force in the personality that strives to be moral and perfect; it is conservative, because handed down from past generations, and seeks to preserve social order. *See also* Ego; Id

synergy A drug interaction in which the effect of two or more drugs taken together is greater than would be expected from the combined effect of each drug taken individually.

synthetic narcotics A subgroup of narcotic drugs; includes Methadone, Darvon, and Demerol. Methadone is used to treat Heroin addictions; Darvon is often prescribed by physicians as a pain reliever.

systemic illnesses Diseases that affect many systems or every system in the body—for example, the common cold.

tapeworm A parasitic flatworm that absorbs food from the intestinal tract.

tar The primary carcinogenic agent in cigarette smoke; formed by the burning of tobacco dust.

tertiary care Medical care involving advanced equipment and procedures—for example, kidney dialysis, or heart and brain surgery; provided only in hospitals. *See also* Primary care; Secondary care

testosterone The male sex hormone; produced in the testes and is responsible for male secondary sex characteristics. In women, small amounts are produced by the ovaries.

tetanus (lockjaw) An infectious bacterial disease marked by spasms and rigidity of the voluntary muscles, especially in the jaw; caused by a poison produced by the tetanus bacillus, which usually enters the body through a wound.

THC (tetrahydrocannabinol) The active ingredient in marijuana and hashish; harmful effects may include damage to the brain and reproductive system, short-term memory loss, and motor function impairment

thermography The infrared detection of "hot-spots" in the body; those with cell or tissue disturbances.

third-party payments Payments of health-care costs by insurance companies or by the government, instead of by patients themselves.

threshold dose The amount of a drug needed to produce an effect.

time structuring Berne's term for a kind of long-term coping that ranges from withdrawal to intimacy. *See also* Withdrawal; Ritual; Intimacy

tolerance The need of a drug user to take more and more of a drug in order to get the original effect.

toxic wastes Industrial chemicals and by-products that are poisonous, corrosive, reactive, or ignitable; are often dumped in landfills, where they seep into and pollute ground water.

trace elements Minerals such as iodine, zinc, fluorine, cobalt, and copper, all needed by the body in amounts of .01 gram or less daily.

trachoma A form of blindness caused by chlamydia and marked by an inflammation of the mucous membrane on the inner surface of the eyelid.

training effect The long-term effect of exercise—especially aerobic exercise: stronger respiratory muscles; an increased number of blood vessels in the lungs; deeper, more efficient breathing; and increased muscular efficiency and endurance.

tranquilizers A group of drugs that are widely prescribed by physicians to treat anxiety and tension. Minor tranquilizers, such as Valium, are the ones most often used; major tranquilizers, such as Thorazine, are only prescribed for severe mental or physical problems.

transactional analysis Berne's method of helping patients understand the ways they structure time and deal with others; emphasizes self-assertion and freedom from control by others.

transference A pattern of behavior by patients undergoing psycho-analysis in which they react to their analysts as they did to authority figures in early life.

transverse presentation A birth in which the baby lies across the opening in the uterus, thereby causing problems in delivery.

transvestite A person who derives sexual pleasure from dressing as a member of the opposite sex.

trial marriage A relationship in which a man and woman live to-gether before making a final decision to marry.

triglycerides The most common forms of fat in the human diet; may consist of saturated, polyunsaturated, or monosaturated fat.

tubal ligation A surgical procedure for sterilizing women. The fallo-pian tubes are cut and tied to keep the egg from being fertilized by sperm.

type A behavior The behavior of people who are competitive, ob-sessed with a sense of urgency, easily hurt, and frequently angry; they often suffer from early heart disease.

type B behavior The behavior of people who are relaxed, easygoing, and free from the need to achieve endlessly; less likely to be found in people with heart disease than type A behavior.

typhus A rickettsial disease marked by high fever, stupor alternating with delirium, intense headache, and a dark red rash.

ulcer A break in the skin or mucous membrane that festers; often a crater-like wound in the stomach wall caused when digestive acids wear away the stomach lining.

umbilical cord A cord arising from the naval; connects the fetus with the placenta within the uterus.

unconscious Freud's term for the vast region of the mind that holds repressed, socially unacceptable impulses, especially those connected with sex and aggression. *See also* Preconscious; Conscious

undernutrition The deficiency of nutrients that accompanies a defi-ciency of calories; especially dangerous in infancy and childhood, since it may cause irreversible mental retardation.

urethra A tube that leads from the bladder to the outside of the body. In males, it forms part of the penis and conveys both urine and semen.

vaccine A preparation containing small numbers of disease agents or their products; injected into the body of a healthy person to stimulate the production of antibodies.

vaginal aspiration (suction curettage) A method of induced abor-tion in which the contents of the uterus are removed, by suction, with an electric pump.

vaginismus A contraction of the outer vaginal muscles that prevents the penis from entering.

vas deferens (pl. vasa deferentia) A long, thick-walled tube that conducts sperm cells from the testes to the ejaculatory duct.

vasectomy A surgical procedure for sterilizing men. The vasa defe-rentia are cut and tied so that sperm cannot pass through the tubes and enter the semen.

virulence The ability of an organism to sicken or kill its host.

virus   A submicroscopic organism that invades a living cell, multiplies within it, and takes charge of the cell's functions.

vitamins   Nutrients that make possible many of the body's chemical reactions, including those that release energy from nutrients other than vitamins. *See also* Fat-soluble vitamins; Water-soluble vitamins; Minerals

voluntary nervous system   The part of the nervous system that controls conscious mental action, like thought, emotion, and language. *See also* Autonomic nervous system

warm-up   A set of stretching and flexibility exercises performed before more vigorous exercise to prevent pulling or tearing of muscles.

water cycle   The constant circulation of water between the atmosphere, the earth's surface, and the water table (below the surface).

water-soluble vitamins   Vitamins such as C. Since the body does not store excesses of them, but excretes them in the urine, it needs to take them in every day.

whooping cough   *See* Pertussis

withdrawal   A form of long-term coping in which people spend as little time as possible with others; may be both physical and mental.

withdrawal symptoms   Symptoms that develop when an addict tries to quit taking an addictive drug; may include anxiety, physical weakness, muscle contractions, abdominal cramps, nausea, weight loss, and increased heart rate.

zygote   a fertilized ovum before cell division begins.

Index

AA (Alcoholics Anonymous), 96
abdominal thrust (for choking), 443–445
abortion, 295, 308–312
  debate over, 310, 312
  illegal, dangers of, 310
  and incest, 310
  methods of, 308–310
  Right-to-Life Movement, 312
  risks from, 309
  spontaneous (miscarriage), 284
  Supreme Court decision, 310, 312
acid (LSD), 73
acid rain, 404
acne
  cause of, 389
  diet and, 389
  suggested treatments for, 389
acupuncture, 395
addiction, 68, 75, 76
  to diet pills, 184
  and pregnancy, 284
  and smoking, 106
  withdrawal symptoms, 68, 76, 78
additives, to food, 161, 162
adolescents
  choices for, 317
  masturbation and, 261
  rebellion and, 325
  stress and, 29
adoption
  attitudes toward, 327
  hard to place children, 327
  process of, 326
adrenal glands, 201
aerobics, 135–138
  general fitness and, 132
  jogging and, 135
  training effect and, 135
agents of infection, 223–229
  causative (etiological), 223
  classification by causal, 231–241
aging, 340–343
  diabetes and, 196
  personality and, 341
  social problems of poverty and, 342
  See also older people, old age
air pollution, 402, 403
  acid rain and, 404
  environmentalism and reduction of,
    414, 415
  infectious disease and, 228
  sources of, 402
  symptoms from, 402
  weather conditions and, 403
alarm reaction (GAS), 34, 35
Alanon, 96
Alateen, 96
alcohol, 12, 14, 82–101
  abuse, 53
  antabuse and, 26
  as big business, 87

blood alcohol level (BAL), 86, 87
  breast feeding and, 291
  college students and, 82
  consumption of, in U.S., 83
  coping and, 46
  crime and misuse of, 428
  depressant nature of, 72, 83–85
  drinking and drugs, 84, 85
  drugs and, 382
  effects of, 83–87
  human costs of use, 88
  impotence and, 278
  as leading drug problem in U.S., 82
  misuse of, 64, 88, 93
  mood-altering effects of, 82
  production of, 82
  pregnancy and, 94, 95, 284
  problem drinkers, 92–98
  Prohibition, 88, 89
  social problems and, 64
  temperence movement, 88
  use of in U.S., 63
alcohol and drugs, effects of mixing
  additive, 84
  antagonistic, 84
  synergistic, 84
alcohol dependence
  stages of, 90–92
  stress and, 90
  symptoms of, 90–92
alcohol misuse, theories of causes, 93
alcoholics, 89, 364
Alcoholics Anonymous (AA), 96
alcoholism, 89, 92–95
  diseases connected with, 92–95
  in elderly people, 341
  impact on family life, 95, 96
  medical treatment of, 89
  nutrition therapy and, 57
  and self-image, 89
  treatments for,
    Alcoholics Anonymous, 96
    behavior modification, 96
    biofeedback, 96
    psychotherapy, 96
algae and eutrophication, 406
allergic reactions, 215
  as cause of shock, 449
  and diet pills, 104
  and rheumatoid arthritis, 217
allergies
  antibodies and, 214
  asthma, 215
  frequency in world population, 214
  inflammation response, 214
  symptoms of, 390
  treatment of, 215
amino acids, 150
amniotic sac, 286
amoebic dysentery, 225
amphetamines, 65, 70

alcohol and, 85
  weight reduction and, 189
anaerobics, 135
anal intercourse, 276
analgesic (pain killer), 68, 69
  and alcohol, effect of mixing, 84
anaplasia, 207
"anatomy is destiny" (Freud), 250
androgen, 279
androgynous personality, 257
anesthesia in childbirth, 288
  effect on fetus, 288
angina pectoris, 204
anopheles mosquito, 240
anorexia nervosa, 183
anorgasmia (frigidity), 278
anoxia, 344, 345
antabuse (disulfiram), 26
antagonism in drugs, 84, 382
anthrax, 226
antibiotics
  acne and, 389
  alcohol and, effect of mixing, 85
  drug interaction and, 382
  leukemia and, 210
  pregnancy and, 284
  sexually transmitted diseases and, 236,
    240
antibodies, 229–232
  and allergies, 214
antidepressants, effect of mixing
  with alcohol, 84
antifertility agent, 306
antigen, 214, 229
  body's response to
    antibodies, 214
    inflammation, 214
antihistamines, 84, 386
  effect of mixing with alcohol, 84
antihypertensive agents, effect of
  mixing with alcohol, 84
antiperspirants, 391
antiprostaglandins, 387
anxiety, 17, 55
aphrodisiacs, 397, 398
apostat, 177
appendicitis, 192, 457
  and obesity, 174
appetite control mechanism, 177
arthritis, 216, 217, 343, 395
  nostrums and, 395
  osteoarthritis, 217
  rheumatoid, 216, 217
  treatments for, 217
arthropods, 225, 240, 241
artificial respiration, 440–442
  in drug overdose, 449
arousal (sexual), 263
aspirin, 63, 380, 382, 386, 387
  and pregnancy, 284
asthma, 215, 304, 454

and the Pill, 304
symptoms of, 215
atherosclerosis, 151, 201–203, 343
  as cause of psychosis, 53
  in senility, 53
athlete's foot, 226, 240
atkins diet, 180
atomic energy, and problems of
  meltdown, 410, 411
  operation, 411
  waste disposal, 410, 411

baby boom, 336, 337
bacilli, 224
bacteria, 224, 225, 228, 389
bacterial disease, see sexually transmitted
      disease
barbiturates, 65, 68, 72
  alcohol and, 84
  dangers of, 72
  effect on nervous system, 72
  withdrawal from, 72
basal body temperature (BBT) method,
      299, 300
  effectiveness of, 300
basal metabolic rate (BMR), 176
basal metabolism, 139
basic four food groups, 162–164
  and fad diets, 180
  a serving of, 164
basic human needs, 23–25, 32
  in reality therapy, 24, 25
battered wives, 425
b-complex vitamins, 163
beer, use of in U.S., 82, 83
behavior, obsessive-compulsive, 50
behavior modification
  alcoholism and, 96
  dieting and, 188, 189
behaviorism, 25, 26
behaviorist theories of violence, 423
  learned response and, 423
bestiality, 265
biofeedback, 96
birth, 286–291
  anesthesia during, 288
  fathering, 289
  fetal positions, 287
  new methods of, 289–291
  places for, 288, 289
  stages of labor, 286, 287
  See also childbirth
birth control
  abortion and, 308–312
  clinics, 302
  dangers of, 295
  in the future, 305, 306
  male contraceptive, 306
  menopause and, 279
  methods of, 295, 297–308
    use effectiveness of, 296
  pills
    cancer and, 213
    interaction with drugs, 382
    smoking and, 110
  reasons for, 295
  responsibility for, 296
  responsible sexual behavior and, 260
  Roman Catholic Church and, 295
birth defects, 282, 284
  alcohol use and, 94, 284

miscarriage and, 284
smoking and, 284
toxic wastes and, 406
birth rates in U.S., 336
birthing centers, 289
Black Death, 223, 343
bleeding, treatment for, 439
blindness
  chlamydia as cause of, 225
  diabetes and, 196
blood alcohol level (BAL), 86, 87
blood transfusions and leukemia, 210
blood vessels, 197–204
Blue Cross, 367
Blue Shield, 367
body cells, and lack of oxygen, 344
body fat and stored energy, 176
body types, 176
boils, 455
bones, broken, 442
bottle feeding, 291
botulism, 193
brain
  cancer, danger signs of, 206
  cerebellum, 14
  cerebrum, 14
  chemistry, 218
  damage, 11
    from alcohol, 12
    and breathing problems, 440–442
    physical disorders of elderly and, 13
  death, 344, 345
  injury and psychosis, 52
  limbic system of, 14
  medulla, 14
  right and left portions of, 195
  stem, 345
  tumors, 11
breast cancer
  danger signs of, 205
  lumpectomy, 212
  mammograms, 212
  mastectomy, 212
  risk factors in, 213
  thermography, 212
breast developers and quackery, 393
breast feeding
  advantages of, 291
  alcohol and drugs and, 291
breasts
  development of, 274
  mammary glands, 274
  size and heredity, 393
breech presentation, 287
bronchitis
  chronic, 109
    and smoking, 109, 215
  treatment for, 215
burns
  causes of, 442
  as cause of shock, 449
  treatment for, 442, 443

Caesarian section, 287, 288
caffeine, 63, 64, 70
  effects of overuse, 72
  products containing, 72
calcium, 153, 157
  importance to body, 153
  sources of in diet, 153

and structure of bones and teeth, 153
calisthenics, 134, 145
calories, 149–151, 165, 178, 180–182,
      188
  daily requirements of, 184
  empty, meaning of, 167
  expended on various activities,
      139–141
    per mile of running, 126
  malnutrition and, 168
  in meat group, 163, 169
  in milk, 163
cancer
  alcohol related, 93
  categories of, 210
  cells, growth of, 207
  circumcision and, 213
  of colon and rectum, 213
  danger signs of (chart), 205, 206
  death rates from, 208, 211
  diagnosis of, 213
  early detection of, 213
  early symptoms of, 209
  esophageal and smoking, 109
  of gastro-intestinal system, 109
  genetic abnormalities and, 195
  genetic predisposition to, 213
  how it grows, 207
  lung, and smoking, 109
  old age and, 341
  Pap test for, 213
  the Pill and, 304
  pipe and cigar smoking and, 113
  risk factors for, 213
  symptoms of, 213
  toxic wastes and, 406
    risk from DDT, 409
  treatment for, 214
  of urinary tract, 109
  of the uterus and cervix, 213
candidiasis and antibiotics, 240
Cannabis sativa, 70
carbohydrates
  as basic nutrient, 149, 150
  complex, 150, 151, 182
  consumption of, 169
  diets and, 180–182
  functions of, 151
  misinformation about, 167
  principle sources of, 151
  simple (the sugars), 150
  as source of energy, 149
carbon, 150
carbon dioxide, 131
carbon monoxide
  in cigarette smoke, 109
  poisoning, symptoms of, 402
carcinogenic substances, 209, 214
  tar in cigarette smoke, 109
carcinoma, 212
cardiopulmonary resuscitation (CPR),
      344, 437, 441, 443
  guide for, 446–449
cardiorespiratory disease, 127
cardiorespiratory fitness
  effect of on heart, 131
  effect of on respiratory system, 131
cardiovascular diseases, 110, 196–204,
      343
  atherosclerosis, 201
  as cause of death in U.S., 197

diet and, 198, 199
  essential hypertension, 201
  heart attack, 203, 204
  prevalence of in U.S., (chart), 202
  stroke, 202
  valve disorders, 201
cardiovascular system
  anatomy of, 199, 200
  physiology of, 199, 200
  problems with in old age, 340
castration, 306
causal agents of disease, 231–241
  bacterial, 236–239
    sexually transmitted, 236–239
  rickettsial, 235, 236
  viral, 231–235
cell pathology, 192
cellular death, 345
cellulose, 150, 159
cerebellum, 14
cerebral cortex, 344
cerebrovascular accident, 202
cerebrum, 14
cervical cap, 302, 303
cervical mucus method, 299, 300
  effectiveness of, 300
cervix, 272, 301–303, 309
  cancer of, 213
chain of infection, 228
chemical transmitters, 218
  diseases of the nervous system and, 218
chemotherapy
  breast cancer and, 212
  leukemia and, 210
  use in schizophrenia, 54
  side effects of, 210, 211
chickenpox, 228, 234
child abuse, 424, 425
  hot line, 425
childbirth
  genital chlamydia and, 237
  genital herpes and, 234
  gentle birthing, 290, 291
  gonorrhea and, 236
  natural, 290
  See also birth
childhood, 320
  adolescence, 317
  cancer, danger signs of, 206
children
  abused, 424, 425
  adoption of, 326, 327
  death and, 345
  effects of undernutrition in, 169
  exposure to cigarette smoke and, 111,
    112, 114
  of heavy drinkers, 97
  home safety for, 453
  hyperactive, 111
  masturbation in, 261
  in one-parent families, 331
  planning the sex of, 251
  role of fathers in raising, 326
  sensitivity to drugs in, 382
Chinese medical practices, 394, 395
  acupuncture, 395
Chinese Restaurant Syndrome
  and MSG, 161
chlamydia, 225
  and sexually transmitted disease, 225
chloramphenicol, 236

chloroform, 288
chlorine, 153, 157
Chlortrimeton, 390
choking
  the abdominal thrust for, 443–445
  prevention of, 444
cholera, 242
cholesterol, 131, 151, 152, 169
  atherosclerosis and, 151
  in meat group, 163
chromosome, 270, 280
  extra, 194
chronic obstructive lung disease,
    (C.O.L.D.), 215, 216
cigarette smoke
  bronchitis and, 215
  as cause of health problems in
    children, 111, 112
  components of, 109
  emphysema and, 215
  gases in, 109
  particulates in, 109
cigarette smoking and cancer, 208, 209,
    212
  risk factor of, 193
cigarettes, 104–120
circulatory system and shock, 449
circumcision, 213, 269
cirrhosis of the liver, 94
classical conditioning, 25
climacteric, 279
clinical death, 344, 345
clinical depression, symptoms of, 51
clitoris, 271–273, 276
Clostridium botulinum, 193
cocaine, 65, 70, 71, 85
  alcohol and, 85
  depression and, 71
  effects of use, 71
cocci, 224
codeine, 75
coffee drinking in U.S., 64
coitus interruptus, 295, 297, 300
cold medicines, 385
  and pregnancy, 284
cold sores (fever blisters), 234
colds, see common cold
collective violence
  war and society, 432, 433
college health service
  evaluation of, 372
college
  stressful situations in, 31
  students
    alcohol and, 82
    drinking and, 82, 97, 98
    drugs and, 65
    living arrangements for, 317–319
    problems facing, 56
    roommates, 317–319
    where to get help, 56
  years as time of choice, 317
colon
  cancer of, 213, 214
  fiber and, 161
colostomy, 214
coma, 345
common cold, 225, 227, 228
  healing process of, 232
  OTC products for, 386
  prevention of, 232, 233

symptoms of, 231–232
  treatment of, 232, 233
common-law marriage, 332
communicable disease, 221–245
  common, 231–240
  control of, 241–243
    host immunization, 243
    mode of transmission, 243
    reservoir, 241, 243
communication, lack of and marriage,
    324
Compazine, 73
competition and stress, 31
competitive sports, 144
complex carbohydrates, 150, 151, 182
conception, 296, 297
condom, 238, 297, 300, 301, 303, 306
  protection against disease, 301
  reliability of as contraceptive, 301
congenital defects, 195
  incidence of, 195
congenital diseases, late appearing, 195,
    196
conscious, the, 16, 17
consciousness, 25
conservationism, 414
  enviornmentalism and, 414, 415
constipation, 387, 456
  OTC drugs for, 387
consumer complaints, how to file, 398
contraception
  biological basis of, 296, 297
  methods of, 295–305
contraceptives
  condom as, 301
  cream or gel, 301
  hormonal, 303
  male, 306
  suppositories, 303
  tampons, 305
cool-downs, 143, 144
Cooper Field Test, 129
Cooper's Point System, 137, 138
coping, 45–51
  active, 46, 47
  conscious, 46, 47
  defense mechanisms and, 48
  dysfunction, 50, 51
  fight-or-flight, 45
  long-term, 48, 49
  problem solving and, 46, 47
  reactive, 45
  short-term, 48
  strategies and overeating, 178
  unconscious, 46
copper, 153, 158
coronary arteries, 203
  disease, 195
    and heavy drinking, 93
coronary thrombosis, 204
corpus luteum, 274
cosmetics, 390, 391
  dangers from misuse, 390
cough medicines, OTC products, 386
coughing, as mode of transmission, 227
couples, unmarried in U.S., 317
  common law, 317
courtship and successful marriage, 322
Cowper's glands, 271, 300
CPR (cardiopulmonary resuscitation),
    344, 437, 441, 443, 446–449

rab lice, 241
reams and gels, spermicidal, 301–303
rime
  rape, 428, 429
  street, 426–428
  victim counseling, 428
ryotherapy, 213
ultural conditioning, 250
ulture, the
  deviant sex acts and, 264
  homosexuality and, 264
  sex roles and, 249–258
  sexuality and guilt and, 260
ulture values
  and stress-related disease, 40
unnilingus, 276
ystic fibrosis, 194

and C (as abortion), 308
andruff, 391
arvon, 75, 110
ay dreams, 262
DT, effects on human health, 409
eath
  average age of, in humans, 338
  brain, 344
  cellular, 345
  clinical, 344
  and the dying, 347
  euthanasia, 351, 352
  fear of, 345, 346
  grief and, 347, 348
  the hospice and, 350, 351
  ignorance of, 346
  impact of, on the dying, 346
  meaning of, 344, 345
    in different cultures, 345
  medical, guidelines to define, 345
  mourning and, 348, 349
  murder as cause of in U.S., 421
  from overdose, 449
  privacy of in U.S., 343
  rates in U.S., 336, 344
  stages of (Kübler-Ross), 347
  and stress, 15
  suicide as cause of, 52
ecibels, 413, 414
  measuring noise pollution, 414
efense mechanisms of body
  antibodies, 229
  antigens, 229
  immunity, 229–231
  white blood cells, 229
elta sleep, 145
emerol, 75
entists, 375, 395, 398
  guidelines for choosing, 375
  quackery and, 395
eodorants, 391
epressants, 69
  alcohol, 63, 64, 72, 83
  barbiturates, 65, 68, 72
  effects of, 72
epression
  alcoholism and, 91
  clinical, 51
  loss and, 51
  nutrition therapy and, 57
  and withdrawal from tranquilizers, 73
eviants, 264
iabetes, 169, 195, 196, 278

age and, 196
cancer of uterus and cervix and, 21, 213
low-carbohydrate diet and, 182
incidence of, 196
juvenile, 196
obesity and, 174
the Pill and, 304
pregnancy and, 295
shock, 196
diabetic coma, 196
diaphragm, 301–303
  keys to effective use of, 302
  jelly and, 297
diarrhea
  causes, symptoms and first aid for, 456
  high-fat diet and, 183
  OTC drugs for, 387
diet
  balanced and long life, 343
  daily and basic food groups, 162
  eating habits and, 165
  groups, 187
  minerals, importance of in, 153
  nutritional conditioning and, 165
  overconsumption and, 169
  pills, 180
    side effects of, 183
  pregnancy and, 285
  Recommended Dietary Allowance
    (RDA), 165
  stressors and, 36
  a suitable, 165
  vegetarianism, 165
  vitamins, importance in, 153
  water, importance in, 153
diets
  Atkins, 180
  high-carbohydrate, 182
  high-fat, 180, 182
  high-protein, 180, 181
  liquid protein, 181
  low-carbohydrate, 180, 181
  low-fat, 180, 183
  macrobiotic, 183
  Scarsdale, 180
dieter's secret prayer, 180
diethyl stilbestrol (DES), 284
dieting as way of life, 174, 175
digestion, fiber and, 159–161
digestive system and disease, 192
digestive tract
  diseases of, 217
dilation and curettage, (D and C), 308
diphtheria, 227, 230, 243
disease
  alcoholism, 89
  classifications of, 192
  of digestive tract, 217, 218
  communicable, 192
  incidence of, 192
  noncommunicable, 192–220
  prevalence of, 192, 193
  prevention and longevity, 342, 343
  stress and, 36–38
distilled spirits, use of in U.S., 83
distress (Selye), 35, 36
diuretics, 387
  effect of mixing with alcohol, 84
divorce, 322, 328–331
  causes of, 329

kinds of adjustment in (Bohannon), 329, 330
rate of in U.S., 328, 329, 331
social trends encouraging, 330
domestic violence, 423–425
  child abuse, 424, 425
  preventing, 425
  spouse abuse, 425
douche, 299
Down's syndrome, 194
drinking
  college students and, 82, 97–99
  heavy, and disease, 93, 94
  irresponsible, signs of, 101
  myths about, 99
  precautions, 100
  responsible, 99
  social respectability of, 82
  teenage, 97
drug(s)
  of abuse, 63
  addiction, 68
  advertisements for, 383, 384
  alcohol, 82, 84
  amphetamines, 65, 70, 85, 189
  barbiturates, 65, 68, 72, 84
  birth defects from, 284
  brand names, meaning of, 380
  breast feeding and, 291
  controlled, 63
  crime and, 428
  cultural approval of, 66
  cumulative effect of, 382
  dependence, stages of, 68
  dose response, 66, 67
  effects of, on nervous system, 66–68
  generic, meaning of, 380
  hallucinogens, 64, 65
  Heroin, 63, 65, 68, 75, 76, 78, 99
  how to take medicine, 387
  illicit, 63
  impotence and, 278
  interaction, 382
  and labor in childbirth, 288
  marijuana, 65, 69, 70, 74, 75, 85, 99
  mental craving for, 68
  methods of administration, 67
  morphine, 63, 75
  over-the-counter, 380, 384–391
  potency of, 68
  pregnant women and, 284
  prescription, 380
  psychoactive, 63, 67
  side effects of, 381, 382
  stages of dependence on, 68
  stressors and, 36
  synergy, 68, 84, 382
  therapy, 78
  tolerance to, 68
  trends, 65
  use, as response to stress, 63
  weight reduction and, 189
  withdrawal symptoms of, 68
  young adults and, 65
drug abuse, 53, 76–78
  causes of, 76, 77
  coping and, 46
  peer pressure and, 77
  prevention of, 76
drug dependency, 57, 382
  nutrition therapy and, 57

pregnancy [handwritten in margin]

drug interaction, 382
D(dreaming) sleep, 145, 146
dying, myths about, 345
dying person's bill of rights, 349
dysfunction (Meninger), 50, 51, 54–58
dysmenorrhea, 387

earache, 454
ectomorphs, 176
ectopic pregnancy, 305
egg cell, *see* ovum
egg sacs, (follicles), 273
ego, 18–23, 31–33, 36
  change and marriage, 319
  and coping with stress, 18
ego development, theory of (Erikson)
  19–23, 36
ejaculation, 260, 278, 297, 300, 307
ejaculatory duct, 271
embryo, 282
emergency medical service (EMS), 437
emphysema, 109, 215
  cigarette smoke as cause of, 215
encounter-group therapy, 56
endometrium, 273, 274
endomorphs, 176
endurance (fitness), 127, 130, 131
energy
  body fat as stored, 176
  calories and, 149
  carbohydrates as source, 149, 150
  food as source of, 125
  measurement of, 149
  needs of body, 181
  sleep and, 145
environment, 402–419
  epidemics and, 229
  infectious disease and, 228
  pollution of, 402–411
  population problem and, 415–417
  urban, 412–414
environmental pollution, 402–411
  air pollutants and, 402
  geographical and weather conditions
    and, 403, 404
  heavy metals and, 409
  pesticides and, 408, 409
  radiation and, 410, 411
  risk factor, 193
  solid wastes, 407
  toxic wastes, 406, 407
  water pollution, 404–406
Environmental Protection Agency (EPA),
  406, 407
environmentalism
  costs of, 415
  National Environmental Policy Act,
    414
  Silent Spring and, 414
  spaceship earth, 415
epidemics, 229, 230
epididymus, 270, 271
epilepsy, 195
epithelial tissues, 210
erectile inhibition (impotence), 278
erection, 269, 277, 278, 396
Erikson, Erik, 19–22, 25, 32, 36
  eight stages of life, 19–22
esophagus, 217
estrogen, 273, 274, 303, 304
etiological agent, 223

etiology, 227
euthanasia, 351, 352
eutrophication, 406
excitement, 276, 277
exercise
  advantages of, 125
  boredom and, 144
  calorie chart for, 185
  cardiovascular disease and, 198, 199
  cool-downs, 143
  dangers of, 138
  fatigue and, 144
  kinds of, 131–138
    aerobics, 132, 135–138
    anaerobics, 132, 135
    isometrics, 132
    isotonics, 132–134
  long term effects of, 132
  logs, 145
  loss of trace elements from, 153
  overload, 143, 144
  sleep and, 145
  stress reduction and, 127
  training effect and, 132, 134–135, 143
  warm-ups, 138
  as way of life, 138
  weight control and, 125, 176
exercise programs, 127–131
  goals of, 131
  measuring fitness, 127–131
exhibitionism, 265
existential therapy, 55
euphoric, 75
eustress and distress, theory of (Selye),
  35, 36
eye makeup, 391

fad diets, 167, 180–183
  dangers of, 180
  diet pills and, 183
  eating habits and, 180
fallopian tubes, 272, 273, 281, 295, 297,
  298, 306
family, the, 316–333
  college years and, 317–319
  divorce and, 327–331
  marriage and, 319–324
  parenthood, 324–327
  regrouping, 331, 332
  separation from and stress, 31
  single parent, 331
  therapy, 57
  violence in, 423–425
family practice, 358
fantasy
  homosexual, 264
  sexual, 262, 263
fasting, and weight reduction, 188
fatalistic suicide, 52
fathers
  role of in childrearing, 326
  single,
    problems of work and family, 331
fatigue
  chronic, 144
  resistance to, 127
fats (lipids), 149–152, 167, 169, 178,
  180–182, 196
  calories in, 150, 151
  consumption of in U.S., 152
  diabetes and, 196

diets and, 180–182
energy and, 150
functions of, 151
importance in diet, 151
in meat group, 163
percentage of in American diet, 152
phospholipids, 150
principle sources of, 151
as source of vitamins, 152
sterols, 150
triglycerides, 150, 151
fat-soluble vitamins, 163
fatty acids, 131
Federal Trade Commission, 385, 399
fellatio, 276
female
  genitals, 272
    cancer of, 205
  secondary sex characteristics, 274
  sex organs
    external, 271, 272
    internal, 272–274, 300
female characteristics, traditional
  249–251, 256
feminine hygiene, 389
feminine sex-role traits, 250
fertility awareness method, 303, 304
  effectiveness of, 298, 300
fertilization, 303, 305
  process of, 280, 281
fertilizers and eutrophication, 406
Fetal Alcohol Syndrome (FAS), 95
fetal positions, 287
fetus, 282, 284, 285, 308–310
  effect of anesthetics on, 288
fetishism, 264, 265
fiber, 159–161, 181
  colon cancer and, 161
  constipation and, 161
  sources of, 160
fight-or-flight reaction, 34
filaria, 226
first aid, 436–457
  general rules for, 439
  kit contents, 437, 438
  problems and treatments, 439–451
  for sudden illness, 454–457
first-degree burns
  causes of, 442
  treatment for, 442
fitness measuring, 127–131
  cardiorespiratory, 127–129
  flexibility, 129, 130
  muscular endurance, 130
  muscular strength, 129
fitness tests, 129, 130
flashbacks, 74
flatworms, 226
flavor enhancers, 161
  MSG (monosodium glutamate), 161
fleas, 225
flouride and tooth decay, 217
flourine, 153, 158
foam, spermicidal, 302, 303
follicles, 273
fomites, 227
foods
  drug interaction with, 382
  fiber content of, 160
  infectious disease and, 228
  social attitudes and, 149

od and Drug Administration, 304
od colors, 161
od poisoning, 228, 229, 456
od processing,
 additives used in, 161, 162
replay, 301
reskin (prepuce), 269
circumcision, 269
ssil fuels and air pollution, 402
eedom and stress, 31
eud, Sigmund, 16–19, 23–26, 55, 250,
 263
 and smoking, 108
eud's theory of personality, 17–19, 32
gidity, 278
uctose (fruit sugar), 150
uit and vegetable group, 163, 169, 178,
 181, 182
 importance of in diet, 163
 recommended daily servings of, 163
ndus, 273
ngal disease, 240
ngal infections, 226
ngus, 225, 226

ll bladder disease and obesity, 174
ames, 48, 49
angrene from diabetes, 196
ases, in cigarette smoke, 109
astritis, 217
astrointestinal cancer, 206
astrointestinal illness, 456, 457
ene patterns, 11
 and brain damage, 11
eneral Adaptation Syndrome (GAS)
 (Selye), 35, 36, 46
 stages of, 35
eneral practice, 357, 358
eneral practitioner (GP), 363, 364
eneric drugs, 380
enes, 194, 195, 270, 274, 280
enetic defects, late appearing, 195, 196
enetic (inherited) diseases, 194–196
enetic traits, 176
enetic variation (mutation), 231
enital (pubic) area, 271
enital chlamydia, 236, 238
enital deodorants, 389
enital herpes, 235, 236
enitals, 238, 239, 261
 female, 272
 male, 269
enocide, 433
estalt therapy, 56
nsing root, 398
ans, 269
lasser, William, 24, 25
ucose
 insulin and, 196
 sources of, 149
lycogen, 150, 181
onorrhea, 236, 238, 305
 pregnant women and, 236
 symptoms of, 236, 238
ossypol, 306
overnment
 drug safety and, 379
 nationalized health insurance, 371
  cost of, 371
 socialized medicine, 370, 371

as third party payer, 360, 361
and tobacco production, 118–120
grains, 163, 169
 importance of in diet, 163
 recommended daily servings of, 163
grief
 physical and mental symptoms of, 347,
  348
 stages of, 348
 of survivors, 347
 usefulness of, 348
 victims of crime and phases of, 428
groin, 269
group practice, 365
gynecologist, 282

habit-forming drugs, 106
hair-care products, 391
hallucinogens, 65
 major effects of use, 74
 see also psychedelics
hallucinations, 71, 73–75
 cocaine and, 71
 and drug overdose, 449
Hansen's bacillus, 228
hardening of the arteries, 151
hashish, 69
hay fever, 214
headache, 454
head injuries and brain damage, 11
health
 alcohol, effect on, 93–95
 holistic concept of, 192
 mental, 11–14, 29
 smoking and, 110, 112–114
health care
 access of minorities to, 358
 costs of, 368–370
  medical technology, 362
 government's role in, 357, 367, 368
 group practice, 365
 new ideas in, 364
 paradoxes of, 357
 place of, 364
 stages of, 363, 364
health care products, 378–400
 advertising and, 379–381
  appraising, 383, 384
  cost of, 380
  guidelines for buying OTC drugs,
   382, 383
 quacks and quackery, 392–399
 specific products, 386–391
health expenditures in U.S., 361
health foods, 395
health insurance, 360
 government's role, 367, 368
 private companies, 367
 types of, 366
Health Insurance Institute, 399
health maintenance organization
 (HMO), 365
heart, 192, 197–204
 effects of fitness on, 131
 fitness of, 126
heart attacks (coronary thrombosis), 203,
 204, 441
 causes of, 445
 CPR, 446–449
 diabetes and, 196
 first aid for, 445–449

obesity and, 174
and the Pill, 304
prevention of, 199
shock and, 449
smoking and, 110
symptoms of, 446
treatments for, 204, 446–449
heartburn, 217
heart disease, 131, 278, 341, 342, 421
 deathrates from in U.S., 203
 overconsumption and, 169
 type A behavior and, 38, 40
heart murmur, 201
heavy metals, 409, 410
 effect on nervous system, 410
 mercury poisoning, 409, 410
Heimlich maneuver, 443–445
hemophilia, 194
heredity
 and breast size, 393
 genes and, 280
 genetic diseases, 194–196
hermaphrodites, 250
hernia, 457
"heroic" means, 350
Heroin, 63, 65, 68, 75, 78, 99
 related deaths, 76
herpes infection
 diseases caused by, 234, 235
 modes of transmission of, 234, 235
 sexually transmitted, 238
herpes simplex and the fetus, 284
heterosexuality, 264
hierarchy of needs (Maslow), 22–25, 36
high blood pressure, 38, 169, 198, 199,
 201, 343
 and cancer of uterus and cervix, 213
 and diet pills, 184
 and the Pill, 304
high-carbohydrate diet, 182
high-fat diet, 182, 183
high-protein diet, 181
histamines, 232
hives, 455
home
 injury in, 451–453
 safety precautions for, 451, 453
homeostasis, 45
home remedies, 357
homosexuality, 264–266
hopelessness scale, 53
hormonal injections, 304, 305
hormonal methods of contraception
 injections, 304
 "morning-after" pill, 304
 the Pill, 303, 304
hormones, 250, 305, 306
 insulin, 196
 male sex, 269
 stressors and, 36
hospice, the, 350, 351
hospitals, 357, 358, 360, 361, 364,
 366–369
 investor-owned (proprietary), 368, 369
 third-party payers and, 360, 361
host, 222, 224, 229, 240, 243
 immunization and, 243
 susceptible, 224
human behavior, modification of, 25
human chorionic gonadrotropin, (HCG),
 282

human interaction (Berne), 56
humanistic psychology, 22–25
hunger, 149
hydrocarbons, 402
hydrogen, 150
hydrogen cyanide, 109
hymen, 271, 272, 389
hyperplasia, 207
hypertension, 195
   essential, 201
   obesity and, 174
hypoglycemia, 182
hypothalamus, 306
hysterectomy, 308
   surgical risk of, 306

id, 17, 18, 25, 32, 33
   basic drives and, 17
   forces of instinct, 32
   pleasure principle, 17
   sex and aggression and, 17
   source of inner stress, 32
illicit drugs, 63–65, 69
   psychoactive, 63
illnesses
   local, 192
   sudden, chart of, 454–457
   systemic, 192
immune reaction, 222
immune system of the body, 214
immunity
   acquired, 222, 229–231
   herd, 230, 231
   natural, 222, 229
immunization, 230
impotence, 278
incest, 265
   abortion and, 310
incidence, 192
indigestion, 387, 388
   OTC drugs for, 387
induced labor, for abortion, 308
industrial by-products, 405, 406
industrialization and population, 336
industry and water pollution, 405, 406
infants
   overfeeding and obesity, 178
   survival and life expectancy, 340
infection
   body's response to, 222
   and brain damage, 11
   process of, 223–228
infectious disease, 227
   body's defense mechanisms, 229
   common communicable, 231–241
      control of, 241–243
   cost in human life of, 223
   frequency of occurrence in U.S., 222
   immunity and resistance to, 229–231
   rats and, 413
infectivity, 228
inflammation response, 232
   acne and, 389
   in allergies, 214
   to infection, 222
   process of, 232
influenza, 233, 234
insanity, 51
instinct, 18, 32
institutional care, 364

insulin, need for, 196
intercourse, 263
   See also sexual intercourse
interferon, 232
interpersonal sexuality, 259, 263–266
   public attitudes, law and, 265, 266
intestines, 217, 218
intimacy, 48, 49, 320
   demand for in marriage, 331
   equal marriage and, 323
intoxication, 63
intrapersonal sexuality, 259–263
intrauterine device (IUD), 297, 304–305
inversion layer, 403
iodine, 153, 158
iron, 153, 158, 163
isometrics, 132, 133
isotonics, 133–135
itching, OTC products for, 388
IUD (intrauterine device), 297, 304
   problems from use of, 305
   use effectiveness of, 305

jogging, 131, 135–137, 163
Jung, Carl, 17

Karvonen formula, 144
Kasch test, 127–129
ketoacids, 196
kidney dialysis treatment, 364
Kinsey's survey, 264
kissing disease, 235
kleptomania, 265

labia
   majora, 271, 273
   minora, 271, 273
labor
   dangers in, 295
   drugs used during, 288
   stages of, 286, 287
lactose, 150
laparotomy, 308
learned response, violence as a, 423
legal drugs, 64
leg lifts, 133
leprosy, 228
lethal dose, 66, 67
leukemia, 210
   danger signs of, 206
lice, 225, 240, 241
life expectancy
   calculating your, 339
   infant survival and, 340
   improved medical care and, 338
liquid protein diet, 181, 189
limbic system, 14
liver disease
   cirrhosis, 94
   hepatitis, 234
local illness, 192
logs for exercise programs, 145
longer life, 336, 342
loss and depression, 51
lovemaking, 276
low-carbohydrate diet, 181
low-fat diet, 183
LSD, 68, 74
lumpectomy, 212

lunacy, 51
lung cancer
   cigarette smoking and, 212
   danger signs of, 205
   risk factor of, 193
lungs, 126, 138, 192
lymphocytes, 210
lymphoma, 206, 210
lysergic acid diethylamide (LSD), 73, 74

mace, 431
macrobiotic diet, 183
mainlining, 67
malaria, 225, 240
male
   reproductive organs, cancer of, 206
   secondary sex characteristics, 269
   sex organs
      external, 269
      internal, 269–271, 306
male characteristics, traditional,
      249–251, 256, 257
male Pill, 306
malnutrition, 168, 169
   nutritional fallacies and, 168
malpractice suits, 362
mammary glands, 274
mammograms, 212
manic-depressive illness, 53, 54
mantra and meditation, 58
marijuana, 65, 75, 99
   and alcohol, 85, 99
   decriminalization of, 69
   major effects of use, 70, 74
marriage, 318–325
   advantages of, 319, 320
   common complaints of, 324
   disappointment in, 322
   equal, 323
   preparation for, 320, 321
   readiness questions, 321
   roommate as preparation for, 318
   successful, 323
   test, 324, 325
masculine sex-role traits, 250
Maslow, Abraham, 22–25, 32, 36
   hierarchy of needs, 22–24
masochism, 265
mastectomy, 212
Masters, William, 276, 279, 293
masturbation, 259–264, 278
   punishment, guilt and, 261
   society and, 261
meals and diet planning, 186
measles, 225, 230, 243
meat group, 163
mechanical methods of contraception,
      301–303
median income by sex and age, 252
Medicaid, 367, 368
medical care
   availability of, 357, 358
   demand for, 363
   high cost of, 360, 361
   medical technology, 362
   specialists, 358, 359, 361
   third-party payers, 360
medical death, 345
medical fraud, 398
medical schools, 363

edicare, 367
edicinals, 63
editation, 58
edulla, 14
egavitamins, 395
elanoma, 209
eltdown, 410, 411
en
  birth control and, 300, 301, 305
  median income of, 252
  sex-role pressures, 253, 256, 257
  sexual problems in, 278
  sterilization of, 306, 307
  suicide among older, 341
enopause, 279
enstrual cramps and Darvon, 75
enstrual cycle, 274, 297–299
enstrual pain, OTC drugs for, 287
enstruation, 273, 274
  and the Pill, 303
ental disorders and homosexuality, 264
ental health
  brain damage and, 11
  coping and, 11
  obesity and, 174
  in old age, 343
  self-esteem and, 11, 421
  stress and, 11, 13
  stressors and, 29
  trust as basis for, 19
ental hospitals, 364
  percent of elderly in, 340
escaline, 73
esomorphs, 176
etabolism
  basal metabolic rate (BMR), 176
  low-fat diet and, 183
etastasis, 207
ethadone, 75, 78
icroorganisms, 222
idbrain, 345
idwives, 289
igraines and the Pill, 304
ilk, 163, 164
  allergic reaction to, 163
  mother's, 291
  tetracycline and, 382
  value of, 163, 164
ind
  adaption mechanism and, 16
  conscious coping and, 46
  memory bank of, 46
  problems of, 51–54
  psychedelics and, 73–75
ind and body relationship, 14–16
ineral deficiency and drugs, 382
inerals, 149, 153, 162, 163
  deficiency symptoms, 157–159
  fad diets and, 181, 188
  functions of, 151
  main roles of, 157–159
  misinformation about, 167
  RDA of, 166
  sources of, 153, 157–159
inimata disease, 409, 410
inipill, 204
inority groups
  access to health care, 358
  medical school and, 359
iscarriages, 111, 284, 305
  alcohol and, 94

mites, 240, 241
mode of transmission of disease
  see transmission
monogamy, 323, 332
mononucleosis, 235
monosaturated fats, 150, 151
monosodium glutamate (MSG)
  in baby foods, 161
  Chinese Restaurant Syndrome, 161
mood, effect of alcohol on, 83–87
mood change
  alcohol and, 91
  hallucinogens and, 74
  marijuana and, 74
  menstrual cycle and, 274
"morning-after" pill, 304
morphine, 63, 75
mothers
  drugs and nursing, 382
  new, 326
  single, problems for, 331
motility, 270
motor control and alcohol, 85, 86
motor functions and marijuana, 70
mourning, 348–350
  the hospice and, 351
  stages of, 348, 349
mouthwashes, 391
mucous membranes, 222, 225, 271
  common cold and, 231
  as defense against disease, 229
mucus, 215
multiple sclerosis (MS), 218
mumps, 230, 243
  juvenile diabetes and, 196
murder, 421
  frequency of, 427
  legal definition of, 422
  street crime and, 426
muscular dystrophy, 194
mutation (genetic variation), 231
mycotic disease, *see* fungal disease
myocardial infarction, 204
myths
  of aging, 341
  about drinking, 99

National Center on Child Abuse and
    Neglect, 425
narcotics
  effects on nervous system, 75, 76
  medical use of, 75
  non-narcotics, 69, 70
  withdrawal symptoms, 68, 76, 78
National Environmental Policy Act, 414
national health insurance, 371, 372
National Health Service (NHS), 370, 371
National Health Service Corps, 358, 359
National Institute on Alcohol Abuse and
    Alcoholism (NIAAA), 88, 89, 97
National Institute of Allergy and
    Infectious Diseases, 233
National Institute of Health (NIH), 64
natural methods of birth control,
    298–301
negative reinforcement, 26
neoplasm, 207
nerve impulses, 198
nervous breakdown, 13
nervous system, 14

abnormalities of, 195
depressants and, 72
diseases of, 218
genetic biochemical problems of, 195, 196
local illness of, 192
narcotics and, 75, 76
stimulants and, 70
neurosis, 50, 53, 57
niacin, 155, 163
nicotine, 63, 64, 70, 106, 109, 110
nitrogen, 150, 181
nocturnal emissions, 262
noise pollution
  measurement of, 414
  stress-related diseases and, 414
non-communicable disease, categories
    of, 194, 195
non-energy nutrients, 153
nonnegligent manslaughter, *see* murder
non-nutrients, 159
non-smokers, 117
nostrums, 167, 393–398
Nuclear Regulatory Commission, 411
nurse-midwives, 370
nurse practitioners, 370
nurses, 369, 370
nursing homes, 340, 364
nursing mothers and drugs, 382
nutrients, 165, 169, 176, 180, 188, 201, 203
  balanced diet and, 149
  basic, 149–159
  basic four food groups, 162–164
  blood flow and, 196
  calories and, 149
  energy and, 149–152
  essential, 159
  non-energy providing, 153, 159
  non-nutrients, 159
nutrition, 148–171, 194
  additives and, 162
  improvement of and long life, 336
  therapy, 57
nutritional fallacies, 167, 168
  and malnutrition, 168
  and fad diets, 178–183

obesity, 177, 178
obstetrician, 282
Office on Domestic Violence, 425
old age
  American culture and, 337
  double standard for women in, 341
  poverty and, 342
older people
  climacteric, 279
  diseases of, 340, 341
  health care for, 364, 367, 368
  home safety for, 453
  menopause, 279
  numbers of, 337
  physical changes among, 340
  proportion of women among, 337
  retirement and, 340
  sex drive in, 279
  social changes among, 340
  suicide among, 341
operant conditioning, 25, 26
opiates, 68, 75

opium, 68
oral contraception, 297
oral-genital sex, 264
oral sex, 276, 278
organ transplants, 204
organic foods, 167, 168
orgasm, 261, 263, 276–278, 301, 396
  problems with, 278
ovarectomy, 306
ovaries, 272, 273, 306
overconsumption, 169
overdose on drugs, 76
  symptoms of, 449
  treatment for, 449
overload, 143
over-the-counter drugs (OTC), 63, 380,
  381, 384–390
  guidelines for buying, 384–386
overweight
  avoidance of and long life, 343
  causes of, 176–178
  chart to determine, 179
  nutrition therapy and, 57
ovulation, 273, 297–299, 304
ovum, 270, 273, 274, 280, 281, 296–298,
  301, 306, 307
oxygen, 126, 131, 132, 134–137, 144,
  150–153, 201, 203, 406
  artificial respiration, 440
  body's need for, 125
  blood flow and, 196
  for heart attack victims, 204
  lack of
    choking, 443
    effect on body cells, 344, 345
  sleep and, 146
oxygen debt, 135, 136

pain, OTC products for, 387
pancreas, 196
Pap test, 213, 239, 305
paranoia, 70
parasite, 222
parenthood, 324–327
parents and child abuse, 424, 425
Parents Anonymous, 425
Parkinson's Disease, 218
particulates in cigarette smoke, 109
peak experiences (Maslow), 23
pedophilia, 265
peer pressure, 31, 77
penicillin, 63
penis (glans), 213, 236, 269, 270, 274,
  276, 277, 300, 301
  enlargers and quackery, 393, 394
peptides, 306
personality, 17, 18, 22, 29, 32
  development of, 18, 24, 25
  dynamics of, 18
  instinct and, 18
  stress-prone, 38, 39
personality, theories of, 17–26
  behaviorism, 25, 26
  Erikson, 19–22
  Freud, 17, 18
  Glasser, 24, 25
  humanistic psychology, 22–25
  Maslow, 22–24
pertussus, 230, 243
pesticides, 408
  effects on human health, 409

peyote, 73
pharmacists, 381, 385
Phencyclidine hydrochloride (PCP), 73
  as anesthetic, 74
phobias, 50
phosphorus, 153, 157
physical fitness and long life, 342
physical health, 11
physical sexuality, 259–266
  emotions and, 260
  interpersonal, 263–266
  intrapersonal, 261–263
  sexual development and, 259–261
physician, 380, 381, 385, 398
  assistants, 370
  choosing a, 372, 373
  communicating with a, 373
  extenders, 369, 370
Pill, the, 303, 304
pinworms, 226, 241
pipes and cigars, 113
  cancer causing agents in, 113
  dangers from inhaling, 117
pituitary gland, 273, 306
placenta, 286, 287, 308, 309
plague, 223, 242, 343
plaque, 110
plasma, 232
plateau phase (Masters & Johnson), 276,
  277, 300
pleasure principle (Freud), 17
poison, 409
  as cause of shock, 449
poliomyelitis, 225, 230, 243
population, 415, 416
  and society, 337
  trends in U.S., 336, 337
post partum depression, 291
pot, 65
  See marijuana
potassium, 153, 158
potency of a drug, 68
poverty
  as cause of street crime, 428
  old age and, 342
  stress and, 13
preconscious, the, 16, 17
pregnancy
  alcohol and, 12, 94, 95
  birth defects, 94
  brain damage, 12
  diabetes and, 295
  diet and, 285
  ectopic, 305
  fertilization, 280, 281
  Fetal Alcohol Syndrome (FAS), 95
  heredity and, 280
  sexual intercourse during, 276
  smoking and, 111, 112, 114
  stress and, 281
  tests, 282
  test tube babies, 281
  three trimesters of, 282–285
  unwanted, 295
  See also pregnant women
pregnant women
  drugs and, 382
  genital herpes and, 235
  need for protein in diet, 150
  rubella and congenital defects, 195
pre-ejaculatory fluid, 271

premenstrual tension, 387
prepuce, 269
prescription drugs, overuse in the elderly
  341
preservatives, 162
pressure points, 440
prevalence, definition of, 192, 193
preventive medicine, 365
primal pain, 57
primal therapy, 57
principle of adaption, 143
private enterprise and medical care,
  357–360
problem-solving techniques, 46, 47
processed foods, 161, 162
proctosigmoidoscope, 213
progesterone, 274, 303, 304
Prohibition, 88, 89
prostaglandins, 387
prostate gland, 270, 271, 277
proteins
  in basic food groups, 163–165
  as basic nutrient, 149, 150
  composition of, 150
  diets and, 180, 181
  functions of, 151
  inflammation process and, 232
  nutritional fallacies about, 167
  sources of, 150, 151, 163
protozoa, 225, 228
protozoan diseases, 240
psychedelics, 69, 73–75
psychoactive drugs, 63, 67
psychoanalysis, methods of, 54, 55
  Freud's work as basis of, 54, 55
psychoses, 50, 52–54, 73
psychotherapy
  alcoholism and, 96
  anorexia and, 83
  nonverbal therapies, 54, 57
  reality therapy (Glasser), 24, 25
  sexual problems and, 279
  talk therapies, 54–57
psychotic disorders, drug treatment in,
  73
psychotropics and alcohol, 84
puberty, 269, 272
pulse, how to check, 441
push-ups, 131, 133, 134
pyribenzamine (Blues), 65

quacks, 392–398
  nostrums and, 393–398
  quick quiz on, 396, 397
quackery, 392
  controlling, 398
  filing a consumer complaint, 398
quarantine, 242
quitting smoking, 113–117

rabies, 225, 226
radiation, 410, 411
  therapy, 213
radioactive materials, 410, 411
rape
  abortion and, 310
  fantasies about, 262, 263
  forcible, definition of, 429
  the "morning after" pill and, 304
  preventing, 428

ality therapy (RT) (Glasser), 24, 25
ecommended Dietary Allowance
  (RDAs), 165, 166
ctum, cancer of, 213, 214
flex and adaption mechanism, 16
flexes, effect of alcohol on, 85
fractory phase, 277
habilitation, 78
inforced learning and smoking, 106
inforcement
  in operant conditioning, 25
  for violence, 423
laxation response, 58
marriage, 331, 332
EM sleep, 145
servoirs of disease, 223, 224, 226
sistance, 229, 231
solution, 276, 277
spiratory muscles, 131
spiratory system
  diagram of, 216
  effects of fitness on, 131, 132
  problems with in old age, 340
  smog and, 402
ythm method, 297–299
boflavin, 155, 163, 164
ckettsiae, 225
ckettsial diseases, 235, 236
ght-to-Life movement, 312
ngworm, 226, 240
ocky Mountain spotted fever, 225, 235,
  236
le models, 253
oughage, 159
undworms, 226
T (reality therapy), 24, 25
bella (German Measles), 225, 230
  danger from in pregnancy, 282
nning, 136–138

dism, 264, 265
line solution, in abortion, 308
nitation
  improvement of, 336
  protozoan infections and, 225
  worm infestations and, 241
turated fat, 150, 151
rcoma, 210
abies, 239, 241
arlet fever, 227
arsdale diet, 180
histosoma, 226
hizophrenia, 54, 57
crotum, 269, 270
ebacious glands and acne, 389
econd-degree burns, 443
econd-hand smoke, 117
elf-actualization (Maslow), 23
  traits, 25
elf-esteem, 23, 29, 36, 45, 48, 51, 54, 261,
  343, 429
  impaired, and violence, 421–424
  intimacy and, 320
  mental health and, 11
  self-control and, 19
  sexual dysfunction and, 277
elf-image, 89, 91
  alcoholics and, 89
  identifying your, 12
  overeating and, 178
  stress and, 29

semen, 271, 277, 299–301, 305, 307
seminal vessicle, 271, 277
seminiferous tubules, 269, 270
senility, 13, 341
sex
  biology of, 268–293
  clinics and quackery, 396, 397
  pleasures of and marriage, 319
sex organs (genitals), 261
  functions of, 269
sex roles
  conformity to, 249, 250
  culture and, 249–251
  role conflict, 251, 253, 256, 257
  stereotypes, 249–251
  traits, chart of, 250
sex therapists, 396, 397
sexist culture, 257
sexual climax and masturbation, 261
  See also orgasm
sexual development, 259–261
  culture, guilt and, 260
  education and, 260, 261
  puberty, 260
sexual dysfunction, 277–279
sexual fantasies, 262, 263
sexual freedom and STDs, 237, 238
sexual intercourse, 259, 274–280,
  297–301, 304
  during pregnancy, 276
  functions of, 195
  lovemaking and, 276
  older people and, 279
  pleasure and, 295, 300
  positions, 275, 276
  premarital, 260
  problems with, in women, 279
  sexual dysfunction, 277–279
  transmission of disease and, 227
sexual response, stages of (Masters &
  Johnson), 276, 277
sexuality, 248–267
  equal marriage and, 323
  physical, 259–267
  sex roles and, 249–258
  social, 249–267
  variant, 265
sexually transmitted diseases (STD)
  chancroid, 239
  chart of, 238, 239
  complications of, 238, 239
  condom, and prevention of, 238
  diagnosis of, 238, 239
  genital chlamydia, 225, 237–239
  genital herpes, 235, 238
  gonorrhea, 236, 238, 305
  granuloma inguinale, 239
  herpes simplex II, 238
  lymphogranuloma venereum, 239
  monilial vaginitis, 239
  non-specific urethritis, 238
  non-specific vaginitis, 238
  pediculosis pubis (crabs), 239
  responsible sexual behavior and, 260
  scabies, 239, 241
  sexual freedom and, 237
  STD "hot line," 238
  symptoms of, 238, 239
  syphilis, 236, 238
  trichomonas vaginalis, 239
  venereal warts, 239

shingles, 234
shock, 196, 443, 449–451
shock (electroconvulsive) therapy, 54
shopping
  advertising and, 170
  guidelines for, 170
sickle cell anemia, 194
  the Pill and, 304
side effects of drugs, 381, 382
silver nitrate solution, 236
sinusitis, 454
sit-ups, 133
skin
  cancer, 205
  defense against disease, 229
sleep
  exercise and, 145
  role of, 145, 146
  stages of, 145
slums, 412, 413
smallpox, 225, 230, 243
smegma, 213
smog
  as carcinogen, 402
  temperature inversions and, 403
smoking, 104–120, 343
  addiction to, 106
  cardiovascular disease and, 198, 199
  coping with stress and, 46, 106
  costs of, 117, 118
  diabetics and, 196
  diseases associated with, 109, 110
  drug taking and, 110
  during pregnancy, risks from, 111, 112
  effects of, 107
  as fire hazard, 452
  as habit, 106
  nonsmokers and, 117
  pipes and cigars
    cancer causing agents in, 113
  reason for, 105, 105
  quitting, motivation in, 113
  society and, 117
  Surgeon General's Report on, 117, 118
sneezing, 227
snorting, 67, 71
Social Security, 337, 367, 368
socialized medicine, 370, 371
  National Health Service (NHS), 370,
    371
sperm, 296, 297, 306–308
sperm cell, 269–271, 280, 281
  motility, 270
  travels of, 270, 271
  viable, 281
spermicides, 299, 301, 305
  creams and gels, 301, 302
  use effectiveness of, 302
  foams, 302, 303
spina bifida, 196
spirilli, 224
spot reduction, myth of, 186
spouse abuse
  hot line, 425
  women's movement and, 425
sodium, 153
S (non-REM) sleep, 145
stages of a woman's life (Sheehy), 20
starch, 150
stereotypes, sex role, 247, 251, 257
sterility, 306

sterilization, surgical, 295, 306–308
  hysterectomy, 308
  popularity of, in U.S., 306
  tubal ligation, 307, 308
  vasectomy, 306, 307
stillbirth, 111
stimulants, 69
  amphetamines, 65, 70, 85, 189
  caffeine, 63, 64, 70, 72
  cocaine, 65, 70, 71
  dependence on, 70
  effects of on nervous system, 70
  nicotine, 63, 64, 70, 106, 109, 110
  synthetic, 70
  tolerance of, 70
stimuli, 16
stomach, 217, 228
  OTC drugs for problems of, 387, 388
stress
  alcohol abuse and, 90
  biochemical changes in (Selye), 33
  causes of, 13, 423
  child abusers and, 425
  college students and, 29, 31
  coping and smoking and, 106
  disease and, 36
  disorders, symptoms of, 37
  drugs and, 63
    among students, 65
  fertility and, 281
  high pressure jobs and, 41
  levels of consciousness and, 32
  management, 47
  mental health and, 13
  in old age, 340, 341
  prevention of, 45
  psychotherapy and, 54
  response, 34
  risk factor, 193
  stressors and, 36
  in teen years, 29
  type A behavior and, 38–40
  type B behavior and, 40
  in young adulthood, 29
  warning signs of, 45
stress control life-style questionnaire
  (Glazer), 39
stress-prone personality traits, 38, 39
stress-related diseases, 36–38
stressors, 29, 34–36
  biophysical, 29
  chemical, 29
  defense mechanisms and, 48
  disease and debility and, 36
  environmental, 29
  negative (distress), 35, 36
  positive (eustress), 35, 36
  psychological, 29
  psychosocial, 29
  social pressures, 29
stretch exercises, 138
stroke, 202, 449
  major and minor, 202, 203
  old age and, 341
  overconsumption and, 169
  the Pill and, 304
  prevention of, 199
  smoking and, 110
sucrose, 150
suction curettage, 308
sudden illness, symptoms of, 454–457

suicide
  hopelessness scale, 53
  modern study of, 52
  among older people, 341
  warning signs of, 52
  in young people, 52, 421
sulfur dioxide, 402
sunburn, 388
  OTC products for, 388
  prevention of, 388
sunlight and skin cancer, 209
superego, 32, 33
suppositories, contraceptive, 303
Surgeon General's Report on Smoking,
  117, 118
surgery, 188, 189, 207, 212, 287
susceptible host, 228
swimming, 136–138
synergy, 68, 84, 382
syphilis, 236–238
  symptoms of, 236, 238
systemic illness, 192

Talwin (Ts), 65
tampons, 389
tapeworm, 226, 241
tar, and cancer, 109
television and violence, 429
temperature inversion, 403
temperence movement, 88
tests
  Cooper Field, 129
  Kasch, 127–129
  marriage, 324, 325
  for pregnancy
    HCG, 282
    urine, 282
testes, 269, 270
testosterone, 269
test-tube babies, 280
tetanus, 230, 243
tetracycline, 236
  drug interaction and, 382
  pregnancy and, 284
tetrahydrocanabinol (THC), 69
Thalidomide, 284
thermography, 212
thiamine, 155, 163
thickeners, 161
third-degree burns, 443
third-party payments, 366
Thorazine, 73
threshold dose, 66, 66
ticks, 225
time structuring (Berne), 48, 49
  transactional analysis and, 56
tobacco, 104–121
  advertising of cigarettes, 118, 119
  consumption of in U.S., 104
  the culture and, 104
  dangers of smoking, 104
  drugs in, 106
  government's role, 118–120
    subsidies, 118, 119
    Surgeon General's Report, 117, 118
    television advertising ban, 118
  pregnancy and, 284
  products, 104
tolerance
  for alcohol, 91

  for drugs, 68
  for stimulants, 70
toothache, 454
tooth decay, 217
  incidence of in U.S., 217
  prevention of, 217
tourniquet, 440
toxic shock syndrome (TSS), 389
toxic wastes, 406, 407
trachoma, 225
training effect, 132, 134–137, 143
  achievement of, 132
tranquilizers, 69
  dependency on, 72, 73
  effect of mixing with alcohol, 84
  in treatment of anxiety, 72
  Thalidomide, 284
transactional analysis (TA), 56
  human interaction and, 56
  time structuring and, 56
transmission, mode of, 224, 228–235
  control of, 243
  epidemics and, 229
  sexual intercourse as, 227
  sneezing and coughing as, 227
  worms as, 241
transverse presentation, 287
transvestism, 265
trial marriage, 332
Trichomonas vaginalis, 240
triglycerides, 150, 151
trimesters of pregnancy
  body changes in, 282–285
  dangers in, 282, 284
  miscarriage in first, 284
tubal ligation, 307, 308
tumors
  benign, 207
  malignant, 207
Type A behavior pattern, 38–40
  heart disease and, 38, 40
Type B behavior pattern, 39, 40
  stress and, 39, 40
typhus, 225

ulcers, 195
  stress-related disorders and, 38
  symptoms and first aid, 456
  treatment for, 218
umbilical cord, 287
unconscious, the, 16, 17
undernutrition, 169
United States Supreme Court
  ruling on abortion, 310, 312
unsaturated fats, 150, 151
urban environment
  noise pollution and, 413, 414
  pests in, 412, 413
  social, 412
urethra, 236, 237, 270, 271
urinary tract infection, 455
use effectiveness of birth control
  methods, 297–305
uterus (womb), 236, 272, 273, 286, 287,
  297, 301–303, 308, 309
  cancer of, 213

vaccines, 230
vaccination, 243
vagina, 236, 272–274, 276, 277, 281,
  299–303, 389

ginal aspiration, 308
ginal opening, 271
ginal spermicides, 297
lium, 72, 84
lve disorders (heart), 201
riant sexuality, 265
s deferens, 270, 271, 295, 306
sectomy, 306, 307
getarianism, 165, 167
  Zen macrobiotic, 165
nereal disease and condom, 301
  See also sexually transmitted diseases
stibule, 271
ctims of crime
  counseling for, 428
  emotional cost to, 431
  grief and mourning, 428
olence
  behaviorist theories of, 423
  causes of, 423
  collective, 432, 433
  coping and, 46
  costs of, 430, 431
  domestic, 423–425
  as learned response, 423
  the media and, 429
  rape, 428, 429
  roots of, 421
  in schools, 429
  stimulants and, 70
  street crime, 426–428
  subculture of, 423
  victims of, 428, 431
ral diseases
  juvenile diabetes and, 196
  See also viruses
ral hepatitis, symptoms of, 234
ruses, 225, 228, 231–235, 238, 239
tamin A, 152–154, 162–164, 166
amin B-complex, 153, 155, 156, 162,
    163, 166
tamin B-6, 155, 163, 166
tamin B-12, 155, 163, 166
tamin C, 153, 156, 162, 163, 166
  common cold and, 233
tamin D, 152–154, 164, 166
amin E, 152–154, 166
tamin K, 152–154, 166

vitamins
  alcohol and, 85
  in basic four food groups, 103
  as basic nutrient, 149, 153, 167
  body functions and, 153
  deficiency and drugs, 382
  enriched products, 167
  fad diets and, 181, 183
  fasting and, 188
  in fats, 152
  fat soluble, 153, 154
  functions of, 151
  importance of, 153
  megavitamins, 395
  RDA of, 166
  water soluble, 153, 155, 156
voluntary nervous system, 14
voyeurism, 265
vulva, 271, 389

war
  casualties in World War II, 432
  society and, 432, 433
warm-ups, 138, 144
water, 149, 153
  average body need for, 153
  basic nutrient, 149
  diet planning and, 186
  loss in dieting, 181
  vital role of, 153
water cycle, 404, 405
  pollution and, 405, 406
  three zones of, 404
  toxic wastes and, 406
water pollution
  environmentalism and reduction of,
    414, 415
  eutrophication, 406
  industry and, 405, 406
  water cycle and, 404, 405
weight, table of, 175
weight control, 173–189
  diets and dieting, 178–187
  food intake and, 176
  fundamental facts about, 174, 176
  metabolism and, 176
  physical exercise and, 176
weight gain and quitting smoking, 116

weight reduction
  behavior modification and, 188
  methods, 189
white blood cells, 232
whole grains, 178, 181, 182
withdrawal symptoms
  in babies, 284
  drug addiction and, 68
  Methodone and, 78
  in users of narcotics, 76
wine, 82
  use of in U.S., 83
women
  abortion and, 308–312
  attitude toward women scale,
    254–256
  contraception and birth control
    methods, 298–305
  sterilization, 306–308
  median income of, 252
  older
    double standard for, 341
    numbers of, 337
    poverty and, 342
  problems with sexual intercourse, 279
  role conflict in, 251
  sex organs
    external, 271, 272, 300
    internal, 272, 273, 306
women's movement, 257
  spouse abuse and, 425
worms, 226, 228

x-rays and pregnancy, 284

yeast, 225
yellow fever, 242
young adults
  drugs and, 65
  sexually transmitted diseases and, 237
  street crime and, 428
  stress and, 29
  suicide among, 52, 421
  violent death among, 421

Zen macrobiotic diet, 165
zinc, 153, 158
zygote, 273, 280